A to Z
CHILD CARE

A READY RECKONER

Everything you wanted to know about child health and diseases

A to Z
CHILD CARE

A READY RECKONER

Everything you wanted to know about child health and diseases

Meharban Singh

MD, FAMS, FIAP, FIMSA, FNNF, Hony. FAAP
Former Professor and Head
Department of Pediatrics and Neonatal Division
WHO Collaborating Center for Training and
Research in Newborn Care
All India Institute of Medical Sciences
New Delhi

CBS

CBS Publishers & Distributors Pvt Ltd

New Delhi • Bengaluru • Chennai • Kochi • Mumbai • Pune
Hyderabad • Kolkata • Nagpur • Patna • Vijayawada

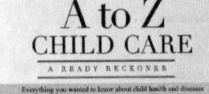

A to Z
CHILD CARE
A READY RECKONER
Everything you wanted to know about child health and diseases

ISBN: 978-81-239-2590-5

Published by Satish Kumar Jain and produced by Varun Jain for
CBS Publishers & Distributors Pvt Ltd

4819/XI Prahlad Street, 24 Ansari Road, Daryaganj, New Delhi 110 002, India.
Ph: 23289259, 23266861, 23266867   Website: www.cbspd.com
Fax: 011-23243014   e-mail: delhi@cbspd.com; cbspubs@airtelmail.in.
Corporate Office: 204 FIE, Industrial Area, Patparganj, Delhi 110 092
Ph: 4934 4934   Fax: 4934 4935   e-mail: publishing@cbspd.com; publicity@cbspd.com

Branches

- **Bengaluru:** Seema House 2975, 17th Cross, K.R. Road, Banasankari 2nd Stage, Bengaluru 560 070, Karnataka
  Ph: +91-80-26771678/79   Fax: +91-80-26771680   e-mail: bangalore@cbspd.com
- **Chennai:** 7, Subbaraya Street, Shenoy Nagar, Chennai 600 030, Tamil Nadu
  Ph: +91-44-26260666, 26208620   Fax: +91-44-42032115   e-mail: chennai@cbspd.com
- **Kochi:** 36/14 Kalluvilakam, Lissie Hospital Road, Kochi 682 018, Kerala
  Ph: +91-484-4059061-65   Fax: +91-484-4059065   e-mail: kochi@cbspd.com
- **Mumbai:** 83-C, Dr E Moses Road, Worli, Mumbai-400018, Maharashtra
  Ph: +91-22-24902340/41   Fax: +91-22-24902342   e-mail: mumbai@cbspd.com
- **Pune:** Bhuruk Prestige, Sr. No. 52/12/2+1+3/2 Narhe, Haveli (Near Katraj-Dehu Road Bypass), Pune 411 041, Maharashtra
  Ph: +91-20-64704058/59, 32392277   Fax: +91-20-24300160   e-mail: pune@cbspd.com

Representatives

- **Hyderabad** 0-9885175004
- **Nagpur** 0-9021734563
- **Vijayawada** 0-9000660880
- **Kolkata** 0-9831437309, 0-9051152362
- **Patna** 0-9334159340

Printed at Gopsons Papers Ltd

to

Parents who are the quintessence of
love and sacrifice for their children

"The prevailing sense of despair at the birth of a female child should be replaced by the awareness and hope, that she is the creator and sustainer of progeny."
                                                                    —Meharban Singh

Preface

The manual has been written to provide culture-specific information on global aspects of common health problems of children from birth through adolescence. The book is loaded with practical and up-to-date information pertaining to all aspects of child care including variations in healthy children, developmental challenges, common day-to-day health problems of children including accidents, poisonings, minor and serious infections, and diseases and disabilities of children. The topics have been arranged in an alphabetical order for ease of retrieval to serve as a ready reckoner. The book has been written in a simple easy-to-understand language without any medical jargon. The book is intended to boost the know-how and confidence of parents to handle day-to-day health problems of their children. The manual is best suited to seek information on first-aid and useful home remedies for treatment of common disorders in children. The home remedies have been taken from reliable sources including standard Ayurvedic texts. Nevertheless, when your child is genuinely sick, you must consult your doctor as early as possible for proper evaluation and management. A glossary of English and Hindi names of grains, lentils, vegetables, fruits, seeds and Indian spices has been provided.

I appreciate the efforts of my daughter Ms Sonia Singh for her help in collection of standard home remedies. The cover design has been created by my grand daughter Ms Ishita Singh. I would like to take this opportunity to thank Mr YN Arjuna, Mrs Ritu Chawla and Mr Tarun Rajput for composing and inserting the manuscript in the word processor and to my friend Shri Satish Kumar Jain for his enthusiasm and commitment to publish the revised book in an improved style and format. I have a fond hope that *A to Z Child Care* would serve as a useful ready reckoner to parents to handle common health issues and problems of their children with confidence and fortitude.

Meharban Singh MD

Child Care Center
625, Arun Vihar, Sector 37, Noida
Tel-0120-4346451, 9818888772
e-mail: *drmbsk@gmail.com*

Contents

ABORTION (Miscarriage)

Fetal death or miscarriage before 22 weeks of gestation or of a fetus weighing less than 500 g is called abortion while later fetal deaths are labelled as stillbirths. Almost 5% of pregnancies end in abortions and some women may have repeated miscarriages. Abortion may occur due to defect in the embryo, placenta or a disorder in the mother. Most abortions occur because of defect in the ovum or sperm. The fertilized ovum or germplasm (zygote) is defective and abortion is nature's way of getting rid of defective fetus. Elderly women (>35 years) or women who had difficulty in getting pregnant are at an increased risk of abortion. Acute viral infection or high grade fever and intake of certain drugs during early pregnancy may lead to fetal death. *In general, a drug which is safe for the mother may be teratogenic (causing malformation or developmental defect in the fetus) and therefore all medications should be avoided during the first 3 months of pregnancy.* At times the placenta is at an abnormal position or is unable to produce enough quantities of female sex hormones to sustain the pregnancy. Smoking, excessive intake of alcohol and substance abuse are associated with an increased risk of miscarriage.

Miscarriage and stillbirths (after 22 weeks of pregnancy) occurring later in pregnancy are usually due to diseases in the mother like toxemia of pregnancy, high blood pressure, diabetes mellitus, thyroid disorders, syphilis or abnormality in the uterus. In women with a lax or weak cervix, miscarriages may occur repeatedly around 20 weeks of pregnancy. These women can be helped by application of a stitch over the cervix with the help of a minor surgical procedure to keep the cervix closed. When labor starts at full maturity, the stitch is removed to allow the mother to deliver the baby. When placenta is low lying (placenta previa), there may be excessive bleeding at the onset of labor leading to stillbirth. High grade fever or acute medical illness during pregnancy, sudden fall or injury and sex during pregnancy (especially during too early or late pregnancy) may cause contractions of uterus leading to miscarriage.

During pregnancy whenever there is blood-stained vaginal discharge or spasms of pain in the lower abdomen, you should immediately consult your doctor and take complete bed rest in the mean time. At times pregnancy is terminated by the obstetrician to save the life of the mother or when fetus has non-treatable genetic defect or developmental abnormality. *Antenatal detection of sex and selective abortion of a female fetus is a criminal offence akin to a murder.*

ACCIDENTS AND INJURIES

Children are prone to physical injuries during their day-to-day play and sports activities. Children are restless, inquisitive and full of energy for kicking, jumping, boxing and pushing around.

Cuts and Lacerations

Incised wound or cuts occur with a knife, blade or scissors. Incised wound has sharp borders while lacerated wound has jagged irregular edges due to injury from a barbed wire. Cuts and lacerations may occur due to sharp edges of toys. A sharp pointed object like a nail can cause a punctured wound on the feet or fingers. It has a small opening but is rather deep and poses a great risk for development of tetanus. A crushed injury or amputation may occur when a finger or toe gets crushed in the door.

First-aid If there is bleeding, apply firm pressure with a clean handkerchief for 4–5 minutes. Do not apply a tourniquet or a tight bandage to stop bleeding. The wound should be cleaned with an antiseptic lotion like savlon or dettol. In a roadside injury, the wound should be thoroughly washed with soap and water. Give paracetamol or ibuprofen to relieve pain. Avoid application of any home remedies like turmeric (*haldi*) over the wound. When a cut or laceration is minor, you can affix a waterproof band-aid over the wound. When cuts or lacerations are large or over the face, consult your doctor as the wound may require stitching. If the wound needs stitching do not give water or milk to the child as the child may have to be anesthetized. When a finger gets crushed in the door, do not try to straighten it. Place the finger in ice cold water or apply a cold pack. If a finger or toe is severed, apply local pressure to stop the bleeding. Put the severed part in a sterile plastic bag, place it in an ice-filled container and rush to the hospital having services of the plastic surgeon. When cut is inside the mouth, on the lips, tongue or inner lining of cheeks (buccal mucosa), give the child a cold drink, ice cream or a cube of ice to suck. Gentle pressure may be required to stop the bleeding. In all cases of open injuries, check with your doctor whether your child needs a booster shot of tetanus toxoid (TT or Td).

Abrasions and Scrape Wounds

Abrasions occur when child falls and grazes the hands, elbows, ankles or knees against the ground. There may be slight bleeding or oozing of plasma. The wound should be washed with soap and water and cleaned with an antiseptic like surgical spirit or savlon. Apply an antiseptic cream and give paracetamol for relief of pain.

Bumps and Bruises

Contused wounds or bumps occur due to falls or blunt injury. The blood vessels under the skin rupture producing a painful pink swelling. The swelling is soft due to leakage of blood and changes color from pink to blue and then various shades of grey during the recovery. When a child gets injured, do not panic but you should remain calm and confident. Instead of reprimanding, reassure and caress the child and tell him that everything shall be alright. Apply an ice bag or a plastic bag with ice cubes or a towel soaked in chilled water over the site of bump for several minutes. It reduces bleeding, swelling and pain. Give paracetamol or ibuprofen for relief of pain. Hot fomentation or application of analgesic cream is advised after 12 hours of injury to reduce pain and swelling.

Sprains and Strains

Sprains occur when ligaments, tendons or soft tissues of a joint are injured. They are most common due to twisting of an ankle or knee joint. When injury occurs due to over stretching or excessive pull of a muscle, it is called as a strain. Strains are common in long muscles specially the hamstrings and quadriceps. Rest and application of cold pack for 10–15 minutes provides immediate relief

A

and reduces the extent of injury. After 12 hours, alternating applications of hot and cold packs (one minute each for a total period of 15 minutes) is useful for facilitating recovery. A crepe bandage should be applied to provide rest to the joint. The injured limb should be kept elevated to reduce the swelling. When upper limb is injured, it should be placed in a sling. Ibuprofen should be given for a week for relief of inflammation and pain. In severe injuries, orthopedic surgeon should be consulted to exclude any fracture and assess the need for application of plaster.

Head Injury

Most head injuries occur due to fall from a cot and are usually minor. The child cries, may develop a bruise or bump but there are no serious consequences. Cold pack can be applied over the site of injury to reduce the swelling due to leakage of blood under the scalp or forehead. Child can be given paracetamol for relief of pain but avoid use of any sedative as it would interfere with evaluation of consciousness of the child.

When head injury is associated with bleeding from the nose or ear, vomiting, temporary loss of consciousness or convulsions, he should be taken to the hospital for investigations and observation. Sometimes the adverse effects of head injury become apparent later on after several hours. If a child is not feeling his normal self and has become drowsy or refuses to drink and eat or is having headache (excessive crying) or vomiting after a few hours, he should be taken to a doctor. The presence of a bump or swelling over the head (without any other symptoms) should not worry you, as it may occur because of collection of blood under the scalp and it does not affect the brain. The swelling would disappear spontaneously in due course of time due to resorption of blood and there is no need to do local fomentation over the head.

During first year of life, never toss your baby in the air or shake his head. The baby's brain is smaller than the size of his skull and brain may get bruised as it falls forwards and backwards with the bouncing movements.

Fractures (Broken bones)

In a serious injury, fall from the roof or an automobile accident, there is a serious risk of fracture of bone/s. In a case of fracture, pain is marked, there is inability to move the limb or the limb may

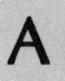

assume an odd or bizarre position. The fracture may be closed (simple fracture) or associated with injury of overlying soft structures (complex fracture) and fractured ends of bones may jut out of the wound.

First-aid The child with fracture should be handled with utmost care. The upper limb should be placed in a sling and lower limb splinted or both lower limbs tied together by placing a soft padding between them. When fracture of neck or spine is suspected, the child should not be moved and he should be handled by a trained paramedical personnel. The child should be placed on a hardboard and lifted without moving him side ways. The injured child should not be given anything to eat or drink after the accident till he has been examined by a doctor. Administration of food or fluids to the child would delay correction of his fracture if this has to be done under general anesthesia.

Home Remedies

- Boil a glass of milk with one teaspoon turmeric powder and sweeten with sugar. Give the warm milk to the child to promote healing.
- Apply warm mustard oil containing turmeric powder over the sprain, cover with cotton and a crepe bandage.
- Take equal amounts of powdered flax seeds (*alsi*) and alum (*phitkari*) and make a paste with mustard oil or melted jaggery (*gur*). Apply over the site of injury and keep it covered with a bandage for 10–12 hours daily for 3–4 days.
- Pineapple juice is useful to promote healing of wound as it contains a photolytic enzyme bromelain.

Prevention of Accidents

Children are prone to accidents due to their carefree behaviour and inability to appreciate dangers. Most accidents are preventable, if due care is taken by the parents and caretakers to keep children under close observation and supervision.

- Infants should not be left alone on a cot unless it has railings or pillows are placed around the baby.
- It is a dangerous practice to shake or toss an infant in the air.
- "Walkers" are notoriously dangerous for causing accidents and should not be used.
- Do not buy toys with sharp edges and projectile toys like guns, pistols, bow and arrows, etc.

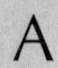

- When children learn to crawl or walk upstairs they should be closely supervised. Stairs should be kept blocked by furniture or a door.
- Balcony should be provided with sturdy railings having closely placed vertical bars. The railings should never have horizontal bars because the child would climb over them.
- Never allow children to play with sharp objects like blade, knife or scissors.
- Discourage the child to play with a swinging door.
- It is dangerous to allow children to fly kites from the roof top.
- Never allow the child to play on the street with heavy traffic.
- Children enjoy climbing trees and walls which should be allowed only under the supervision of an adult.
- Never place the child between you and the steering wheel while driving. Infant should be placed in a special baby seat or taken in the lap while sitting on the back seat. The child should not be allowed to stand on the back seat facing the rear window (like a dog!).
- Adolescents are prone to automobile accidents because of their love for speed and craving for macho image. Teenagers should be provided with road safety guidelines and should be allowed to drive motor bikes only when they are legally allowed to do so.
- Keep a first-aid box handy at home. It should be stocked with roll of cotton wool, sticking plaster, waterproof band-aid strips, cotton and crepe bandage, arm sling, hand towel, antibiotic cream, antiseptic wash (savlon, dettol), iodine containing lotion (betadine), calamine lotion, scissors, safety pins, tweezers, pain killers (paracetamol, ibuprofen), antihistamines (phenergan, benadryl), ice bag in the fridge, ORS sachets, etc.

ACIDITY AND HEARTBURN (Dyspepsia)

Dyspepsia is uncommon in children but may occur due to over-eating, consumption of oily or fried items, junk food, excessive intake of chillies and condiments. Intake of certain drugs especially steroids and non-steroidal anti-inflammatory drugs (NSAIDs) may cause acidity. There is pain, discomfort and burning sensation over upper abdomen and behind the chest

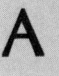

bone (sternum) with sour eructations, or belching. It may be associated with reflux or regurgitation of stomach contents into the food pipe or esophagus. There is excessive secretion of saliva (water brash) to dilute acid contents of stomach.

Treatment The offending drug/s should be stoppd. Intake of water, milk, curd and bland diet helps. Avoid intake of tea, coffee, cold drinks, condiments, chillies and cheese. The child should not lie down in bed immediately after a meal. Avoid intake of lemon juice and sour fruits. Administration of antacids and drugs blocking production of acid in the stomach (omeprazole, pantoprazole) provide prompt relief.

Home Remedies

- Boil half a teaspoon of dried Indian gooseberry (*Amla*) with a half teaspoon of dried *Harad* powder in a cup of water. Filter and cool. Sip slowly on and off to relieve heartburn.
- Suck a piece of liquorice (*Malathi*) or drink a concoction of liquorice made in water.
- Eating a ripe banana with a cup of milk is soothing for the stomach lining.
- Taking one teaspoon of psyllium husk (*Isaphgol*) with a half cup of milk relieves acidity and reflux.

ACNE (Pimples)

Acne is a skin eruption that affects 80% of adolescent boys and girls because of surge of androgenic hormones. They are more severe in boys than girls. It is more common in children with oily skin with overactive sebaceous or oil glands. Skin lesions (comedones) start from forehead and face around 10–12 years of age and may spread to front of chest, shoulders and back. Comedones may get clogged with dust or dirt to form blackheads. Certain medications (steroids, anticonvulsants) may aggravate skin lesions. The lesions may develop superadded bacterial infection leading to formation of pustules followed by formation of pitted scars on healing.

Treatment Strict personal hygiene should be maintained and child asked to wash his face with soap and water at least 4 times in a day especially when he comes back home from school, tuition class,

A

Home Remedies

- Wash the face with fresh butter milk followed by warm water for 3–4 times in a day and dab dry with a soft absorbent towel.
- Make a thin paste of jambul (jamun) seeds by rubbing it on a stone and apply it over the pimples. Let it dry for 1–2 hours and rinse it off with warm water.
- Make a face pack of either gram flour or lentil (*masoor*) powder with a half a teaspoon of turmeric. Apply on the face on alternate days for half to one hour and rinse it off with warm water.
- Grind a teaspoon of dried onion seeds with a little milk and add half a teaspoon of fresh lime juice. Apply it over the pimples at night and wash it off in the morning.
- Boil neem leaves in water over slow fire. Cool, strain the leaves and make a paste. Apply daily on the pimples and wash off after half an hour.
- You can prevent and treat blackheads by using homemade facial scrubs on a regular basis. Facial scrubs help in removing dead skin cells and dirt from clogged pores. The face can be steamed before using the facial scrub.
- Grate one raw potato and rub it over the blackheads for 15 minutes. Let it dry and then wash the face with warm water.
- Crush fenugreek leaves (*methi*) and make a paste with water. Apply over the backheads and leave it on for 15 minutes before rinsing.
- Make a paste of coriander leaves (*dhania*) and turmeric powder. Rub over the blackheads and leave it on for 15 minutes before rinsing.
- Apply aloe vera (*kawaar gandhal, kanwaar paatha*) juice or pulp over the blackheads. Leave it on for 15 minutes before rinsing and washing with a facial scrub.
- Beat one egg white and add one teaspoon of honey. Apply this mixture on the face and leave it on for 20–30 minutes before rinsing with warm water.

playground, dance class and social visit. No oil-based skin care products or creams should be applied on the face. The pimples should not be touched, scratched or squeezed with fingers as it will lead to formation of unsightly scars. Whenever there is superadded bacterial infection, oral and topical antibiotic gel or cream (clarithromycin, erythromycin, clindamycin) is advised to control it. There is no role of any dietary restrictions. In severe cases, expert opinion of a skin specialist should be sought.

ACUTE OTITIS MEDIA (AOM)

A

Children are prone to develop middle ear infection (otitis: ear infection, media: middle ear) following an attack of cough and cold. There is a channel or tube (Eustachian tube) which connects middle ear with back part of the nose to maintain air pressure and balance. When tube gets blocked due to inflammation, middle ear infection sets in. Children are prone to develop middle ear infection when they are fed in a lying-down position (without keeping the head raised) when milk may enter the Eustachian tube and block it. Acute otitis media is more common in children with bottle feeding, cleft palate and enlarged adenoids. Children with recurrent upper respiratory infections and poor immunity (poor nutrition, Down syndrome) are more likely to develop middle ear infection.

Salient features The condition should be suspected when a child with common cold develops fever and pain in the ear. Infant is likely to have marked irritability, excessive crying and may pull at his ears. The older child would complain of pain in one or both ears. Nose is usually blocked and may be perpetually blocked in a child with enlarged adenoids. Eardrum may be retracted (blocked Eustachian tube with resorption of air in the middle ear), congested and bulging. When eardrum perforates, pus is discharged through the ear which is associated with relief of earache. It may be associated with significant hearing loss which usually improves following recovery.

Treatment Every child with cough and cold should be checked by the pediatrician for making an early diagnosis of AOM before perforation of drum occurs. Paracetamol or ibuprofen can be given for relief of pain and fever. Application of heat over the ear with a pad of cloth warmed over hot water bottle or a heated electric press provides relief. Nasal congestion and blockage of Eustachian tube should be relieved by instillation of saline water nose drops, steam inhalation and administration of nasal decongestant. When eardrum is intact, there is no role of ear drops. Appropriate antibiotic should be administered for 7–10 days on the advice of your doctor. When eardrum is congested and bulging, an ENT specialist should be consulted for drainage of pus. In a case of persistent AOM, when eardrum is retracted, child is asked to practice Valsalva maneuver, i.e. by keeping the nose and mouth closed, the child blows the air into the ears. He can be asked to

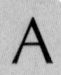

A

make soap bubbles, blow candles or inflate balloons to equilibrate air pressure in the middle ear. Whenever there is perforation of the eardrum, swimming should be avoided or done after wearing ear plugs.

ADENOIDS

Adenoids are small pads of lymphatic tissue, one on either side, which are located near the posterior or back openings of the nose. Just as tonsils serve as sentinels to prevent entry of germs through the mouth, the adenoids guard against the entry of pathogens through the nostrils. In some allergic children, adenoids get enlarged, thus preventing the entry of air through the nose. The child is unable to breathe through his nose and keeps his mouth open both during the day but more commonly at night. The child keeps the neck extended during sleep (which partially relieves airway obstruction), and breathes through the open mouth with a drooping jaw. There is excessive drooling of saliva and loud snoring. The oral cavity and tongue becomes dry because of mouth breathing and there is foul breath. Adenoids may produce characteristic facies (dull or "unintelligent looks") with open mouth, drooping of jaw, drooling of saliva, expressionless face and protruding upper teeth. Enlarged adenoids may block the Eustachian tube (channel between back of the nose and middle ear) leading to repeated attacks of earache because of infection of the middle ear (acute otitis media). A blocked Eustachian tube prevents entry of air into the middle ear causing partial vacuum with a feeling of retracted drum on one or both sides.

Treatment Unlike tonsils, adenoids are not visible through the nose. Their size can be assessed by taking X-ray of the neck (lateral view). Steam inhalation and use of anti-allergic medicines (antihistaminics) may provide some relief. Nasal puffs containing antihistaminic and steroids are available which can be used at night for relief of intractable nasal congestion. When child is uncomfortable due to excessive enlargement of adenoids, there is

Home Remedies

Steam inhalation can be done by adding eucalyptus, mint leaves, holy basil leaves (*tulsi*) or caraway seeds (*ajwain*). In an older child *Jal Neeti* can be done under the supervision of a yoga teacher.

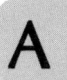

marked snoring and frequent episodes of ear infections, adenoids can be surgically removed by an ENT specialist. The older practice of removing adenoids and tonsils en bloc is no longer recommended. Tonsils should be removed only if they are excessively enlarged and associated with frequent episodes of streptococcal throat infection.

ADOLESCENCE AND PUBERTY

It is a period of transition from childhood to adulthood because of sudden surge of sex hormones. Adolescence is associated with rapid physical growth (weight gain and increase in stature), sexual maturation and emotional development. There is a wide age range when puberty (sexual maturation) begins and it is influenced by heredity, nutrition and general health. Girls mature sexually and emotionally 2 years earlier than boys. That is also the logic as to why in an arranged marriage it is preferred that the girl should be at least 2–3 years younger than the boy. A large majority of girls begin their sexual development at the age of 10 years (budding of breasts, appearance of pubic hair) and have their first menstrual period (menarche) around 12 years of age. During first year, the periods may be infrequent, irregular and painful. At this stage, the body shape of a girl assumes a "feminine figure" with full grown breasts, narrow waist, wide hips and big bums. When breast enlargement starts before 8 years of age or menstruation is delayed beyond 15 years, it is a cause for concern and consultation should be sought with an obstetrician. The average boy starts to have pubertal changes 2 years later and achieves sexual maturity during 14–18 years. The initial sign of sexual maturation in boys is increase in the size of testes and scrotal sac followed by increase in the size of penis. This is followed by appearance of pubic hair, hair in the armpits and over the face (moustache followed by beard) and cracking and deepening of voice. When pubertal changes appear before the age of 10 years or they are delayed beyond 16 years (no testicular enlargement or pubic hair) in boys, it is a cause for concern and a consultation should be sought with a pediatrician.

Health Needs

Due to rapid physical growth spurt, adolescent child should be given a balanced nutritious diet with additional calories, proteins, vitamins and minerals. Teenagers are prone to develop nutritional deficiencies if they are not provided with adequate amounts of balanced diet. Iron deficiency anemia is extremely common among adolescent girls. They should be given supplements of iron, folic acid and calcium. Adolescent girls must have optimal health and nutritional status before they get married so that there are no nutritional constraints to the fetus during pregnancy. Due to excessive intake of junk food and sedentary life style, obesity is emerging as an important public health problem among adolescents.

Teenagers need constant emotional support and guidance by the parents because of increased risk of violent or delinquent behaviour. Due to peer pressure, they are prone to develop various addictions, like smoking, drinking alcohol and substance abuse (see **Box**). A good communication between teens and their parents, a sense of belonging to their social circle and strong moral values (*sanskar*) provide insulation and protection against negative peer pressure. There is high incidence of depression and suicides among adolescents. Unless properly cautioned and guided, teenagers are at an increased risk to develop STDs (sexually transmitted diseases) and unwanted pregnancy by indulging in unsafe and unprotected sexual activities.

Common markers of substance abuse

- Spending time alone with lack of communication and social withdrawal from family members.
- A change in the choice of friends and way of dressing.
- Lack of energy, irregular eating habits, poor sleep and deterioration in school grades.
- Bloodshot eyes and frequent "colds" or nose bleeds.
- Unexplained mood changes like irritability, hyperactivity and depression.
- Running away from home or attempting suicide.

Health Problems

Adolescents develop curiosity about sexual matters and they have sexual fantasies. Boys may experience night emissions or "wet dreams" in their fantasies. Masturbation is common at this stage to achieve sexual gratification. It is normal and without any adverse effects as long as it does not arouse any guilt feelings or sense of shame. Most adolescents have a profuse strong smelling perspiration in their armpits, which may cause unpopularity with their schoolmates. They should maintain a good standard of personal hygiene by taking daily or twice a day bath and using body deodorants. Acne or pimples on the face due to excessive secretion of sebum may cause embarrassment and disfigurement especially if they are squeezed. Girls may have painful and irregular menses (dysmenorrhea) especially during first 1–2 years of their onset. They can be relieved by hot fomentation and intake of analgesic-cum-antispasmodic medication, to relieve pain and discomfort due to cramps. Unless sexual hygiene is maintained, adolescent girls are prone to develop pelvic inflammatory disease (PID) and infertility later in life. During menses, tampon (intravaginal pad) should be avoided because of potential risk of causing toxic shock syndrome (TSS) due to staphylococcal infection. Headaches are common due to anxiety, stress and migraines. There is increased incidence of tuberculosis during adolescence. Thyroid disorders (both hypo- and hyperthyroidism) may occur during adolescence. Mitral valve prolapse (floppy valve syndrome) is common among adolescent girls. Teenage children are prone to suicide attempts because of endogenous depression, academic failure and rejection in romantic relationships.

Vaccinations

Catch-up vaccines are given if any of the routine vaccines have been missed. A booster dose of hepatitis B vaccine, MMR, chicken-pox vaccine, typhoid vaccine and flu vaccine (once a year) are given during 5–10 years of age. A booster dose of Tdap or Td is given around 10 years. Tetanus toxoid or Td boosters are given every 10 years. In girl children, human papillomavirus (HPV) vaccine can be given during 9–14 years of age in 2 doses (0 and 6 months) for prevention of carcinoma cervix. In girls above 14 years, 3 doses are given (0, 1–2 months and 6 months).

Emotional Support

There must be a healthy and mutually respectful adult-to-adult relationship between parents and their teenagers. Children should feel free and confident to confide their problems and concerns to their parents (usually daughter to the mother and son to the father). Most adolescents feel rebellious regarding the constraints, strict

A

discipline and rules imposed by the society and their parents. Nevertheless, teenagers need guidance and want that there should be consistent rules of code or conduct which they can follow. The rules, however, should not be arbitrary, inconsistent or over bearing. It is but natural for parents to know where the teenager is going for a party, who are his friends, where he can be contacted in case of an emergency and when he is expected to come back home. Whenever there is a delay or change in plan, the teenager must call home well in time to intimate and explain the reasons for delay. It is equally important that parents should also tell their children where they are going, how to reach them in case of an emergency and when they are expected to be back home. Parents can teach good habits and discipline to their children by their own example of good conduct and not by any sermons or commands. Teenagers should not be bullied or ordered by the parents and they should not be taken for granted. Most parents do expect that their adolescent children must behave with due politeness and courtesy towards them and other family members, friends, teachers and relatives. And they should understand their obligations to assist their parents in the family chores and should have a sense of dignity and responsibility to feel as an integral part of the family to share both happiness as well as challenges in life. Teenagers should be encouraged to take part in outdoor activities instead of brooding or fantasizing all the time. They should be helped and guided to widen the scope of their interests by developing hobbies and activities to enhance their creativity and skills. They should be encouraged to spend their leisure time in body building, competitive sports, reading, music, dancing, painting, writing, social welfare activities, etc. so that they have no time for being idle and aimless.

ADOPTION

Adoption is a boon for couples who do not have children of their own or when a single parent wants to adopt a child. About 1–2% couples are infertile and despite several therapeutic interventions and recourse to various assisted reproductive technologies (IVF, GIFT, ZIFT, TOT, etc.) and surrogate motherhood, they are unable to beget children of their own. According to "Hindu Adoption and Maintenance Act 1956", there is a legal provision for needy parents to adopt children who are not biologically related to them.

What are the options for seeking children for adoption?

The child can be taken for adoption from among children of relatives who are willing to offer their child for adoption. More commonly, the child is taken for adoption from an orphanage, foster home or from a hospital where children are abandoned by their unwed mothers or due to other social reasons. You can register with any one of the specialised adoption agencies, preferably nearest to your home or online at www.adoption-india.nic.in.

What is the procedure for adoption?

In order to take an informed decision, the adoption agency provides pre-adoption counseling to address the concerns and apprehensions of adoptive parents. You can check your eligibility for adoption on the website of Central Adoption Resource Authority (CARA), Ministry of Women and Child Development or contact them at e-mail: cara_wcd@nic.in. Social worker or public health nurse provides guidance to the family for completing the formalities for adoption. The adoptive parents should apply for adoption by filling the necessary form which is signed by both the adoptive parents. The adoptive couple is required to produce a medical certificate regarding their inability to produce a child, marriage certificate, proof of age, income certificate or statement of bank balance. The social worker provides pre-adoption counseling and assesses the suitability of the adoptive parents. Initially the child is handed over to the adoptive parents for foster care on a trial period. During this period, the social worker is asked to assess the suitability of adoptive parents and quality of care provided to the child by home visits. If a child is not able to adjust or the care provided by the adoptive parents is unsatisfactory, the agency has the right to take away the child and deny adoption. When child is well adjusted and adoptive parents are found to be caring and considerate, legal adoption is confirmed. After legal adoption, the child gets all the rights and privileges which are granted to the biological child.

Should a child be medically screened before adoption?

When a child is picked up for adoption from an orphanage or a foster home, the adoptive parents can get the child examined by a pediatrician for its suitability for adoption by assessing his/her nutritional status, physical growth, neuromotor development, presence of any chronic or contagious disease and immunization record. Laboratory investigations are carried out for complete blood count, X-ray chest, Mantoux test, markers of sexually transmitted diseases like VDRL, HBsAg, HIV and if indicated TORCH prolife.

Should an adopted child be told that he is not the biological child of the parents?

Every child who is adopted must be told, as early as the child can comprehend (usually after 5 years or school entry), that he or she is adopted and foster parents are now the real parents. When the adopted child comes to know about this fact from sources other than the adoptive parents, it may cause severe psychological trauma due to betrayal and breach of trust, and may ruin relations between the foster parents and the child forever.

AIDS (Acquired Immunodeficiency Syndrome)

AIDS is a life-threatening disease caused by human immuno-deficiency virus (HIV). In Asia, India alone accounts for 60% of all patients of AIDS. Children account for about 10% of all cases of AIDS. It is estimated that about 10 million children are infected by HIV in the world and they are destined to die within the next 5 years.

Mode of infection Most children get infection from their HIV-positive mother during pregnancy and delivery. The mother-to-child transmission risk varies between 20 and 35%. There is an additional 15% risk of transmission of HIV infection through breast milk. About 80% HIV infections in children occur during perinatal (before, during or soon after delivery) period and the remaining by transfusion of potentially infected blood and blood products to children suffering from hemophilia, thalassemia major and other hemato-oncologic disorders. Transfusion of unscreened blood carries a grave risk of transmission of not only HIV but many other blood-borne diseases like hepatitis B virus, hepatitis C virus, syphilis, and malaria. In adolescent children, there is an additional risk of HIV infection by use of infected needles by drug abusers

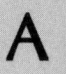

and by indulging in unprotected homosexual or heterosexual activity. AIDS is not a contagious disease and it is not transmitted by living or playing with an AIDS patient or through touch or kissing. Unlike malaria or dengue fever, HIV infection is not transmitted through mosquito bites.

Clinical features HIV-positive mothers have an increased risk of abortion, poor fetal growth and premature delivery. Rarely, a baby may the born with congenital defects like small box-like head, increased distance between the eyes (hypertelorism), flat nose, long slit-like eyes and patulous lips. However, most babies born to HIV-positive mothers are normal at birth. The manifestations of the disease usually appear between 6 and 18 months and most affected children die by 5–8 years of age. There is profound damage to their body organs concerned with defence mechanisms or immunity. These children develop frequent and persistent episodes of fever, diarrhea, respiratory infections, fungal infections (thrush in the mouth, food pipe, anus), tuberculosis, enlargement of lymph nodes, liver and spleen. They are prone to develop unusual bacterial, viral, fungal and parasitic infections. Their weight gain is poor with various grades of undernutrition. Some patients may develop AIDS-associated cancer and encephalopathy.

Diagnosis Elisa and Western blot tests may be positive in a newborn baby, even when baby is not infected, because maternal IgG antibodies against HIV are passively transferred through the placenta from the mother to her baby. These passively transferred antibodies gradually wane off and disappear by 15 months of age. When these antibodies persist beyond 15 months, it is indicative of active HIV infection of the infant. Early diagnosis of HIV infection in an infant can be made by demonstration of HIV-specific IgM antibodies, p24 core antigen or demonstration of HIV-DNA by PCR technology. These children show evidences of defective cell-mediated immunity (reduced number of lymphocytes and CD4 cells) while their serum immunoglobulin levels are usually elevated in response to occurrence of frequent infections.

Treatment These children need tender, loving care with compassion and concern because they are likely to lose their

A parent(s) in infancy because of AIDS. They should never be isolated or shunned because they are not contagious (unlike cough and cold) and there is no risk of infection to other children and caretakers, who can safely caress, cuddle, kiss and feed them. It is important that the child and family should not be ostracized by the society due to the stigma of AIDS. The child can attend a creche or play school without any risk to other children or caretakers. However, precautions should be followed while collecting and handling specimens of blood and for disposal of syrings and needles.

A number of antiretroviral drugs are available but they are expensive and associated with side effects. Drug therapy is associated with in increase in CD4 cell counts, reduced morbidity, increased survival and improved quality of life. Breastfeeding is recognized to pose additional 15% risk of transmission of HIV. Breastfeeding should preferably be avoided and infant given animal milk or formula feeds with a cup and spoon. During weaning, high caloric nutritious feeds should be given to prevent malnutrition and intercurrent infections. Maintenance of strict oral hygiene and topical application of antifungal lotion can prevent oral thrush. Intercurrent infections should be prevented, recognized early and treated promptly.

Immunizations Live vaccines (like BCG, oral polio vaccine) should be avoided in children with manifest AIDS as diagnosed by IgM-specific HIV antibodies and PCR studies. Affected children (and their healthy siblings as well) should be given killed or inactivated polio vaccine (IPV). Administration of oral polio vaccine to healthy siblings may infect the child with AIDS. In addition to the routinely administered killed vaccines, optional vaccines like pneumococcal, meningococcal and influenza vaccines should be given to all children with HIV infection. When HIV-infected child develops serious viral infections like measles and chickenpox, specific immune globulins may be life saving.

Prevention There is no protective vaccine as yet available against AIDS. Administration of antiretroviral therapy to HIV-positive mother during late pregnancy and delivery, and to her infant during first 4–6 weeks of life can reduce the risk of transmission of HIV infection. Elective cesarean section, before rupture of membranes, and avoidance of breastfeeding are associated with reduced risk of vertical transmission of HIV from mother to her infant. Public education and crusade should be launched against drug abuse, dangerous sexual practices and risks posed by professional blood donors. Sex and family life education should be imparted to adolescent boys and girls in high schools to spread the message of safe sex and contraception by use of condom to prevent both sexually transmitted diseases (STDs) and unwanted pregnancies. Contraceptive pills do prevent conceptions but they do not provide any protection against STDs.

AIR TRAVEL

The safest period to fly during pregnancy is the middle of pregnancy between 14 and 28 weeks of gestation when there is least risk of miscarriage and premature delivery. Most airlines do not allow pregnant women to travel by air during the last month (after 36 weeks of gestation) of pregnancy because of risk of premature labor and delivery. It is preferable to ask for an aisle seat and seat belt should be fastened below the abdomen and across the top of your thighs. You should drink plenty of water and make frequent movements at the ankle joints. It is a good idea to stretch and take occasional walks up and down the aisle during a long flight.

First-aid medicine kit

- Antifever and anti-pain medicines (paracetamol, ibuprofen).
- Antivomiting drugs (domperidone, ondansetron hydrochloride).
- Antidiarrheal medicines (norfloxacin, ofloxacin, cefixime) and sachets of oral rehydration salt (ORS).
- Cough and cold medicines
- Abdominal colic (dicyclomine hydrochloride, drotaverine hydrochloride).
- Anti-allergic drugs (chlorpheniramine maleate, cetirizine dihydrochloride).
- Antacids.
- Any drug/s which are routinely given to the child for any chronic disease.
- Antiseptic cream.
- Band-aid and crepe bandage.

A

Air travel is safe in children at all ages. When a child is critically sick and being transferred by air to a referral hospital, he must be accompanied by a doctor or a health care professional. In healthy children, specially those with a cough and cold, there may be severe pain in the ear/s during take off and landing because of sudden changes in air pressure in the middle ear. Infant should be put to breast or offered bottle feeding or a pacifier during take off and landing to prevent earache. The older child can be offered a candy or a chewing gum to suck and ears should be plugged with cotton. Whenever you are travelling with kids for a vacation or family get-together, you must carry the doctor's prescription and essential first-aid medicine kit (see **Box**).

It is desirable to have a medical or health care insurance for the family when travelling overseas. Most pharmacies in the Western countries, unlike Indian drug houses, are very strict in selling drugs over-the-counter and dispense than only against doctor's prescription.

ALLERGIC CONJUNCTIVITIS

Allergic conjunctivitis may occur due to exposure to airborne allergens (pollen, molds, animal dander, etc.) or topical medications. It is more common in summer and spring. It may occur in association with allergic rhinitis or hay fever. There is marked itching, watery discharge from eyes and redness in one or both eyes. The condition responds to local instillation of eye drops containing sodium cromoglycate and ketorolac. *Steroid containing eye drops should never be used unless advised by an ophthalmologist.*

ALLERGIC RHINITIS (Hay fever)

Allergic rhinitis occurs due to exposure to airborne allergens (dust, pollen, spores, pollutants, dust mites, etc.) which may be seasonal (hay fever) or throughout the year (perennial). The common symptoms include marked sneezing, itching, blockage and watery discharge from the nose. It may be associated with itching, redness and watery discharge from the eyes. Unlike viral cold or flu, fever is absent. In some children, allergic manifestations may spread to involve the respiratory passages leading to an attack of bronchial asthma. Treatment includes avoidance of known allergens (when feasible) and use of antihistamines for relief of symptoms. In children

A

above the age of 5 years, steroid nasal sprays provide prompt relief but they must be used under the guidance of a pediatrician.

ALLERGY

It is an unusual response or reaction to substances which are otherwise harmless. The allergic tendency is usually hereditary or there is familial predisposition when it is called atopy. The atopic individual readily becomes sensitized to common protein allergens at normal levels of exposure. Allergic disorders are relatively less common in exclusively breastfed babies. The allergic response may occur to any item which is inhaled (dust, pollen, molds, fungus, dust mites, animal dander, smoke, cockroaches, mosquito repellants, etc.), consumed or taken (oral and injectable drugs, milk, nuts, eggs, fish, chocolates, food color, preservatives, etc.), applied on the skin (soap, powder, cosmetics, hair dyes, oil, synthetic fabric, etc.) or due to insect bites (mosquitoes, bed bugs, bees, wasps, etc.). The common allergic disorders include skin allergy (atopic dermatitis or eczema, urticaria or hives, contact dermatitis, etc.), allergic rhinitis or hay fever, bronchial asthma, drug allergy, food allergy and allergic reaction to insect bites. Apart from specific features of various allergic disorders, the laboratory markers include raised eosinophil count and serum IgE level. The treatment of various allergic disorders is discussed under specific disorders. A variety of antihistaminic drugs are available to treat allergic disorders and most potent being steroids which should be taken only on the advice of a doctor. The first generation antihistaminics (chlorpheniramine maleate, diphenhydramine hydrochloride, pheniramine maleate) produce a number of side effects including sedation, while second or third generation antihistaminics (hydroxyzine hydrochloride, cetirizine hydrochloride, loratadine) are relatively safer with minimal or no sedation.

ALOPECIA (Baldness)

Alopecia or scanty scalp hair in children is uncommon. There is a mistaken belief that shaving of scalp hair is followed by profuse growth of hair which is untrue. The common causes of scanty scalp hair include, poor nutrition, deficiency of protein and trace minerals (zinc, copper) and essential fatty acids (omega-3 fatty acids), hypothyroidism, chronic debilitating diseases, localized

A

diseases of scalp (fungal infection) and developmental disorders (ectodermal dysplasia, progeria). Some children with abnormal behaviour may pluck their hair and eat them which may cause obstruction in the stomach. Alopecia may occur due to traction when "pony-tail" is made to keep them tidy. Alopecia commonly occurs following chemotherapy for cancer which recovers after cessation of therapy. Alopecia or scanty hair are managed by treating the underlying local or systemic disorder. The child should be given balanced high protein diet with supplements of vitamins and trace minerals. Avoid pulling or tugging the hair or forcing them into restrictive styles like ponytails or curling. Comb the hair gently and avoid over brushing the hair. Coconut and *Amla* hair oils are credited to improve the texture and growth of scalp hair. Behaviour therapy helps in children with the habit of plucking and eating their hair. Dandruff and fungal infections of scalp should be treated on the advice of skin specialist. Surgical technique of hair transplantation is becoming popular but is generally practiced in adults. Common home remedies for treatment of sparse hair or alopecia are listed in the **Box**.

Home Remedies

- Massage the scalp with sesame oil every night and cover with a cap. Wash in the morning with a herbal shampoo and rinse with water containing apple cider vinegar (15 mL in one liter of water).
- Take equal quantity of olive oil and oil of rosemary (or 2 parts of almond oil and one part of rosemary oil) in a bottle and shake vigorously. Massage into the scalp at night and put on a cap. Wash the hair with a herbal shampoo in the morning.
- Mix a tablespoon of honey, juice of one medium-size onion and 15 mL vodka. Rub the mixture into the scalp at night and cover with a cap. Wash with a herbal shampoo in the morning.

AMBLYOPIA

Amblyopia or visual inattentiveness is defined as decrease in visual acuity that occurs in early life due to lack of clear image falling on the retina. The eyes are normal looking and no abnormality is found on examination by an ophthalmologist but child ignores to use or focus with the amblyopic or "lazy" eye. There may be variable (eye/s may converge inwards or diverge outwards) non-paralytic squint on one side or alternately on both sides. The condition is treated by covering or patching the normal eye to stimulate proper visual development of the amblyopic eye.

Amblyopia should be differentiated from partial or total loss of vision (blindness) in early life due to short sightedness (myopia), developmental disorders of eye/s, infections, tumor, injury, retinopathy of prematurity (ROP), and vitamin A deficiency. The common correlates of blindness in young children include squint (nonaligned or crossed eyes), nystagmus (jerky movements of eyes) or roving eye movements, clumsiness, timidity, poor school performance, blinking of eyes, keenness to sit in the first row in class or watch TV from a close distance. Children with blindness are more responsive to sound or touch and may get easily startled. They may have delayed neuromotor developmental milestones. Whenever a child has lack of social smile by 6 weeks of age, he must be taken to an ophthalmologist for complete evaluation of eyes.

AMEBIASIS (Amebic dysentery)

Amebiasis is caused by parasite *Entamoeba histolytica* and infection occurs by consuming contaminated food and water. The disease is more common in regions with poor standard of personal and food hygiene, over crowding and inadequate sanitation. Acute infection causes loose motions with blood and mucus in the stools (dysentery). Abdominal cramps, flatulence and frequent urge to pass stool (tenesmus) are common. Unlike bacterial or bacillary dysentery, fever is absent or minimal and stool mostly comprise of mucus and blood with little fecal matter. At times the infection becomes chronic with recurrent episodes of abdominal pain, loose motions and constipation. Rarely, the infection may spread to other parts of the body through bloodstream and produce amebic abscess most commonly in the liver.

Treatment Amebic dysentery is treated by administration of metronidazole or tinidazole under the supervision of a pediatrician. Amebic liver abscess is treated by aspiration under ultrasonographic guidance and administration of effective drugs. The disease can be prevented by maintenance of strict personal hygiene, avoidance of food items from road side vendors and drinking safe water.

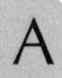

AMENORRHEA

Cessation of menstrual periods is called amenorrhea and usually signifies pregnancy and menopause (after 45 years). During first 6 months–1 year of onset of menstruation, the periods may be scanty, irregular with delay of several days off and on. Menstrual periods may become scanty when there is chronic systemic illness, disordered eating, poor nutrition, pelvic inflammatory disease and hyper- or hypothyroidism. Amenorrhea with dysfunctional uterine bleeding, hirsutism (facial hair), pigmentation over the neck and axillae, and acne (pimples) is suggestive of polycystic ovarian disease (PCOD). When onset of menses is delayed beyond 15 years, the child should be examined and investigated by an obstetrician.

AMNIOCENTESIS

The technique used for collection of amniotic fluid during pregnancy for diagnostic purposes is called amniocentesis. The procedure is performed to assess the maturity of fetus, determine the severity of Rh hemolytic disease and for prenatal genetic and chromosomal studies. The procedure is simple and best performed around 15–16 weeks of pregnancy. The procedure should be performed with due aseptic precautions under ultrasound monitoring to minimize the risk of damage to the placenta or fetus. The procedure is usually safe and common complications include bleeding, infection and premature onset of labor.

ANAL ITCHING

The commonest cause of anal itching is pinworm or threadworm infestation. The itching mostly occurs at night when worms try to wriggle out of the anus. White thread-like moving worms can be seen when bottom is examined with a torch light at night. In girl children, the worms may enter the vaginal orifice causing sudden episodes of shrieking at night. Other causes of anal itching include constipation, anal fissure (injury due to hard stools), rectal prolapse, fungal infection, diaper rash, and poor bottom hygiene. There is no scientific basis for the common belief that anal itching is caused by excessive intake of sweets or mangoes. Apart from specific treatment of the underlying cause, symptomatic relief is provided by local application of a moisturizing or a calamine-based soothing cream or coconut oil. It is important to remember that when child is suspected to have pinworms, all family members should be treated otherwise reinfection commonly occurs.

ANAPHYLAXIS

Anaphylaxis is an immediate hypersensitivity or allergic reaction which may be life-threatening. The allergen is usually a drug (often through injection or orally), blood product or food protein (milk, grains, nuts, eggs, fish) which forms a complex with a specific IgE antibodies which is then bound to the surface of certain cells (mast cells, basophils) which trigger the allergic response. Sudden release of chemical mediators (histamine, leukotrienes) cause dilatation of blood vessels, leakage of plasma from capillaries, swelling of voice box (larynx) and swelling or spasm of air passages.

The onset of symptoms is sudden and dramatic. There is tingling or fainting sensation with a "lump" in throat followed by hoarseness of voice and difficulty in breathing due to spasm of bronchi. Edema of voice box may cause hoarseness and noisy breathing. Skin rash with itching may appear. Sudden abdominal cramps and diarrhea may occur due to involvement of intestines. Shock may supervene due to cardiovascular collapse.

Treatment Administration of adrenaline (0.01 mL/kg 1:1000 solution) intramuscularly is life saving. It can be repeated every 15–30 minutes. In mild cases, oral antihistamines and steroids are useful. Children with known food allergy, with history of previous attacks of anaphylaxis, must carry a pre-loaded adrenaline syringe (EpiPen, Ana-Kit), so that life-saving shot can be taken by the child or given by the parents in case of an unexpected emergency.

ANEMIA

Anemia is defined as low level of hemoglobin in the blood, either because there are a few red blood cells or there is less hemoglobin in each cell or both. Hemoglobin level of less than 11.0 g/dL in preschool children and less than 12.0 g/dL in school going children is suggestive of anemia.

Causes The most common cause of anemia is iron deficiency. It is a common condition in infants and adolescents. Milk is relatively deficient in iron. Prolonged milk feeding without complementary semisolid iron-containing weaning foods is the commonest cause of iron deficiency anemia. Parasitic infections, such as malaria and worm infestation (especially hookworm) and frequent respiratory and gastrointestinal infections further aggravate iron deficiency. Dietary deficiency of folic acid and vitamin B_{12} causes a different type of anemia (megaloblastic anemia) which is associated with reduced number of platelets (thrombocytopenia). Other important causes of anemia include blood loss (especially due to excessive menstrual blood loss in adolescent girls), breakdown of red blood cells inside the body (hemolytic anemia especially due to thalassemia major). Life-threatening anemia may occur due to lack of production of red blood cells (aplastic anemia) and blood cancer (leukemia).

Clinical features The child would look pale, although some fair-skinned children may look pale without anemia. Pallor is usually seen over the face, palms, nail bed and tongue. The child may be lethargic, irritable or cranky and may have poor appetite. The child may like to eat inedible objects, like clay and mud (pica). The child may not be playful and active because of easy fatigability. The child may develop breathlessness on walking, running and playing. Anemic children are more susceptible to develop frequent infections. Iron deficiency during early life has been shown to slow down neuromotor development and reduce learning capacity.

Treatment After 6 months when complementary feeds are started, child should be given home-based weaning foods rich in iron. Cereal, pulses, legumes, dark green leafy vegetables, beetroot, certain fruits (banana, apple, pomegranate), egg yolk and jaggery (*ghur*) are good sources of iron. Non-vegetarian foods (especially muscle, blood and liver) are excellent sources of iron, which is more readily absorbed. Iron absorption is enhanced by intake of vitamin C rich food (citrus fruits, sour vegetables). Medicinal iron can be given in the form of drops, syrup or tablets on the advice of a physician for prevention and treatment of iron deficiency anemia. Iron is best given in-between the meals in 2–3 divided doses. Iron therapy must be continued for at least 2–3 months to correct anemia and replenish the body stores of iron. Some children may not tolerate medicinal iron and may develop either constipation or loose motions. Tolerance is often improved by changing the medicinal iron salt. Intake of iron syrup may

A

lead to black staining of teeth and passage of greenish-black-colored stools. Administration of water or offering an apple after oral administration of iron syrup, reduces the risk of discoloration of teeth.

ANOREXIA (Loss of appetite)

Hunger is a basic survival urge controlled by hypothalamus in the brain. Appetite is adversely affected when child is having febrile illness or discomfort in abdomen. Food fussiness or refusal to eat is a behaviour disorder and should not be confused with loss of appetite. The common causes of genuine anorexia include infections, painful conditions in the mouth (teething, ulcers, thrush) or pain elsewhere (especially abdomen), cardiorespiratory insufficiency (rapid breathing), chronic systemic disease (tuberculosis, liver or kidney disease, cancer) and use of drugs especially antibiotics. Other causes of anorexia include anxiety, stress, depression, smoking and drug abuse. Anorexia is managed by identification of the underlying cause and treating it. Appetizers and micronutrients may be given for symptomatic relief on the advice of a doctor.

ANOREXIA NERVOSA

It is a rare psychological eating disorder among adolescent girls who have an abnormal fear of obesity, distorted body image and they practically starve themselves by refusing to eat. There is intense fear of becoming obese despite progressive weight loss. Amenorrhea is common which may be primary (delayed onset or scanty menses) or secondary. There is loss of sexual libido and infertility. These children may have excessive physical activity, excessive interest in studies, preoccupation with preparation of food and bizarre eating behaviour. The child may starve herself or eat in binges and then purge herself of food by self-induced vomiting or the use of cathartics. The commonly associated psychological symptoms include social isolation, depression, anxiety, obsessional symptoms and perfectionistic traits. They are prone to suicide and adverse health consequences due to chronic starvation. The child needs intense psychological support, behaviour modification, and compassionate handling. Many patients need intensive treatment after admission to the hospital for nutritional rehabilitation.

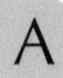

ANTENATAL CHECK-UP

When a married woman misses her period, it usually signifies onset of pregnancy. She should consult an obstetrician for confirmation of pregnancy by doing a urine test. It is desirable to have at least 5 antenatal check-ups (onset of pregnancy, 2–3 months, 5–6 months, 7 months, 8 months and 9 months). Height, weight gain during pregnancy, growth of uterus, swelling of feet, and blood pressure are checked during each visit. Hemoglobin, blood group, urine for proteinuria and blood glucose are checked routinely to exclude pregnancy-induced hypertension, toxemia of pregnancy and gestational diabetes mellitus. Other laboratory investigations include tests for syphilis, HIV, intrauterine infections, and thalassemia trait. Ultrasound examination is done to time (assess gestation) and confirm pregnancy, assess the growth of fetus, location of placenta and exclusion of developmental defects. Mother should take adequate diet containing green leafy vegetables, high protein foods and seasonal fruits. She should drink plenty of water and take adequate rest. Supplements of vitamins, iron, folic acid, zinc and calcium should be taken during pregnancy. Medications should be taken only on the advice of an obstetrician and should preferably be avoided during first 3 months of pregnancy because of potential risk of causing congenital malformations in the fetus. In selected cases, when there is a developmental, genetic or chromosomal defect in a previous sibling, specialized tests like amniocentesis and chorionic villus sampling are done for antenatal diagnosis. When diagnosis of a life-threatening or disabling developmental or genetic defect is made, option can be given to the parents for medical termination of pregnancy.

APHTHOUS ULCERS

Some children are prone to develop recurrent episodes of painful ulcers in the mouth. They are usually due to a viral infection (Herpes simplex) and generally more than one family member is affected. Prolonged use of antibiotics, nervous tension or stress and injury to the oral mucosa by the bite or toothbrush may predispose to development of ulcers. The ulcers have a greyish-white base with angry-red margins. The ulcers may be present over the tongue, inner surface of lips, gums and inside of the cheeks. They are extremely painful and cause drooling and

A

Home Remedies

- Burn alum in a non-stick pan and make a powder. Mix it with glycerine and apply over the ulcers.
- Boil few guava and neem leaves in water to make a decoction. Strain it and keep in the refrigerator. Use it 3–4 times a day as a mouth rinse.
- Herbal tea made with few crushed henna leaves and liquorice (*malathi*) can be used for gargles and mouth rinse.

---

difficulty in feeding. Paracetamol may be given if pain and discomfort are marked. Local application of an antiseptic-cum-anesthetic gel or boroglycerine or toothpaste provides symptomatic relief. Chlorhexidine mouth rinse is useful to promote recovery. The child should be given soft bland diet without spices and chillies. Relief of constipation and intake of B complex vitamins may reduce the risk of ulcers. A number of home remedies are useful for treatment of mouth ulcers (*see* **Box**). Regular brushing of teeth (without causing injury to the gums) and maintenance of strict oro-dental hygiene are effective to prevent their recurrence.

APPENDICITIS

Appendix is a finger-like appendage on the intestine at the junction between small and large intestine. Acute appendicitis is inflammation of the appendix due to infection. There are no known predisposing factors but there may be genetic or familial predisposition. There is sudden onset of fever, vomiting, loss of appetite and pain in the centre of abdomen above the navel. After few hours, the pain shifts to the right lower abdomen, which becomes extremely tender on touch. Whenever abdominal pain is associated with fever and typical migration story (pain from centre of the upper abdomen moving to right lower abdomen), the child must be seen by a pediatric surgeon to rule out the possibility of acute appendicitis. When diagnosis is confirmed, the treatment is surgical excision of appendix, which can also be done through a button hole with the help of a laparoscope without any surgical scar.

ARTHRALGIAS AND ARTHRITIS

Pain in the joint/s without any signs of inflammation (like swelling, redness and warmth) is called arthralgia. In arthritis,

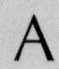

the affected joint/s is swollen, warm, red, tender to touch, and movements are restricted and painful. Arthritis may occur due to involvement of the affected joint/s as a result of injury, bleeding, infection or inflammation. The involvement of joint/s may be one of the manifestations of a systemic disorder like rheumatic fever, rheumatoid arthritis, serum sickness, collagen vascular disorder, etc. Joint pains are usually worse in the morning on getting up from sleep followed by gradual relief as the day dawns. Joint pains are worse in winter or temperate climate compared to summer or tropical climate. The term "rheumatism" should be avoided and should not be confused with acute rheumatic fever or rheumatoid arthritis.

Treatment During injury or sprain of a joint, a cold pack should be applied for 5–10 minutes to reduce local bleeding. When single joint is affected, local application of a counter-irritant cream, hot fomentation and crepe bandage provide relief. Administration of paracetamol or non-steroidal anti-inflammatory drug (NSAID) is useful for symptomatic relief. When multiple joints are involved, child must be seen by a pediatrician for investigations and appropriate management.

ASTHMA (Asthmatic bronchitis, bronchial asthma, wheezing)

Asthma is an inflammatory disease that affects the small airways (bronchioles) that carry air in and out of the lungs. It is characterized by recurrent episodes of cough, breathing difficulty and wheezing in a child who has an inherited susceptibility to manifest atopy or allergy to a variety of environmental allergens. The antigen–antibody reaction in the air passages leads to release of histamine which cause inflammation and spasm of muscles of bronchioles. There is swelling of lining of the airways with production of sticky mucus or phlegm and constriction or spasm of muscles of small airways.

Asthma Triggers

A large number of triggers are known to initiate an attack of asthma. Bronchial asthma is usually caused by allergens which are inhaled into air passages. The commonly inhaled allergens include dust, dust mites, pollutants, pollen of flowers or weeds, cockroaches, molds, fungi, yeast, hair or dander of pet animals or

A

birds. The attack of asthma is often triggered and aggravated by environmental pollution (dust, automobile exhaust, pesticides, fire crackers, etc.), smoke (over crowding, conventional *chullah, hawan*, poor vetilation, cigarette smoking by parents), cooking odors, air fresheners, perfumes, deodorants, *agarbatti, dhoop*, soaps, hair oils, cosmetics, talcum powder, insect sprays and mosquito repellants. During the last decade, the incidence of asthma has almost doubled among urban children because of increasing pollution, smoke and smog in the cities. Food allergens are uncommon triggers of bronchial asthma and they include artificial colors and preservatives in soft drinks, fruit juices, dry mixes for making cold drinks, ketchup, jam, chicklets, gems, candies, lollypops, chips or crisps, etc. Allergy to fresh fruits and vegetables is rare but is well documented with dry fruits or nuts especially if they are contaminated with molds. Viral infections and certain drugs (aspirin and non-steroidal anti-inflammatory drugs) are common triggers for asthma. Exercise, exposure to cold, change of weather and emotional stress of examination may trigger an attack of asthma in susceptible children. The parents should be vigilant and maintain a diary to identify various factors and situations which lead to wheezing.

Common Manifestations

The disease may start at any age. The child gets frequent attacks of viral or allergic colds (sneezing, watering of nose and eyes, itching of nose, redness of eyes) which is followed by bouts of intractable spasmodic cough, wheezing and breathing difficulty. The cough is persistent, "chesty" or wet, spasmodic and worse at night and early morning. The cough may be triggered by feeding and bouts of crying or laughing. The cough is often followed by vomiting which is associated with relief due to expulsion of sticky or tenacious phlegm. The attack may be associated with fast breathing with retractions of chest wall. Breathing out is more difficult and often prolonged. Wheezing (whistling sound especially while breathing out) is best heard when ear is placed on the chest wall (over the front or back) of the child. In severe cases, wheezing may be audible from a distance. In many cases, spasmodic cough is a dominant feature while wheezing or breathing difficulty is minimal. These children are diagnosed to have cough-variant asthma. There is genetic background or family

A

history of bronchial asthma, recurrent episodes of common cold, sneezing or drug allergy. The child may show personal manifestations of atopy, i.e. atopic dermatitis or eczema, urticaria, hay fever, food allergy and drug allergy. Obesity is known to aggravate asthmatic manifestations.

Conditions that may be confused with asthma

It must be remembered that all cases of wheezing are not due to asthma and asthma can occur without obvious wheezing. In children below 2 years, wheezing may occur due to acute bronchiolitis (RSV infection), bronchopneumonia, congestive heart failure, gastroesophageal reflux disease (GERD), cystic fibrosis, and foreign inhalation. Wheezing in infancy is more difficult to treat due to greater narrowing of bronchioles.

Treatment

Bronchial asthma is a chronic disease and all the likely triggers in the environment and food should be eliminated. A large number of drugs are available to relieve the acute attack of asthma. They must be administered early to avoid hospitalization. The *reliever drugs* include short-acting β_2-agonists (salbutamol, levosalbutamol, terbutaline), xanthines (theophylline), anticholinergics (ipratropium bromide) and corticosteroids. In a severe attack, oral administration of steroids provides prompt relief. Inhalation therapy is preferred because of its greater efficacy and lower incidence of side effects. Depending upon the age of the child, several modalities are available for inhalation therapy (see **Box**).

There is a wrong belief that inhalers are habit forming but they may become ineffective if canister is empty or when they are used

Available modalities for inhalation therapy	
Age	Recommended device
0–4 years	Nebulizer with a mask, MDI* with a spacer and mask, aerochamber with a mask
5–8 years	Rotahaler, MDI with a spacer
> 8 years	MDI, Rotahaler

*MDI: Metered dose inhaler. Nebulizer is more effective and can be used at any age.

Correct method to use a metered dose inhaler (MDI)

School going children

- Child is asked to completely exhale or take the breath out completely and hold the mouth piece of the MDI tightly with lips.
- The actuator of the inhaler is pressed while child takes a deep breath to inhale the aerosole.
- Most school going children, with some practice and guidance, can coordinate pressing of the inhaler with their breath to effectively inhale the medication directly without using the spacer device.
- Two puffs of beta-2 agonists can be taken every 5–10 minutes during first one hour to treat a severe attack of asthma.

Preschool children

- Due to poor hand-breath coordination, a spacer device with a mask is used.
- The mask is tightly placed on the face to cover the nose and mouth of the toddler.
- Children between 4 and 5 years can be asked to hold the outlet of the spacer between their lips.
- The actuator of the inhaler is pressed and child is asked to breathe normally. It takes about 10–15 seconds for completely inhaling the medication released in the chamber. The second puff of the medication can be taken after 15 seconds.
- A smaller volume (250 mL) spacer is used in young children and a large volume (750 mL) spacer for older children.
- MDI with a spacer is as effective as a nebulizer and easier to use because procedure takes about 30 seconds (compared to 12–15 minutes with a nebulizer). But 5 doses of MDI are equivalent to one dose of medication administered through a nebulizer.
- The spacer should be washed with a detergent every week and air dried.

without due regard for the correct procedure (see **Box**). Nebulization with an electrical device can be used for nebulization of bronchodilators and steroids. They are more effective than metered dose inhalers. A mask should be used to cover the nose and mouth for effective nebulization in preschool children while an older child is able to inhale the medicine through his mouth. Nebulization is ineffective when nebulizer outlet is merely placed infront of the nose of the child (see **Box**).

A

Correct use of a nebulizer

- Nebulization is more effective and can be used at any age.
- Medication is delivered with the help of an electrically operated device and can be used both at home and hospital. In hospital setting, the device is operated by using oxygen flow at a rate of 6–7 liters/min.
- In a preschool child, a mask is used to cover the nose and mouth. In older children, the child is asked to hold the mouth device between his lips.
- The drug volume should be at least 3 mL by adding normal saline. Three doses of drugs should be nebulized after every 20 minutes during first hour of therapy.
- Patient should be asked to inhale through his mouth. Although it may be difficult to control breathing pattern during an acute attack but deep and slow breathing is advocated.
- Drug should be nebulized over a period of 10–12 minutes. If the procedure is taking more than 15 minutes, either instrument is malfunctioning or supply of air/oxygen is defective.
- A good mist formation suggests that the procedure of nebulization is satisfactory.
- After relief of acute attack, the instrument and mask should be washed with a mild detergent followed by sterillium, to keep it ready for the next use.

Prevention

Asthma is a chronic disease with frequent relapses which may be seasonal or throughout the year (perennial). All the possible triggers in the environment and food should be eliminated. A diary should be maintained to identify the trigger/s which irritate or aggravate the attack, so that they can be eliminated. The environment of the child especially bedroom should be kept dust free and well ventilated. Avoid use of carpets and heavy curtains. Instead of brooming, vacuum cleaner should be used. The filter of the air conditioner should be cleaned frequently. The home should be kept free of dust mites (expose bed sheet to sunlight once a week), cockroaches and other insects. Pets and stuffed toys should preferably avoided. Children with asthma should avoid smoky, stuffy, over crowded and polluted places. The use of insect sprays or mosquito-repellants, strong perfumes, deodorants, *agarbatti, dhoop,* etc. should be avoided when child is around. The physical activity should be limited to the tolerance level of the child.

Home Remedies

- Avoid intake of cold water, ice-cream, fried foods, milk, yoghurt, rice, banana, slimy vegetables like okra (*bhindi*), *arbi*, and colocasia (*kachaloo*), etc.
- Add half teaspoon of ginger juice, half teaspoon powder of cloves (*laung*) and cinnamon (*dalchini*), and one teaspoon of honey in a cup of boiling water. Drink at night everyday.
- Boil 6 cloves (*laung*) in a cup of water. Take one teaspoon of concoction with honey 3 times/day.
- Soak overnight 1–2 figs (*anjeer*) in a cup of water. Take the figs and drink the water first thing in the morning. Figs are rich in trace minerals zinc and copper.
- Take a teaspoon each of long pepper (*mugh or pipli*), dried powdered ginger (*sonth*) and cloves (*laung*). Powder them together, mix honey and make a paste. The paste can be licked 4–5 times a day or whenever there is a bout of coughing.
- Dried Indian gooseberry (*Amla*) powder (half spoon) mixed with one teaspoon of honey should be taken every morning with warm water.
- Herbal tea made with fennel (*saunf*) and cloves (*laung*) is soothing for persistent cough by breaking up the thick tenacious mucus.
- Drink a glass of hot milk with a teaspoon each of turmeric and honey twice a day for one month.
- Mix half teaspoon each of bitter gourd (*karela*) and holy basil (*tulasi*) paste in 5 mL honey and take it every night for one month.
- Massage mustard oil with a little camphor vigorously over the chest during an attack of asthma. It loosens up the accumulated phlegm and helps in its expectoration.

The body resistance against infections and allergy can be boosted by intake of balanced nutritious diet and intake of supplements of micronutrients (vitamin A, vitamin C, vitamin D, zinc, calcium and selenium) which are credited to have anti-infective, anti-allergic and anti-oxidant capabilities. Omega-3 fatty acids and their active metabolites (DHA and EPA) are anti-inflammatory in nature and have been shown to reduce the severity of allergic diseases including bronchial asthma. Yoga and breathing exercises help to improve the vital capacity of lungs. Leukotriene receptor antagonists (montelukast, zafirlukast) can be used for prevention of mild to moderate attacks and exercise-induced asthma. In children with persistent and severe bronchial asthma, long-acting inhaled steroids (fluticasone) and a long-acting β-agonist (salmeterol formoterol) can be used for prophylaxis on a long-term basis.

A

Frequently Asked Questions (FAQs)

What general guidelines and dietary restrictions should be followed by children with bronchial asthma?

Asthma is caused by an allergic response to dust, dust mites, pollen, grass, fungi, molds, etc. It is not possible to totally avoid exposure to these allergens but an attempt should be made to minimize the exposure. Avoid use of carpets and heavy curtains in the bedrooms of the patient. The mattresses, blankets and pillows should be kept in dust-free covers. The filter of air conditioners should be washed frequently and room temperature should be kept above 26°C. The home should be kept free of dust mites (by exposing bed linen to sunlight once a week), molds, cockroaches and other insects and rodents. Children with asthma should avoid smoky, stuffy, over-crowded and polluted places. The use of deodorants, perfumes, *agarbatti, dhoop*, insect sprays and mosquito-repellants should be avoided when asthmatic child is around. Bathroom, kitchen, and fridge should be kept clean and free of cockroaches and molds. The child should be shifted to another place when white washing, painting, repairs and pest control measures are being planned.

Food items have relatively less risk of causing or aggravating reactive airway disease but may trigger bronchospasm either directly or by virtue of development of viral infection. The child should be advised to avoid intake of chilled water, ice-cream, food items containing synthetic colors, flavors and preservatives, like cold drinks, tetrapack fruit juices, tang, ketchup, jams, pickles, canned food, chicklets, gems, candies, lollypops, chips or crisps, etc. In Ayurvedic system, the food items which are slimy in nature are credited to produce phlegm and should be avoided. They include milk, curd, rice, banana, okra (*bhindi*), *arbi*, and colocasia (*kachaloo*).

What is the role of skin testing for identification of an allergic child?

Skin testing is cumbersome and not routinely undertaken in children. When conducted, allergic response is elicited against a large number of allergens. The desensitization process becomes time consuming, unreliable and hazardous. It is possible to estimate the level of food-specific IgE antibodies in the blood but

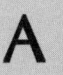

they are also of limited utility. Identification of possible triggers by constant vigilance and maintaining a diary is more useful and cost-effective.

What drugs should be avoided by an asthmatic child?

Aspirin and non-steroidal anti-inflammatory drugs (NSAIDs) should be avoided because they are known to increase bronchial reactivity and bronchospasm in susceptible children. Paracetamol is the antipyretic and analgesic of choice in asthmatic children having fever and discomfort. Non-selective beta blockers and certain formulations in eye drops should be avoided by asthmatic patients.

Can a change of residence help an asthmatic child?

In some children, the change of residence may help, if the new place is not having the allergens which are bothering the child. However, the benefits may be temporary and symptoms may reappear after sometime after exposure to some other allergens. There are social and financial implications of change of residence, the decision should be taken with caution and due consideration. When a change of residence is feasible, it is suggested to move initially on a "trial basis". The trial move should last for at least 3–4 months before taking a final decision.

What is the role of cough syrups and expectorants?

These medicines have no role in the management of bronchial asthma and they should be avoided. The act of coughing and vomiting helps the patient to get rid of excessive secretions of mucus and phlegm. The use of antihistaminics should be avoided during an attack of bronchial asthma because they are likely to aggravate breathing difficulty by making bronchial secretions more viscid and tenacious. The child should be encouraged to drink plenty of liquids to maintain adequate hydration to prevent drying of bronchial secretions. Drinking warm water with honey often terminates bouts of coughing in asthmatic children.

When two inhaler medications are being taken by the child, what should be the sequence of their administration?

When a patient is taking both a bronchodilator and corticosteroid aerosol, the bronchodilator (salbutamol, terbutaline, ipratropium bromide) should be taken first. After about 3–5 minutes, when bronchi would have relaxed and dilated, aerosol of corticosteroid should be taken for its more effective delivery and penetration to the distal smaller airways or bronchioles.

Are inhalers habit forming?

There is a wrong belief that inhalers are habit forming. They are effective and life saving. They may become ineffective, if canister is empty or when they are used without due regard for correct procedure. The empty canister is likely to float on the surface of water.

Can asthmatic child take part in competitive sports?

The asthmatic child should be encouraged to lead a normal life and take part in all outdoor activities. The physical education teacher or coach should be informed about the asthmatic condition of the child. The level of their performance in sports should be guided on the basis of the physical capability. In some children, physical activity and exercise are known to precipitate an attack of asthma. These children should take leukotriene modifier and long-acting inhaled β-agonist before taking part in sports and physical training to prevent wheezing and shortness of breath. Swimming is an excellent sport for asthmatic children. Yoga and breathing exercises (*pranayam*) are useful to improve lung functions. Human potentiality is profound and some of the world's best athletes and sports legends have been asthmatic. Van Dykan, a world famous asthmatic youth earned many gold medals in the olympic swimming competitions.

How to identify an attack of asthma at its earliest?

Identification of triggers, early symptoms (cough at night or early morning, getting out of breath easily, throat irritation and fatigability) and twice daily (morning and evening) monitoring of peak expiratory flow rate (PEFR) with a peak flow meter can recognize an impending attack of wheezing.

Children above the age of 5 years can be taught how to use a peak flow meter. The child is asked to stand erect and take a deep breath to inflate the lungs fully. The mouthpiece of the flow meter is taken in the mouth and lips are tightly closed over it. Air is then exhaled out with a force by taking a maximum outbreath. The procedure is repeated 3 times and the highest

Normal PEFR values in children			
Height (inches)	PEFR (liters/min)	Height (inches)	PEFR (liters/min)
43	147	55	307
44	160	56	320
45	173	57	334
46	187	58	347
47	200	59	360
48	214	60	373
49	227	61	387
50	240	62	400
51	254	63	413
52	267	64	427
53	280	65	440
54	289	—	—

reading is recorded. Average PEFR values of the child, when he is well, should be established as a personal norm. The predicted average PEFR values in children of different heights are given in the **Box**. Depending upon the actual PEFR of the patient, three categories are identified as follows:

Green zone: Peak flow of more than 80% of the predicted average or child's known average PEFR when well. A reading in this zone means patient is doing well on current medications or without medications.

Yellow zone: Peak flow between 50 and 80% of the predicted or child's average PEFR. It suggests a mild attack requiring increase in inhalation therapy on ambulatory basis.

Red zone: Peak flow of less than 50% of predicted PEFR or child's average. A reading in this danger zone suggests that child is having a moderate to severe attack of bronchial asthma and he should be immediately admitted to the hospital for further management.

Do children "outgrow" from their asthmatic tendency?

Yes, most children who do not have atopic tendency, do improve as they grow. About one-third of children outgrow their asthma by 5 years and one-half are free from asthmatic attacks by 8 years of age. About 10% of affected child continue to have their asthmatic attacks during adolescence and later in life. Children with more severe and persistent or perennial symptoms are less likely to lose their asthma but they tend to show some improvement when they reach puberty. It is also true that some children after having recovered from their asthma in childhood may regain their asthmatic tendency in adult life.

Is bronchial asthma curable?

We have excellent life-saving *reliever drugs* to provide relief from an attack of asthma and *controller drugs* to reduce the frequency of attacks. The disease can be effectively controlled but unfortunately there are no foolproof modalities to provide cure. Despite several claims in different systems of medicine, to the best of our knowledge, there is no sure shot curative remedy with any of them. Even the well publicized unique method of administering medicines by asking the patient to swallow a "medicated live fish" by Gouds on June of every year in Hyderabad is of doubtful utility. Some indigenous practitioners are known to prescribe powdered "corticosteroids" on a long-term basis which lead to development of side effects like moon facies and excessive weight gain. Avoidance of allergens which trigger the attacks is most useful to provide relief and long lasting remission. However, one should never forget that faith, suggestion, will power and "time" are great healers and miracles do happen.

ATOPIC DERMATITIS (Eczema)

Allergic menifestations over the skin of children with familial or hereditary predisposition for allergy or atopy is called atopic dermatitis. The disease may start in infancy and is more common in formula fed or bottle fed babies. Administration of fruit juice may trigger the allergic manifestations but usually no predisposing factors are found. In infants, skin rash is distributed over the cheeks, behind the ears and scalp. The diaper area is usually spared. In older children, flexor surfaces of extremities (creases of elbows, wrists and knees), neck, axillae and groins are affected. Skin lesions consist of papules (pin head-sized solid elevations on skin) and vesicles (fluid-filled papules) with weeping or wet lesions which develop scales, scabs or crusts. Secondary infection may develop due to scratching and rubbing. The child is uncomfortable and cranky because of intense itching. The disease runs a

A

prolonged course with remissions and relapses for several months and years. Laboratory investigations usually show increased number of eosinophils and elevated levels of IgE antibodies in the blood. Children with dandruff (seborrhea of scalp) may develop similar skin manifestations but they do not show any laboratory markers of atopic dermatitis.

Treatment Skin hygiene should be maintained by regular baths and control of itching. A non-irritant soap or cleansing lotion should be used to clean the affected areas of skin. When superadded bacterial infection has occurred, antibiotics should be taken on the advice of a doctor. Local application of a steroid cream followed by a moisturizing lotion or cream is associated with prompt relief. Itching can be controlled by administration of an antihistamine (promethazine, hydroxyzine). If any trigger is suspected or identified, it should be eliminated.

ATTENTION DEFICIT HYPERACTIVITY DISORDER (ADHD)

This descriptive name is more appropriate than the old nomenclature of "minimal brain dysfunction". The disorder affects 3–5% school going children. Boys are affected 5 times more often than girls. Its prevalence is relatively less in India compared to the West. The exact cause of disorder is unknown but there is increased familial tendency or genetic predisposition. There is some derangement of chemical neurotransmitters (dopamine) in the brain. There is controversial link between diet and hyper-activity in children. There is no evidence that excessive intake of sugar is associated with hyperactivity. However, food additives, food colors, preservatives, caffeine and vitamin C-rich foods may trigger hyperactivity. There is some correlation between ADHD and low intake of omega-3 fatty acid and DHA.

How to suspect it?

The developmental milestones are usually normal and some children may have above normal intelligence. School problems and learning disabilities due to hyperactivity and poor attention span are seen in 10–30% children with ADHD. The affected children are restless, hyperactive, inattentive, impulsive, unable to sit still and are perpetually "on the go" as if "driven by a motor". They are constantly on the move, fidget, squirm, aimlessly touch and poke their fingers into everything. They are unable to sit through a TV program or listen to a story due to short attention span. They have an impulsive behaviour, blurting out answers before completion of questions and have trouble waiting for their turn or standing in a queue. Their behaviour becomes worse in crowded places and infront of guests. They are aggressive in their behaviour and uncooperative with their classmates and have difficulty in cultivating friendship. They may have antisocial behaviour like disobediency, defiance, lack of discipline, destructiveness, fire setting, and inflicting harm to others.

What other conditions can mimic ADHD?

Children with temper tantrums and "spoilt" child due to over-indulgence are often wrongly labelled to have ADHD. The diagnosis should be delayed till child goes to a regular school when concept of rules and discipline is more likely to be followed by children. Normally outgoing, ebullient, wiry and energetic children should not be wrongly labelled as ADHD. Hyperactivity and inattention are also recognized features of low intelligence, epilepsy, poor vision, hearing disability and intake of certain medications which should be ruled out. It is important to remember that a highly intelligent child may become hyperactive or inattentive because he is bored with the teacher or mother. The child should be evaluated by a psychiatrist and clinical psychologist for making a definitive diagnosis.

Treatment

Parents and teachers should be counseled to handle these children with due care, sensitivity and compassion. These children should not be spanked or penalized for their "naughty" behaviour. It must be realized that child's behaviour is not intentional, it is involuntary or spontaneous. These children should be kept busy and given supervised tasks to improve their attention span. The child should be encouraged to take part in physical activities, sports, yoga and meditation. Paradoxically, neurostimulant drugs (methylphenidate, amphetamines) which are known to cause hyperactivity and restlessness, provide relief to these children. Medications are given to children who are severely affected and are above the age of 6 years. They should be taken under close supervision of a doctor because of potential risk of serious side effects. Tricyclic antidepressants are used in children with poor response to stimulant medications.

AUTISM SPECTRUM DISORDERS

It is a group of pervasive developmental disorders, like autistic disorder, Asperger's syndrome, Rett's disorder, Kanner's autism and childhood disintegrative disorder. They are characterized by qualitative impairment of social interactions, abnormalities in speech or communication and stereotyped repetitive behaviour. The condition is believed to affect 2 per 1000 children in the west. The disorder is 4 times more common in boys than girls. The condition may be likened to a major psychiatric disorder like infantile "schizophrenia" and its exact cause is unknown. There is probably an abnormality in the neurotransmitters or brain chemicals and has a genetic or familial predisposition. Recent studies have shown reduced activity in the pre-frontal and parietal cortex with reduced number of Purkinje cells in the cerebellum and a less number of tightly packed neurons in the limbic area of brain. Lack of interaction and emotional support by one or both working parents is a recognised predisposing or precipitating factor. There is no evidence that thiomersol contained in MMR vaccine has any role in the causation of autism. Incidentally, thiomersol is no longer used as a preservative in MMR or any other vaccine.

Salient Features

Autistic children are difficult to diagnose and they are often confused with mental retardation. These children may have normal development during infancy and then regress in their social interactions and communication skills. The manifestations are usually evident by the age of 2 years.

- The autistic children live in their own world and do not like to play with other children. They lack emotional warmth and social interactions.
- There may be delay in development of speech (no babbling by one year and not speaking two word phrases by 2 years) or gradual loss or regression of speech and social skills after having achieved it.
- Speech may be absent or they may have gibberish and repetitive language (echolalia) of their own.
- They have brief eye contact or no eye contact and do not like to be held or cuddled.
- They live in their own world without any social interactions (like bye-bye at one year) and do not respond to their name when called from behind.

- They may have strange compulsive and repetitive behaviour like rocking, bouncing, head banging, throwing toys, swinging, spinning objects, flapping or twisting of hands, and asking repetitive questions.
- They are "oversensitive" to special sensory inputs of sound, smell, touch, taste and vision. They are fascinated by visual stimuli like flickering of light or moving objects (like fan, top or *lattu*). They have a habit of sniffing, licking or smelling objects and walking on their toes. They have relative insensitivity to pain.
- They are not interested in interactive games (like peek-a-boo) and pretend playing or make-believe games and have a short attention span. They lack in social interactions, facial expressions, gestures and non-verbal communication.
- They may have immense liking towards some inanimate object (like teddy bear) and may react violently to any change in their environment and daily set routines or rituals. The sleep may be severely disturbed.
- During follow-up, some children may develop evidences of mental subnormality and seizures. These children may become aggressive and display destructive and self-injurious behaviour.

Treatment

The child and family dynamics should be evaluated by a psychiatrist and an experienced child pychologist to make a correct diagnosis and exclude other conditions especially mental retardation. Evaluation is done by using a checklist for autism in toddlers (CHAT), screening tool for autism for 2-year-old (STAT) and social communication questionnaire (SCQ). There is no specific therapy for autism spectrum disorders.

- These children should be handled with utmost care, emotional support and compassion under the guidance of a specially trained psychologist. Intensive and early interaction, speech therapy, behaviour modification, occupational therapy, play and social skill therapy and sensory integration activities are most useful. They need a structured and supportive environment with plenty of individual attention and group interactions.
- A number of dietary restrictions are advocated but their role is controversial. It is recommended to avoid intake of food additives, preservatives and junk food. Excessive intake of

sugar and chocolates should be avoided. There is some evidence that avoidance of milk and gluten containing foods (wheat, rye, oats) may offer some therapeutic benefit. The intake of cruciferous vegetables (containing sulforaphane) like broccoli, mustard leaves (*sarson ka saag*), cauliflower, cabbage, turnip, radish and kale (*karam ka saag*) should be avoided. Nutritional supplements containing pyridoxine (vitamin B_6), magnesium and dimethylglycine (DMG) are credited to show some benefit. Intake of omega-3 fatty acids and DHA are useful to control hyperactivity.

- Drugs have no specific role but may be used as adjuncts to control associated symptoms. Anti-anxiety (diazepam), anti-aggressive (clonidine, risperidone), anticonvulsants (carbamazepine, phenytoin sodium) and sedatives (chloral hydrate, haloperidol) medications may be given as and when required, the side effects of drugs should be closely monitored.
- A variety of alternative treatments like yoga, reiki, dance, foot reflexology and acupressure have been tried with variable results.

AVULSION OF TOOTH

Tooth may get knocked out of the mouth during a fight or an accident. Nothing needs to be done if it is a temporary or milk tooth because its palce will be taken up by the permanent tooth in due course of time. When a permanent tooth is knocked-out, it can be reimplanted if proper precautions are taken. Hold the tooth by its crown (the part which is visible in the mouth or used for chewing) under the running tap for 10 seconds to wash the root. Do not scrub or rub the root to avoid any damage to the attached tissue which is required for reattachment. Insert the tooth back into its socket, place a folded gauze piece or a clean soft cloth over it and ask the child to bite it gently to keep it in place. If you are scared to implant the tooth, it should be placed in a cup of cold milk (without sugar) or in saliva and child taken promptly to a dentist. Reimplantation is usually successful if it is achieved within 30 minutes of avulsion. The child should be advised to take liquid or soft diet for the next 2–3 days and avoid eating any solid food. When tooth reimplantation is rejected, the dentist can provide a dental bridge or dental implant.

BABY BATH

Babies are born wet and naked in a room which is maintained at a temperature to provide comfort to the mother while ignoring the biological needs of the baby. At birth, the baby should be immediately dried and effectively covered to prevent exposure and fall in body temperature. Babies are coated with a protective cheesy light-yellow-colored material called vernix particularly in the folds of neck, armpits and groins. It provides protective covering to the delicate skin of the baby and no vigorous attempts should be made to remove it. The skin should be gently cleaned off any blood, mucus or meconium (some babies may pass meconium in the womb) by a soft and sterile towel. The baby should be effectively covered and clothed and kept next to the mother to provide her warmth to stabilize baby's body temperature. *There is no need to bathe the baby at birth which should be postponed to the second or third day.* In many hospitals, no baby bath is given during the hospital stay of the baby.

Sponge Bath

The dip baths are avoided as long as the umbilical stump is attached to the navel. The baby can be sponged daily till cord falls. Take lukewarm water in a basin with two soft cotton or flannel towels. Place the baby on a large fluffy towel in a warm and comfortable room. Keep the baby wrapped in a towel and expose only those parts of his body, which are being sponged. The face should be cleaned first by using a damp cloth without any soap. The remaining areas of the skin are sponged by using a damp towel soaked with mild liquid soap solution. During sponging, special attention should be paid to creases like neck, behind the

46

ears, armpits and groins. After cleaning, all traces of soap are removed with a wet towel. Diaper area should be washed in the end, first with a soapy sponge followed by a towel soaked in plain water. In addition, during diaper change; the bottom and groins should be gently but thoroughly cleaned and kept dry to prevent nappy rash.

Dip Bath

The baby is given dip baths when umbilical cord has fallen and navel has healed. Depending upon the weather, birth weight and health status of the baby, there is no need to give a bath every day. The bath should be given in a room which is warm and free of draught. The fan should be switched off. All the items needed during and after the bath should be collected and kept by your side (**Box**).

Items required for baby bath

- Bath tub or a wide plastic basin of a bright color.
- Bucket of lukewarm water or put the geyser on.
- One large fluffy towel and two baby napkins and soft towels.
- Baby oil, shampoo, soap or cleansing soap solution, talcum powder, moisturizing lotion, and hair brush.
- Cotton balls and cotton buds.
- Surgical alcohol or spirit.
- Baby dress, napkin and safety pin.

The plastic basin or baby tub is filled up to half or two-thirds with lukewarm water. The baby's skin is very delicate and only a mild soap or cleansing soap solution should be used. The newborn baby can be straddled or placed on your arm or legs and his head should be supported. After a couple of months, the baby can be placed in the water tub while supporting his back and head on your left arm and hand. The baby's bottom should be cleaned, if it is soiled with poops before placing the baby in the tub.

First the baby's head should be washed by using a non-tear baby shampoo. The lather should be rinsed off by pouring water with a mug after placing your hand over his forehead so that soapy water drains out from the sides and does not enter the eyes. Rinse it several times to remove all traces of shampoo. Dry the scalp with a towel before proceeding further. If some soap manages to enter his eyes and baby cries, clean them with a damp towel soaked in plain warm water till all traces of soap are removed. Baby's face should be cleaned next taking care to thoroughly clean the creases behind the ears and neck. Clean the eyes, wiping gently from nose outwards, using a sterile cotton wool ball moistened with warm water for each eye. Avoid use of any soap an the face. This is followed by washing the trunk and extremities by paying special attention to armpits, groins and hands. The diaper area should be thoroughly washed with soap and water in the end. Most babies enjoy taking bath and hate being taken out of the tub. A couple of plastic toys floating around in the tub water adds to the fun and joy of the bath. *Never leave your baby in the bath tub alone even for a moment to attend the door bell or do any other chore.*

After the bath, the baby should be covered in a large fluffy towel. The skin should be dabbed dry with a soft baby towel instead of firmly wiping it. There is no virtue in using talcum powder except to provide pleasing smell to the baby. *Never sprinkle powder over the baby because baby can get choked by inhaling it or it may enter the eyes.* Take a small amount of powder on your finger tips and dab it over the neck, chest, armpits and groins. A moisturizing cream or lotion can be applied to the whole body. The baby is dressed.

Brush the scalp hair with a soft baby brush. There is no need to apply any hair oil after the bath. Most babies love to take a feed after the bath and go off to sleep due to relaxation of massage and bath. Depending upon the behaviour and liking of your child, you can establish his daily routine regarding the time for his bath, feed, sleep, play, potty, etc.

BAD BREATH (Halitosis)

Foul breath is relatively uncommon in children as compared to adults. It occurs predominantly due to poor oro-dental hygiene because of lack of proper brushing of teeth and cleaning the tongue. Mouth breathing due to persistent blockage of nose (Adenoids) is a leading cause of foul breath. Other causes of bad breath include caries or cavities in teeth, prolonged febrile illness or persistent infection in the lungs. The condition is treated by removing the underlying cause, ensuring oro-dental hygiene, chewing of cardamom (*ilaichi*) or clove (*laung*) or parsley leaves and xylitol containing gum. Herbal tea made from fenugreek (*methi*) seeds and cardamom is a useful remedy.

B

BALANCED DIET

All individuals especially children, pregnant women and nursing mothers need a balanced nutritious diet having all the essential nutrients. The diet should have adequate proportion and balance of body-building proteins, energy giving carbohydrates and fats and micronutrients like vitamins (vitamins A, B complex, C, D, E, K) and minerals like calcium, iron, iodine and zinc. The diet gets balanced when a child is given a good mixture of cereals like wheat and rice, *dals*, legumes, green leafy vegetables, seasonal fruits, milk and milk products. The non-vegetarians can take eggs, mutton, poultry products and seafood. Lean meat (poultry products and fish) is preferred over mutton because latter contains more saturated fat and is not very heart-friendly. Soft drinks, fizzy colas, canned juices, candies and junk food are loaded with empty calories and lack in adequate amount of essential nutrients.

BALANITIS

Inflammation of the urethral tip in boys is called balanitis. There is redness and pus discharge from the urethral meatus. It may be associated with difficulty and discomfort in passing urine (dysuria) or frequent urge for urination. The prepuce may be tight with difficulty in retracting the foreskin. Ascending infection may lead to inflammation or infection in the urinary bladder (cystitis).

Treatment Urine should be examined to exclude urinary tract infection (UTI) and identification of pathogenic bacteria. The urethral site should be washed with soap and water by retracting the foreskin. Antibacterial cream should be applied at the site of inflammation 3–4 times in a day. When there is associated UTI, oral antibiotics are given under the guidance of a physician. If preputial opening is narrow, dilatation of the orifice or circumcision (excision of foreskin) can be done by a pediatric surgeon under local anesthesia.

Baldness (*see* Alopecia)
BED WETTING (Nocturnal enuresis)

Depending upon the family constitution or genetic background, some children are dry at night after their first birthday but most are likely to achieve the bladder control by the age of 3 years. By and large, most children become dry at night by the time they start going to a regular school. About 5 percent children do not achieve bladder control at night by the age of 5 years and are labelled to have nocturnal enuresis. The condition is more common in boys than girls. Enuresis may be primary, i.e. the child never achieved bladder control or after having achieved the bladder control at night for a period of 6 months or more, the child starts wetting the bed again (secondary enuresis).

The exact cause of enuresis is not known. It seems children with enuresis have a small capacity of urinary bladder and they are blessed with a deep or sound sleep. The sensation of full bladder does not wake them up and they void during sleep (whether it is day time or night sleep). Children with secondary enuresis may have an underlying stress or emotional distur-bances. The common causes of stress include birth of a new sibling, a move to a new home, a change to a new school or exposure to a scary movie or video. There is increased familial tendency of bed wetting in certain families indicating hereditary or genetic basis. Most children with bed wetting do not have any urinary symptoms during day time. When there are associated urinary symptoms during the day time like frequency of passing urine, difficulty in voiding or lack of control, and passage of excessive quantities of urine, the child should be investigated for underlying kidney disorder. Bed wetting may undermine the self-esteem of some children and interfere with their social interactions and peer relationships. School-age children who continue to wet at night are reluctant to accept invitation from their friends to sleepover or join overnight school excursions, educational trips or summer camp.

Treatment

Most children with bed wetting respond to general measures without use of any medicines. The child should be asked to restrict his fluid intake to at least 3 hours before going to bed. He should be advised to take early dinner and avoid taking rice, curd and milk at night. Intake of sesame seeds (*black til*) in jaggery (*gurh*) is useful to reduce urine output. The child should be asked to empty the bladder before going to sleep and repeat several times while falling asleep that "I will not wet my bed today". These positive thoughts get lodged in his subconscious mind to strengthen his will power to achieve bladder control. He should be asked to maintain a calendar of dry and wet nights. The child should be

B

encouraged and rewarded for dry nights by words of praise, pat on the back, golden stars or gifts. He should be constantly encouraged and supported by positive thoughts to control the habit. Parents should avoid nagging, scolding or belittling the child when he fails in his attempts to achieve a dry night. Instead he should be inspired and reassured that "you have the ability and if you exercise your will power, you can control it". During the day time, the child should be encouraged to drink plenty of water and asked to hold the urine as long as possible till the urge to pass urine cannot be further controlled. This procedure enhances the capacity of the bladder.

Most children are able to achieve bladder control at night by following the above mentioned general measures. The use of "moisture alarm" or "potty pager" and drugs have a limited utility due to high risk of relapse. The "moisture alarm" consists of a small sponge pad that is worn under the panties. There is an electrical sensor in the pad which is attached to an alarm box. When sponge pad becomes wet, the alarm is triggered thus waking up the child. After several nights of alarm use, the child gets conditioned to wake up before voiding or before the alarm rings. Some "deep sleepers" may not wake up to the sound of alarm, wherein a parent should take the responsibility of awakening the child when alarm goes off. If a "moisture alarm" device is not available, even an ordinary alarm clock can be tried. Over a couple of days, you should try to identify the usual time when the child wets his bed, which is often fixed and constant. The child can be conditioned to wake up before the accident by setting the alarm 15–30 minutes before the anticipated time of wetting the bed.

Home Remedies

- Give one walnut and a teaspoon of raisins or jaggery (*gurh*) at bed time daily.
- Ask the child to chew cinnamon bark and take 1–2 bananas daily.
- Crush two Indian gooseberries (*amla*), add one tablespoon of honey and a pinch of turmeric. Give one teaspoon of the mixture every morning.
- Boil some mustard seeds or fennel (*saunf*) or black sesame seeds in milk and give it to child daily at night.
- Massage the lower abdomen with warm olive oil at night.

B

The use of medicines should be avoided or delayed till the age of 8 years. They have a limited role because of risk of side effects and high chances of relapse on stopping therapy. Tricyclic antidepressants and nasal spray of desmopressin may be used under the guidance and supervision of a pediatrician.

BEE AND WASP STINGS

Honey bees and wasps (Hornet, yellow jacket) usually produce minor allergic symptoms. When there are multiple stings, especially in young children, it may produce life-threatening manifestations. Even a single sting in the mouth, tongue or throat may cause swelling and obstruction of the airway. There is local pain or burning sensation, redness, swelling and itching. Rarely generalized rash, anaphylaxis and circulatory collapse may occur.

Treatment Remove the stinger by scraping with a credit card, nails or tweezers. Wash the sting site/s with soap and water. Apply ice pack over the site of bite for 10–15 minutes followed by application of a soothing cream or calamine lotion. Pain can be relieved by administration of paracetamol or ibuprofen. Consider administration of booster dose of tetanus toxoid (TT or Td) if more than 10 years have elapsed after the last shot. When life-threatening symptoms develop, the child should be taken to the hospital or administered of epinephrine (EpiPen) at home.

Home Remedies

- Make a thick paste of baking soda or common salt in water and apply over the site of bite.
- Apply a cotton wool swab soaked in vinegar or lime juice over the bite site/s.
- Cut a fresh slice of lime and hold it against the sting site.
- Sliced onion or garlic can be rubbed over the sting site/s.
- Crush 1–2 leaves of holy basil (*tulsi*) and press against the site of bite/s.
- Crush one clove of garlic and add half teaspoon of common salt. Apply the poultice over the site of bite and wrap with a bandage or band aid.

B

Prevention

- When going out door for trekking or hiking, especially in areas with thick vegetations, wear full sleeve shirt and trousers.
- Wear socks and shoes when outdoors.
- Apply insect repellant containing diethyltoluamide (DEET) to the exposed areas of skin.
- Avoid use of strong smelling products like soap, shampoo, oil, powder, deodorants, perfumes, etc. because they attract insects.
- When attacked by a swarm of bees, move back slowly and do not wave your arms around or swat at them in a panic.
- If there is a bee nest near the vicinity of home, get it removed by a professional.
- If you have pets, they should be regularly treated for fleas.
- Bed bugs and mites should be eliminated by frequently changing the bed sheets and blankets and exposing them to sunlight.

BEHAVIOUR PROBLEMS

Children are innocent (and ignorant) and carefree without any ill will, jealousy or malice towards anyone. They are full of life and energy and "live in the present moment" without any memories of the past and fear for the future. They are confident, fearless and have full faith and trust in their caretakers. They are indeed spiritual in their characteristics and have all the attributes that saints and holy people endeavor to acquire. They have no desires or ambitions and are fully absorbed in the "moment" with innocence and pure love. Early childhood is usually blissful with no responsibilities but all the fun and frolics.

Producing children does not need any skills and is achieved as a natural biological instinct. But upbringing of children is an art which demands active efforts, concern, sensitivity and skills of parents. Depending upon their genetic background or constitution, children are born with different temperaments and personality characteristics. Childhood is the most vulnerable and formative years of one's life. Children develop various attributes of their behaviour (whether good or bad) depending upon what they watch and go through in life.

B

Children learn what they live with!

If a child lives with criticism,
he learns to condemn.

If a child lives with hostility,
he learns to fight.

If a child lives with ridicule,
he learns to be shy.

If a child lives with shame,
he learns to feel guilty.

If a child lives with tolerance,
he learns to be patient.

If a child lives with encouragement,
he learns confidence.

If a child lives with praise,
he learns to appreciate.

If a child lives with fairness,
he learns justice.

If a child lives with security,
he learns to have faith.

If a child lives with approval,
he learns to like himself.

If a child lives with acceptance and friendship,
he learns to find love in the world.

If a child lives with serenity,
he learns to have peace of mind.

— Dorothy L Nolte

Children are truly at the mercy of their caretakers to look after their physical, mental, social and emotional needs. Parents, teachers, siblings and friends have a profound effect on the development of behaviour pattern and personality of children. The seeds of integrity, character and discipline are sown in childhood. They are planted by parents and tilled by teachers. The successful adults do have pleasant memories of happy childhood while maladjusted adults are constantly haunted by the emotional scars of early life. Parents must understand the constitutional make up and aptitude

B

of their children and provide them with right stimulation, supervision and support to bring out the best in them (**Box**).

Common Behaviour Problems

Fears and phobias

Depending upon the genetic stock, some children are brave while others are timid, some are easily scared while others are fearless. When parents have strong fears, they are likely to transmit them to their children. The common fears and phobias in children include fear of school, strangers, darkness, height, water and ghosts. Usually these fears are transitory and they gradually disappear as the child grows. The child may develop fear of dark or ghosts if you tell frightening stories to your child at bed time. The child may develop nightmares after seeing a horror movie or a scary TV program. Children develop fear of hospital or injection if you frighten them with injections to mend their behaviour. When fears are imaginary and without any rational basis, they are called as phobias. They have no reality and they exist only in the mind.

Fears are often caused due to lack of confidence in the child. Parents as caretakers have to provide them with assurance, support and trust. You should never belittle the child, chide him or tease him for his fear. Fear is very real for the child. Do not argue or reprimand him but let him talk about his fear. Give him extra love, protection and moral support. You can narrate to him

---

What parents ought to do?

- Children need role models more than critics.
- Parents must set a good example for their children to emulate.
- Say "No" when it is appropriate because children do respect a firm denial.
- Give protection and security but give him freedom to explore the world and never try to possess him.
- Treat and respect the child as you do to a grown up and never humiliate him.
- Assign household chores and responsibilities to your children.
- Children do what their parents do, not what their parents say.
- Be cautious and considerate what you say to your children. They do remember your bad and rude words when they grow up.

B

stories of brave people to boost his morale and self confidence. If he is afraid of dark, take him along with you in the dark and give him extra hug. You can leave a night light on in his bed room until he gets over his phobia of darkness. There is always a basis or trigger for every fear, and you should try to identify it in order to institute corrective action. In conclusion, when a child is loved and made to feel secure, when he is constantly reassured and encouraged and he gets engrossed in his studies and play activities, he will gradually get over his inner fears and imaginary worries.

Jealousy and rivalry

Most human emotions inspire us to do well in life. Healthy jealousy and rivalry encourage us to do better and excel others in this competitive world. Sibling rivalry is common when a new baby is born who takes away the major attention of the parents. Unfavorable comparison between siblings is a common cause of jealousy. The girl child may feel extremely jealous of his brother who gets more attention and greater freedom for outdoor activities.

It is important that the parents should prepare the elder child for the arrival of his sibling well before his birth. He should be made to feel proud as a big brother/sister. He should be given the privileges of the big brother/sister instead of developing feelings of jealousy and insecurity. You cannot correct feelings of jealousy

Tips to handle sibling rivalry

- Prepare the elder sib before the birth of next baby.
- Give extra attention to the older child because he understands while the newly born baby is not bothered.
- Hold him, hug him, praise and reward his good and grown up behaviour.
- Keep some gifts at hand to give to the elder child when visitors bring gifts for the new baby. Let him also play with the toys of the younger sibling and make him learn the art of caring and sharing.
- Visitors should be told to pay equal or even greater attention to the elder sibling.
- Do not remind him that he is now old or grown-up but involve him for doing some chores of the new baby under your supervision.
- Do not leave him alone with the baby and make sure that he does not harm the baby.

by explaining to the child that it is bad to be jealous. This will make the child more tense and confused. He may become irritable, cry endlessly, lose interest in his toys and may become violent and destructive. Parents should handle sibling rivalry with common sense and patience (**Box**).

At times jealousy may provide motivation to do better and achieve the desired target. For example, a girl who is obese could be motivated to become slim like her friend. The child may start doing better in studies by emulating a bright child. When a child is endowed with self-confidence and has caring and considerate parents, he is less likely to be bothered by any imaginary or real rivals in life. A child who feels important and loved, and his parents have the confidence that he is making best efforts to compete in life in accordance with his capabilities, he is unlikely to suffer from any jealousy due to success of others.

Destructiveness and bullying

Children are curious and careless, they are likely to pick and throw anything that they can lay their hands on. Toddlers are known to poke their fingers everywhere and would turn all the items on the dressing table upside down. They are curious to dismantle a toy or a household gadget despite warnings from parents. They need constant supervision and guidance to prevent unnecessary breakages. The breakable items should be kept out of their reach. As they grow and gain understanding, they learn to hold breakable and precious items with due care. Instead of constantly telling your child, "don't do this, don't do that", you must tell him what he should do to exploit his energy and impulses into creative activities. To satisfy their curiosity and innate desire to destroy, they should be allowed to handle inexpensive objects, old magazines and newspapers, old calenders, wooden blocks and junk items. He should be encouraged to make castles of sand and given clay for modelling so that he can exploit his capabilities to create, destroy and rebuild. Most children pass through this phase of development and learn to respect their own belongings and property of others.

It is important for children to learn the value of property and rights of other people. Some adolescents may break window panes or smash the wind screens to demonstrate their macho image. The exuberant energy of children at this age should be channelized into creative and constructive activities and competitive sports. Some delinquent children may deliberately destroy property by setting fire or by indulging in *dadagiri*. Such aggressive and unreasonable behaviour is an indication that something seriously has gone wrong in the upbringing of the child. This behaviour may be an outcome of inter-parental conflicts or over indulgence by parents. Some of these children are also victims of substance abuse. These children need professional help for correction of their defiant and anti-social behaviour.

Cheating, stealing and lying

Children learn what they see. If parents do some minor cheating and lying in their day-to-day activities, children are likely to learn them. The common examples are not receiving a phone call by saying, "tell him, I am not at home" or cheating in a game of cards. The parents often take the child to a doctor by assuring him that no injection will be given when the purpose of the visit is to get him his vaccination shot. They promise to buy him a toy or take him for a ride in the car as a reward for his good behaviour but they never live up to their promise. Instead, it is important for parents to set an example and serve as role models to their children. Accept your mistakes and apologize if you want your child to accept his mistakes. Be humble when you talk to the servants of the house if you wish your child to be a good human being.

Children do not know the values of truth and honesty unless they are told about them. Simple stories for children extolling the virtues of truth, honesty, friendship, humility, cooperation, etc. and condemnation for vices like anger, greed, jealousy, envy, and arrogance are extremely useful to imbibe and inculcate good attributes and desirable qualities of life. Children often lie to escape punishment or gain an advantage. Sometimes they are afraid to tell a truth because of fear of punishment. The child may be worried to show his school report card due to embarrassment of poor grades. The child may cheat at a game in order to win. The child may pick up an eraser or pencil of a school-mate as a prank or revenge. You must try to understand the genesis and basis of his behaviour instead of calling him a thief or a liar. He should not be humiliated for his act. Instead he should be encouraged and inspired to follow the path of honesty and truthfullness. Once you repose your faith in him and he realises the value of being trusted, he will gradually give up the habit of cheating and lying.

The shy and timid child

The child who is constantly over protected and over indulged by parents is likely to become withdrawn and shy. He cannot face the hard realities of outside world because his life at home is too cushioned. He is constantly protected from all dangers and given little opportunity to develop self-confidence. It is desirable to protect children from dangers of traffic, heights, balconies and open windows by providing adequate safety measures rather than by giving constant negative warnings. If you constantly say to the child "don't do this", "don't do that", "you will hurt yourself", "watch out otherwise you will fall", etc. he is constantly scared and confused. The child is likely to become timid because he does not want to upset or annoy his parents. Timidity is usually reflected in school or at playground or with strangers. Most of these children may be aggressive or bossy at home but extremely nervous; shy and timid in the outside world. They become introvert and withdrawn and may not be able to greet or utter a single word infront of strangers. It is important to follow a balanced approach in upbringing of children and they should not be cushioned by over protection and over concern. They must be encouraged to become independent to face the harsh realities of life. It is important that the child should unfold and evolve his talents and abilities in a natural way. He should be inspired and encouraged to take part in sports activities. He should be enthused to take part in music, dance and other cultural activities. Above all, he should be made independent and self-reliant by taking part in his day-to-day activities.

BIRTHMARKS (Nevi)

Birthmarks or nevi are flat or elevated patches in the skin involving either blood vessels (vascular) or due to change in pigmentation of the skin. They may be present at birth or appear subsequently during childhood. They are usually benign and may be present in about 10% of newborn babies. Their cause is unknown and they are not inherited. According to folklore, birthmarks are caused by unfulfilled wishes of the mother during pregnancy or due to sudden strange and frightful experience by the expectant mother.

B

Vascular Nevi

Salmon patch (stork bite, nevus simplex)

They present as dull pink areas of skin over the nape of neck (site from where the fabled stork carries the baby), forehead and upper eyelids (angel's kiss). They are seen in over 40% of newborn babies and gradually fade away during infancy but pink areas over the upper part or of the neck may persist.

Portwine stain (nevus flammeus)

They present as maroon-red or purple-red patches on one side of the face, scalp, neck or limb. They may be associated with vascular malformation of the brain on the same side (Sturge-Weber syndrome) or underlying subcutaneous tissues and bone of the extremity. Skin defect can be minimized by use of cosmetics or by pulse-dyed laser therapy.

Strawberry mark (cavernous hemangioma, hemangioma simplex)

They appear as dark-red or pinkish skin patches raised above the surface of skin like a strawberry. They are compressible on pressure. They are usually present over the face, neck or shoulder. During first 5–6 months, they grow in size along with growth of the baby. They gradually disappear over the next 2–3 years leaving behind pale and puckered skin. When large in size, they can be treated by local application of skin cream containing corticosteroids and oral or topical propranolol.

Pigmented or Pale Nevi

A large number of birthmarks with different colors (brown, coffee with milk color, blue, black, etc.) may be seen at birth or appear subsequently during childhood. They may be flat or slightly raised above the surface of the skin.

Café-au-lait (coffee with milk) spots are brown or tan-colored skin patches of various shapes, sizes and number. When café-au-lait spots are more than 6 in number or large in size, they may be associated with CNS abnormalities due to neurofibromatosis.

B

Mongolian blue spots are common at birth in newborn babies of races with dark skin or mongolian origin (East Asian, East African, North American). They present as blue-gray or blue-black spots or a large patch over the lower back and buttocks giving an appearance of a bruise. They spontaneously disappear as the child grows and no pigmentation is seen after the age of 4 years.

Moles (Melanocytic nevi)

Moles are dark-brown or tan-colored spots due to overgrowth of melanocytes in the skin. They are extremely common. They may be flat or slightly raised, round or oval in shape and vary in number from 10 to 40. They are usually benign and persist throughout life. When a mole is atypical (dysplastic nevus) with an irregular border with a sudden change in color, shape or size and appearance of itching, it may progress to development of cancer (malignant melanoma). They can be treated by freezing (cryotherapy), laser therapy and surgical excision.

Nevus anemicus are pale or white (decreased or absent skin pigmentation) birthmarks of different sizes and shapes. There is no specific treatment and they are managed by application of cosmetics or laser therapy.

BIRTH REGISTRATION

When a baby is born in a hospital, birth registration certificate is given by the hospital authorities mentioning the name of the parents, date and time of birth and sex of the child. Hospital authorities get the birth registered with the municipal authorities. When delivery occurs at home, parents should get the baby's birth registered at the Municipal Office. Birth certificate should be kept in a safe custody because it is needed as a proof of age at the time of admission to the school and on other occasions later in life. Many parents follow the old custom of getting an horoscope or *janam patrika* made by a *pundit* (or with the help of a computer these days) which is based on exact date, time and place of birth as well as the constellation of stars under which the child was born. It appears that the age old Indian horoscope is an equivalent of what scientists have now created as a human genome! You can certainly get on horoscope prepared but birth certificate from municipal authorities is mandatory.

BITING

When teeth erupt and child is breastfeeding, some babies may start biting the nipple while breastfeeding. The child bites either due to irritation of the gums or because of frustration of not getting enough milk. Don't laugh or approve this behaviour and you should firmly say "no biting" and calmly disconnect the prankster from the breast and divert his attention by playing or talking to him. Do this each time he bites so that he gets the message of your disapproval.

After one year, occasional biting to show pleasure is common. You should discourage it by saying that it hurts. In some children, biting increases in frequency and intensity during 2–3 years. It may be a sign of frustration and unhappiness when child is too much restricted or forcibly disciplined. At times lack of discipline, over attention or over indulgence is the cause of biting. It may be a demonstration of jealously or aggressive behaviour. When the child is unhappy and tense most of the time and keeps biting you or other children without any provocation, it is abnormal.

Most of the time, biting is a temporary developmental phase and it passes off in due course of time. When biting episodes are excessive or unprovoked, you should handle them firmly. When you can predict that child is going to bite, try to ward off the attack by protecting yourself or the other victim. If he succeeds in biting, you must give a firm message that you don't like it and he should not do it again. Hold him, look into his eyes sternly and tell him not to do it again because it hurts. Never bite him back or slap him because he may keep the fight on or he may consider it a game of biting and slapping. Never laugh when child bites or call him a "doggie", which gives indirect approval to his biting behaviour. Try to find the underlying cause for jealousy and resentment so that it can be resolved. He should be provided with greater opportunities to play and learn to cooperate with other children. He should be appreciated and encouraged for his good behaviour. Biting usually disappears by the age of 3 years when child can express his frustration by speaking and he has developed better control to restrain his impulses.

BLINDNESS

Newborn babies respond to bright light by blinking and turning their head towards diffuse light. The baby can appreciate different colors but red and black colors are perceived best. Infants are usually fascinated by stripes, checkerboards, bull's eyes and squares. Around 4–6 weeks, the child is able to fix his gaze and look into your eyes and gives a social or interactive smile when talked to. The lack of social smile by 6 weeks of age may indicate either defective cognition (mental subnormality) or lack of vision. When a baby is unable to see, he will not blink in response to bright light, may have purposeless roving eye movements and persistent squint or crossed eyes. He may not give any blink response when you suddenly bring your finger towards his eyes. A blind infant is extrasensitive to noise and gets easily startled by sudden noise. The child with visual defect may show evidences of clumsiness, timidity, poor school performance, keenness to sit in the first row or watch TV from a close distance. Whenever there is a doubt about the visual acuity of the child, you should consult an ophthalmologist for detailed examination of eyes and evaluation of vision by a variety of modern tests like optokinetic nystagmus, and visual evoked responses (VER).

Blindness may date back to birth or appear subsequently anytime later in life. Blindness dating back to birth may occur due to developmental defects (nondevelopment of certain parts of eyes, intrauterine infection, glaucoma, cataract) and retinopathy in a prematurely born baby. When a prematurely born baby is given oxygen therapy or provided assisted ventilation, he must be examined by an ophthalmologist in the neonatal intensive care unit (NICU) for early diagnosis and treatment of retinopathy of prematurity (ROP). Defective vision or blindness may occur subsequently in life because of short sightedness (myopia), infections (brain and eye infection), tumor, trauma and vitamin A deficiency (keratomalacia or softening of the cornea). The child with defective vision should be assessed by an ophthalmologist for early identification of the underlying cause and its appropriate management including early surgery or use of glasses.

BLINKING OF EYES

Blinking of eyes is an involuntary protective mechanism to prevent injury to the eyes against bright light, strong wind, dust or foreign body. It helps to keep the eyes moist. Normally eyes blink at a rate of 10–20 blinks/minute but blinking rate is much less in young infants. Excessive blinking is most commonly due to nervous tics or habit disorder. Common predisposing factors include stress, anxiety and fatigue. The condition is more common in boys than girls. Blinking may start as a prank or following irritation or infection in the eyes. When child finds that blinking is eliciting lot of attention by the parents, the habit continues. Brief episodes of blinking with staring look and inattention in adolescent girls is suggestive of petit mal epilepsy which should be excluded by doing an EEG. When blinking is associated with facial and vocal tics with use of obscene gestures and words, it is suggestive of Gilles de la Tourette syndrome which is usually a life long condition.

Intelligent neglect and lack of concern by parents would break the habit in a few days or months. When blinking is associated with excessive watering of eyes, irritation, redness or visual difficulty, you should consult an ophthalmologist.

BOILS (Furuncles, impetigo)

A boil is a localized, tender, pus-filled vesicle surrounded by angry red base. It may occur as a consequence of accidental pulling out of a hair root or due to poor personal hygiene especially during summer and rainy season. Boils may occur at any site in the body but are more common over the buttock. The boils located over the nose, face and head are considered dangerous because infection may travel to the brain. Boil with deep infection under the skin may form an abscess. When a pus point forms, the abscess may rupture spontaneously or on application of pressure. Boils may be associated with pain, malaise and fever.

Home Remedies

The availability of effective oral antibiotics and antibiotic containing skin creams have made home remedies unnecessary.

- Make a decoction of dried neem-leaf powder or dried neem bark by boiling them in water. Give half a cup of the decoction daily for cleansing the body system. A teaspoon of honey can be added to make it palatable.

- Grind fresh tender neem leaves into a paste and apply over the boils.

- Make a paste of fresh ginger and turmeric by grinding them together. Apply over the boils 2–3 times everyday.

Treatment Paracetamol or ibuprofen can be given for relief of pain and fever. The child should be given a bath preferably twice a day with an antiseptic soap (savlon and dettol). Ointment containing an antibiotic (sodium fusidate, muciprocin) can be applied 2–3 times daily over the boils. In case of multiple boils, oral antibiotics can be taken on the advice of a doctor. Belladonna plaster can be applied to facilitate ripening of the abscess. Drainage of pus is mandatory when an abscess has formed.

BOTTLE FEEDING

Most babies can be fed with exclusive breastfeeding up to 6 months of age. When semisolid weaning foods are introduced around 6 months of age, breastfeeding should be continued and there is no need to start bottle feeding. At a later date, generally after first birthday, when breast milk supply wanes off, milk feeds can be started and given with a cup or glass. *There is thus no need to introduce bottle feeding in the care of healthy term babies.*

At times despite sincere efforts and due to certain medical and social conditions in the mother, complementary or sometimes total feeding with an animal milk or formula may be required in the following situations.

1. Adopted baby.
2. Inadequate lactation.
3. Twin or triplet babies.
4. Seriously or critically sick mother.
5. Mother receiving anti-cancer drugs.
6. Working mother who is unable or unwilling to breastfeed.
7. Social constraints.

When for a genuine personal or medical reasons, bottle feeding needs to be given, the mothers should not feel guilty or unnecessarily upset. The babies can be fed satisfactorily with formula feed or animal milk when due precautions are taken to ensure proper cleanliness and sterility of feeding utensils and bottles.

The Choice of Milk

Any liquid milk which is procured by the family for household use can be given to the baby without dilution. Children should be given full cream milk except when overweight. Dried milk powders are often preferred because of less chances of contamination and adulteration, ease of storage and uniformity of composition but they are expensive. Most infant formulas are fortified with iron and vitamins. In order to make their composition as close to human milk as possible, most baby formulas are fortified with docosahexaenoic acid (DHA) and arachidonic acid (AA). Milk powders should be reconstituted as per the instructions printed on the container. In general, one level (not heaped) measure of powdered milk is dissolved in one ounce (30 mL) of pre-boiled or filtered warm water to obtain full-strength milk. Reconstitution of milk powder into a larger volume of water is the commonest cause of poor weight gain by the baby. Hands should be washed thoroughly with soap and water before preparing a feed. The powdered milk can be directly taken in the feeding bottle instead of using another container for reconstitution of milk. It is more convenient and there is lesser risk of contamination. In order to promote breastfeeding, the production, marketing and promotion of breast milk substitutes (powdered milks) are governed by Infants Milk Substitute Act, 1992. The Act does not allow advertisement of infant milk substitutes, infant foods or feeding bottles. According to the Act, no baby food (not even cereal-based) can be promoted for children below the age of 2 years.

Fresh liquid milk is suitable and more cost-effective for feeding babies but it is difficult to store during summer months without an ice box or refrigerator. The milk should be boiled and cooled every time before use. During first 2 months of age, pure cows' or buffaloes' milk may be diluted in a ratio of 3 parts of milk and one part of water to reduce protein load to the kidneys. When milk is delivered home by the milkman, the dilution should be left to him! Animal milks have greater quantity of proteins which are of different types (casein which is difficult to digest compared to easily digestible lactalbumin or whey protein of human milk) and are less sweet because of lower content of lactose. Mother can add sugar to sweeten the milk according to baby's liking. The milk should be strained before pouring into the feeding bottle otherwise the cream may block the hole in the teat. After 2 months of age, most babies can be fed with a full strength animal milk.

How much milk to offer?

Breastfed babies regulate their feed intake depending upon their needs and mother does not need to worry about any guidelines or calculations. During bottle feeding, offer 30–45 mL of milk during first week of life. Whenever baby completely empties the bottle, additional 15 mL of milk should be offered during the next feed. The volume of feed should be gradually increased by one ounce (30 mL) after every month or so. The best guide that the baby has taken a full feed is indicated by the observation that some milk remains in the bottle when baby has stopped sucking. The left over milk must be immediately discarded (or consumed by an adult) and feeding bottle should be rinsed with water to prevent bacterial growth. The maximum amount that a baby drinks during one feed is a full bottle of 8 ounces (about 240 mL). After one year, baby should be given maximum of three bottles of milk feeds and the rest of his nutritional requirements should be met by giving cereal-based semisolid foods, lentils, vegetables and fruits.

Technique of Bottle Feeding

A straight wide-mouthed feeding bottle should be used because of ease of cleaning. The hole in the rubber teat should be created with a red hot sewing needle. It will burn the rubber to make the hole which will remain patient. When a feeding bottle with milk is inverted, there should be a fine spray of milk for 1–2 seconds and then milk should flow in regular drops and not as a stream. When milk flows as a constant stream, the hole in the teat is too big and if drops fall too slowly, the hole is too small. In both situations, the baby is likely to swallow too much air while feeding and develop colic or regurgitation of feeds. Mother should pour milk on the back of her hand to make sure that milk is not too hot. Use pre-boiled or filtered warm water (which can be kept stored in a flask) for reconstitution of milk. Feeds should be offered on demand as in case of breastfeeding. A common sense approach should be followed instead of any strict routine or ritual. The baby should be fed when he is hungry and allowed to sleep as long as he wants. After some time, baby would establish his own routine and mother can adjust her daily routine accordingly.

The child should preferably be taken in the lap while bottle feeding. Mother should pay full attention and interact with her

B

baby while bottle feeding. She should provide close skin-to-skin contact and intently look at her baby while bottle feeding. The bottle should be tilted enough so that nipple is completely filled with milk to avoid swallowing of air by the baby. The nipple should be removed from the baby's mouth when it gets collapsed to relieve negative pressure or vacuum in the bottle. She should interact with the baby while feeding to ensure that the baby takes a complete feed before he falls asleep. After the feed, the baby should be made to sit or put on the shoulder to eructate the swallowed air. After burping, the baby may be placed on his back or right lateral position with head end slightly raised. *It is dangerous to support the feeding bottle with a cushion or pillow and leave the baby and bottle alone for self feeding. There is a potential risk of choking and aspiration and the baby may suck lot of air when bottle rolls down.* During bottle feeding, the baby's head should be kept slightly raised, otherwise milk may enter the Eustachian tube (channel between the back of the nose and middle ear) and lead to middle ear infection (acute otitis media or AOM). After the age of 9 months, most babies can hold the bottle and self-feed without any risk of choking. After the first birthday, attempts should be made to feed the baby with a cup or glass. Use of attractive and a decorative cup or a baby glass with motifs may motivate the baby to accept this method of self feeding. Most babies drink water from a cup or a glass as early as 6 months but refuse to take milk from a cup or glass because they identify milk with a feeding bottle. *A sipper should never be used either for giving water or milk because of potential risk of infection.*

Feeding during Sleep

It is not a good practice to offer a bottle feed during sleep. It may lead to development of dental caries as milk remains in contact with teeth while the baby is asleep. Feeding during sleep is also associated with risk of development of ear infection as the milk may trickle into the Eustachian tube and cause infection of the middle ear (AOM). Occasional bottle feeding during sleep may be given if baby had been fussy, irritable or unwell due to teething or minor illness but it should not lead to development of a bad habit with adverse consequences.

Sterilization of Feeding Bottles and Teats

Bottle feeding is a potential source of infection (especially diarrhea) unless due care is taken to maintain sterility. Mother should have at least four feeding bottles and enough teats. The left over milk must be discarded or consumed by an adult and the bottle should be rinsed and cleaned with a detergent or soap solution by using a brush. The left over milk is a potential breeding ground for bacteria and should never be reused or remain in the bottle till the next feed. Teat should be cleaned with a tooth brush and common salt to remove any milk curds or cream from its hole. Keep a separate saucepan or a large utensil for boiling the bottles. Bottles and teats must completely dip in water and should be boiled for at least 10 minutes. After boiling and cooling, water should be drained and pan with bottles and teats should be kept covered. Four feeding bottles and teats can be sterilized twice a day to cover 8 feeds during 24 hours. Electrical bottle sterilizers are available and are convenient to use. The bottles and teats can be sterilized by immersing them in a solution of sodium hypochlorite (Milton). One table spoon (15 mL) of Milton is added to a liter of water and bottles and teats are kept soaked for 3–4 hours. The bottle and teat should be drained off Milton solution and rinsed thoroughly with boiled or filtered water before use.

The liquid milk must be boiled and cooled before each use. The water used for reconstitution of powdered milk must be filtered (or passed through RO system) or boiled for at least 5 minutes to ensure that it is sterile and safe. After taking or making the feed in the bottle, teat must be kept covered with a plastic lid to prevent contamination by flies unless baby is given the feed immediately. The responsibility of washing, cleaning and sterilization of feeding bottles and teats should not be given to a maid or an *ayah* and mother must personally look after this most important aspect of bottle feeding to prevent the risk of contamination and infection.

Feeding with a Cup and Spoon or *Paladay*

Due to potential risk of infection and "nipple confusion" with bottle feeding, it is recommended to give complementary feeds to babies with a spoon or *paladay* (small cup with a rounded snout which is normally used as a *diya*). Most babies (even small and preterm babies) accept feeding with a spoon or *paladay* without any difficulty. The infant should be held in the lap, head slightly raised and edge of the spoon or *paladay* is touched to the lips of the baby. As soon as the milk touches the lips and tongue, the baby makes swallowing efforts to drink the milk. When baby is satisfied, he will turn his head away or stop swallowing the milk which collects in the throat. The procedure is safe but time consuming. Mother needs to use lot of patience to feed the baby with a spoon or *paladay* but efforts are well rewarded because risk of bacterial contamination is extremely low by this method and it is easier for the baby to accept breastfeeding concurrently or subsequently because there is no "nipple confusion". The feeding cup and spoon or *paladay* should be washed with soap and water immediately after each use and kept effectively covered.

Hazards and Benefits of Bottlefeeding

Bottle feeding is unnatural and animal milks or milk formulas are not suitable to serve the nutritional and biological needs of human babies. Bottle fed babies are more vulnerable to develop gastrointestinal infections, respiratory infections, allergic disorders and ear infections. Due to frequent infections and over dilution of formula, the child may have poor weight gain and under nutrition. In well to do families, aggressive bottle feeding is associated with increased risk of obesity, diabetes mellitus, high blood pressure and coronary artery disease later in life.

In well off families, especially when help of a maid is available to look after and feed the baby, bottle feeding does provide greater respite, freedom and option to the mother to join her office earlier, have a better social life and there is no need for any dietary restrictions or nutritional demands and greater freedom for resumption of normal sexual activity.

BOTTOM CARE

Bottom is constantly soiled by urine and stools and must be kept clean all the time. If the diaper area remains soiled by stools for a long time, the baby may develop nappy rash. In girls, there is a potential risk of development of ascending urinary tract infection. In boys, soakage of penis with urine and stools may lead to development of scarring of the foreskin (prepuce) or phimosis with difficulty in passing urine.

After each soiling, clean the bottom with moistened cotton wool or a soft cloth. The cleaning must be done gently because the area is extremely delicate. *In girls, the bottom must be wiped from front towards the back so that there is no risk of contamination of the urethral opening and vagina by the feces.* As the child grows, bottom can be washed under the tap with warm running water. Bottom should be dab dried gently with a soft towel. The nappy area can also be cleaned with skin care wipes which are soaked in a baby lotion that provides a protective layer of moisture on the skin. There is no need to apply any baby powder or use it sparingly over the groins. If baby has developed nappy rash, apply a soothing skin cream as advised by your doctor. The nappy rash recovers much faster when baby is kept naked and bottom is exposed to air and sunlight.

BOWED LEGS

Most normal babies have curved legs at birth. When a baby lies flat on the bed with feet touching each other, there may be a gap of up to 5 cm between the knees. When child starts walking, the bowing or curvature of legs becomes less and child often develops knock-knees after 2 years. In some families, there is a greater tendency to have bowing of legs but it is usually not a cause for concern. When bowing of legs is marked and persists beyond 2 years, rickets (vitamin D deficiency) and development bone defect should be ruled out. When bowing is marked or limited to one side, and associated with rotation, torsion or angulation of tibia, you should consult an orthopedic surgeon.

BOWEL AND BLADDER CONTROL

Bowel Control

During early life, passage of urine and stools are involuntary activities without any control either to initiate the act or to stop it at will. When rectum is full of feces, further increase in pressure in the intestines following a feed leads to opening up of the anal canal and passage of stools. Some infants may pass a motion after each feed. There may be some straining efforts on the part of the baby especially if stools are dry or hard. As the child grows, there

B

is some regularity in passing stools, either after the morning feed or afternoon meal. Before the urge to pass stool, the child may become still, stop playing with his toys, strain a little or go red on the face. The mother should be observant and sensitive to identify the subtle signals of the baby indicating his toilet needs as he grows. After 1–2 years, the child may come towards you, look intently into your eyes and strain a bit. He can be promptly made to sit on a potty to avert soiling of underclothes. During potty sessions, the child can be kept busy with toys or a picture look. When efforts at potty are rewarded, the child should be appreciated to strengthen the process of conditioning. After a successful potty session, the toddler should be encouraged and praised for his grown-up behaviour. Aggressive toilet training tactics should be avoided as they may make the child rebellious.

Around 2 years of age, some fussy children develop a "possessive" feeling and they "don't let go" or relax to evacuate. At times, passage of hard stools may lead to formation of a crack or fissure in the anus with coating of stools with streaks of blood. The process of defecation in these children may cause intense pain with further holding of stools and development of severe consti-pation (obstipation). Medical advice should be sought to resolve this vicious cycle of withholding stools or psychological constipation.

When adequately trained, most children become independent to look after their toilet need by 3–4 years of age. The child would inform the mother or "take her permission" to sit on the potty and would be able to wash the bottom when water is poured by the mother. In girls, it is important that the water is poured from front and she is trained to wash the bottom from front-backwards. When bottom is washed from back-forwards (from anal opening towards the vulva) in girls, there is a potential risk of fecal bacteria entering the urethral orifice to cause ascending urinary tract infection. After washing the bottom, the child should be trained to wash his hands with soap and water and explained the importance of personal hygiene.

Bladder Control

Bladder control is achieved a little later than bowel control. Newborn babies pass urine almost after every feed 8–12 times in a day. As the child grows, the bladder capacity increases and he is able to hold urine for a longer period. *Most babies cry before passing*

B

urine due to unpleasant sensation of a full bladder, stop crying and become dazed while passing urine and start crying again after having passed urine due to discomfort of a wet nappy. Most infants are likely to pass urine on waking up and then after every 2–3 hours. The observant mother should be able to recognize the subtle signals on the part of child before voiding. The baby may indicate his need for passing urine by touching or holding the genitals or by jumping up and down. If unattended, he may give a shriek and wet his pants or create a mess by splashing his hand in the pool of urine. When child is held over the wash basin or placed on the potty at the appropriate time, he is likely to void and get gradually conditioned. If he is unwilling to sit on the potty, avoid forcing his to do so. It is preferable to wash some extra nappies rather than to use aggressive tactics and create unnecessary fuss or a scene.

Children do have their own likes and dislikes and they like to do things in their own way and will. The use of unnecessary force and coercion may lead to development of rebellious attitude. In the fight of wills, children are more likely to win than the parents. After the age of 2 years, the child can be taken to the bathroom to void. Boys get trained to urinate while standing by watching their schoolmates or elder brother. No special efforts are required to train them in this art. When proper training is given, most children are likely to become dry by the age of 2–3 years. Occasional accident may occur when the child is engrossed in play, is unhappy or unwell or when he is in an unfamiliar environment. Most children are likely to have satisfactory bowel and bladder control by the age of 3 years when they are ready to go to play school.

BREASTFEEDING

Breastfeeding is the birth right of every baby. Nature has so designed that when a baby is born, a ready-made drink in the form of breast milk flows like a divine nectar. Breast milk is the ideal food for all babies whether big or small and sick or healthy. Milk of different mammals is specific to serve the biological needs of their offsprings by virtue of unique biological and biochemical composition. For example, milk of a cow or buffalo is meant for her calf, milk of a mare is meant for her colt, milk of an ass is best for her pony, so on and so forth. *Indeed, breast milk is not only species specific, it is baby specific. The milk of a mother is best suited to serve the biological needs of her baby!* Every mother wants to breastfeed her baby because it is natural and instinctive. She must be provided with necessary guidance, support and encouragement by her husband, family members and health care professionals. By and large, every mother can successfully breastfeed and provide a best start in life to her baby. *Like mother's love, there is no substitute for mother's milk.*

Virtues of Breast Milk

Breastfeeding provides unique health benefits not only to the baby but also to the nursing mother too.

Health benefits to the baby

1. Breast milk is a complete food and it provides all the nutrients that a baby needs during first 6 months of life. Breast milk is more easily digestible due to presence of digestive enzyme lipase and high quality of whey proteins. Healthy term breastfed babies do not need any supplements of vitamins and minerals during first 6 months of life (except vitamin K and vitamin D).

2. Breast milk contains a number of anti-infective substances, protective antibodies and friendly lactobacilli (probiotics), which protect the baby against development of diarrhea, respiratory illness (cough and cold) and other infections (especially ear infection). Breastfeeding has been shown to reduce the risk of death due to diarrhea by 14 times, acute respiratory infections by 4 times and other infections by 3 times.

3. Breastfed babies are less likely to suffer from allergic disorders like asthma and eczema. Rarely, breastfed babies may develop an allergic disorder when mother consumes allergenic food like cow's milk, eggs, nuts and citric fruits.

4. Breastfeeding provides immunological and health benefits to the baby for the lifetime. Breastfed babies have been shown to develop better protective response to various vaccines compared to bottle-fed babies.

5. Breastfed babies are less likely to suffer from caries teeth, diabetes mellitus, obesity, high blood pressure, heart attacks and certain cancers during adult life.

6. Breastfeeding provides emotional security and promotes close bonding between the mother and her baby. Breastfeeding provides maternal warmth, physical closeness and comfort to the baby.

7. Breastfeeding stimulates all the five special senses of the baby, i.e. touch, sight, smell, hearing and taste.

8. Breastfed babies are smarter and have been shown to have 8 points higher intelligence quotient (IQ). High concentration of two long chain fatty acids (arachidonic acid and docosahexaenoic acid or DHA), lactose and sialic acid promotes brain growth.

9. There is no risk of adulteration, dilution, contamination of breast milk.

10. The risk of cot deaths or sudden infant death syndrome (SIDS) is less in breastfed babies.

Health benefits to the mother

1. During breastfeeding, there is release of oxytocin (a feel good hormone) which promotes ejection of milk. Oxytocin helps to contract the uterus so that there is reduced risk of bleeding and anemia after delivery.

2. Breastfeeding delays ovulation and onset of menstruation which provides natural means to ensure spacing of children. Nevertheless, the protection against pregnancy is not fool proof and mothers who are breastfeeding must seek proper contraceptive advice.

3. Breastfeeding is convenient and less time consuming. There is no need to buy feeding bottles and animal or powdered milk and no time is wasted for sterilization of bottles and preparation of feed.

4. Mothers who breastfeed their babies have a reduced risk of development of breast and ovarian cancer and osteoporosis.

5. Mothers who breastfeed their babies have a sense of accomplishment and satisfaction and feel more relaxed and calm in discharging their mother-craft duties.

6. There is a misconception among several women (and their husbands) that breastfeeding spoils the figure. On the contrary, breastfeeding helps to maintain and regain the pre-pregnancy body weight earlier because energy stores laid down during pregnancy are consumed faster during lactation. As far as the shape of breasts is concerned, there is no difference whether mother breastfeeds or gives formula feed to her baby.

7. There is economic saving to the family and society because money and resources are not wasted for purchase of feeding bottles, bottle sterilizer, bottle warmer, animal milk or formula. There is reduction in medical costs because of lower incidence of various infections in breastfed babies. However, nursing mother should consume additional 500 kcal/day, extra proteins and supplements of micronutrients especially vitamin A, vitamin D and calcium to maintain her own health and ensure production of good quality of milk.

Preparation for Breastfeeding

The preparation and motivation for breastfeeding should begin during antenatal visits. The cleaning of nipples and their eversion if retracted and treatment for cracked nipples must be instituted during pregnancy so that the baby does not face any difficulties during breastfeeding. The absence of any sucking difficulties during early nursing is of great importance to establish cordial mother-child relationship and reduce the incidence of lactation failure. There is no correlation between the size of the breasts and adequacy of lactation. Breast milk is produced in the special glands in the breast which are present in good number in all women irrespective of the size of breasts.

Physiological Basis of Lactation

Sucking is the best stimulus to enhance lactation. When a baby sucks vigorously, several hormones are released to produce the milk and eject it out. Sucking movements stimulate nerve fibers in the nipple. These nerve fibers transmit messages to the hypothalamus in the brain. The pituitary gland responds to these messages by release of two hormones, prolactin and oxytocin. Prolactin stimulates the breast to produce more milk. Oxytocin stimulates the tiny muscles surrounding the milk ducts of the breast. The contraction of these tiny muscles squeeze the ducts and eject the milk into the reservoir under the areola. When a baby sucks frequently and vigorously, the milk production and ejection are enhanced. When a baby is sick or small and unable to suck effectively due to mechanical difficulties (cleft lip or palate, retracted or cracked nipples), the milk production falls. Pain and anxiety also interfere with these hormonal mechanisms leading to unsatisfactory lactation.

Promotion of Lactation

During pregnancy, breasts enlarge in size under the influence of sex hormones and become functionally mature to secrete milk when baby is born. During pregnancy, mother should be motivated and emotionally prepared to breastfeed her baby. She should be told about the virtues and advantages of breastfeeding not only to her baby but also for her own health and well-being. *Breasts must be examined during antenatal check ups to exclude and manage any problems like cracked or retracted nipples.* During lactation mother should take plenty of liquids, drink extra milk and take a nutritious diet to provide additional 550 kcal and 20–25 gm proteins per day to meet the nutritional cost of lactation. And since breast milk is rich is calcium (300 mg/liter) and several other vital nutrients for the baby's growth, adequate intake of calcium, vitamin A, vitamin D, omega-3 fatty acids, DHA and other micro-nutrients is essential to ensure successful lactation and production of good quality of breast milk.

Healthy and normal babies (even when born by elective cesarean section) should not be kept in the nursery but should lie next to the mother. Ensuring early skin-to-skin contact and eye contact with the baby enhances lactation. Early (within one hour of birth) and frequent feedings with complete emptying of each breast are associated with increased production of milk. The act of sucking is associated with release of two hormones (prolactin and oxytocin) which are known to enhance milk production and promote ejection of milk. Milk production is related to the concept of supply and demand, more vigorously and frequently a baby sucks, more milk is produced. When a mother is relaxed, confident and keen to breastfeed, she is likely to produce more milk. Adequate support, guidance and encouragement from husband, family members and health care professionals is associated with enhanced milk production. Anxiety, lack of confidence and pain (due to cracked nipples or engorged breasts) are known to adversely affect the milk yield. An anxious brain may switch off the mechanism which controls the release of hormones for production and ejection of milk. Adequate rest, sleep, relaxation and frequent nursing with complete emptying of each breast, are associated with satisfactory yield of milk. Early introduction supplementary bottle feed may lead to poor lactation because baby finds it easier to feed from a bottle and refuses to make efforts to breastfeed. Mother should be advised to avoid the use of a dummy nipple or pacifier which can also adversely affect the milk production.

The Role of Galactagogues

The substances which are credited to enhance milk production are called as galactagogues or lactagogues. In our traditional system, a large number of food items are credited to promote lactation. Home remedies for improving milk yield include consumption of fenugreek (*methi*) seeds, *tulsi* seeds, *pupali*, fennel (*saunf*), cumin seeds (*jeera*), cinnamon (*dalchini*), poppy seeds (*khas khas*), garlic, carom seeds (*ajwain*), ginger, gum acacia, coriander seeds (*dhania*), alfalfa, unripe papaya, oats, etc.—virtually anything in the kitchen. The aforementioned food items are usually consumed in the form of *laddoos*, *kheer* or porridge, *burfi*, *halwa*, *mukhwas*, sprinklers or decoction like herbal tea. The very fact that the list of galactagogues is so large, it suggests that there is no fool proof remedy. They are all based on folklore, faith and cultural wisdom. In modern system of medicine, there is no potent or effective galactagogue. Metaclopramide (a drug used for vomiting) has been tried with a variable efficacy for promotion of lactation.

When to give the first feed?

Baby should be put to the breast as soon as mother has recovered from the fatigue of labor. After a normal delivery, the baby can be offered the first feed within one hour while most babies born by elective cesarean section can be put to the breast within 4 hours of

B

birth. There is no need to give any other milk or drink like glucose water, tea, honey or *ghutti* and baby should be put to the breast without giving any pre-lacteal feed.

What is colostrum?

The thick-yellowish milk, which is produced during the first 2–3 days of delivery, is called colostrum. It is very rich in proteins, protective antibodies and vitamin A. *It must be given to the baby because of its high nutritional qualities and disease fighting capabilities.* There is a cultural practice in some communities to express colostrum and discard it, which is strongly condemned. During initial 2–3 days, milk yield is low (especially after the birth of first baby) but it is enough to meet the nutritional needs of the baby because colostrum is concentrated and rich in nutrients. And healthy term babies do have enough stores of energy (glucagon in the liver) and they do not need any complementary feeds. The practice of introducing bottle feed (especially to cesarean born babies), during first 1–2 days when lactation is gradually building-up, is an important cause of lactation failure. Bottle feeding leads to "nipple confusion" because baby uses different technique to feed from rubber teat of a bottle compared to breastfeeding and therefore the baby is not keen to suckle from the breast. There is reduced hormonal stimulation to the breast because of reduced sucking efforts on the part of the baby which may lead to lactation failure.

Art and technique of breastfeeding

Breastfeeding is natural and instinctive and most mothers are able to breastfeed without any difficulties. There are many ways to breastfeed and every mother develops her own style to suit her baby. There are certain principles and guidelines that will help the mother to breastfeed her baby with ease and comfort. She should master the art of breastfeeding by patience, perseverance and development of self-confidence.

1. The mother should sit comfortably on a chair, on the bed or squat on the floor to feed her baby. It is important that she must feel comfortable and her back must be supported. She may also feed while lying down, if baby was born by cesarean section or she is unwell.

B

2. The baby is held in the arm so that his head and neck rest in the hollow of her elbow, the back is supported on her forearm and buttocks by her hand. When she is feeding the baby on the right breast, her right arm should be used to cradle the baby and vice versa.

3. The mother should bring the baby's entire body snugly towards her, so that baby's tummy touches her mother's tummy. The baby's head and neck must be comfortably supported in the hollow of mother's elbow.

4. The baby should be raised to the level of the breast so that baby's mouth can easily grasp the nipple and areola. Mother can place a pillow below her arm or raise her thigh to lift the baby, if she is sitting cross-legged on the floor. To bring the baby snugly close to her, the mother may need to tuck her baby's arm away so that it does not come in the way. Mother can use her free hand to support her breast or to fondle her baby once the baby is well "attached" or "latched" for feeding.

5. When the lips or cheek of the baby touches her breast, the baby will automatically open his mouth and "root" towards the nipple. *The baby should grasp the nipple and part of areola of the breast in his mouth.* This is called "attachment to the breast". The lactiferous sinuses which store the milk are situated just underneath the areola. In order to effectively suckle the milk from the breast, both nipple and the areola should go into the baby's mouth. Proper "attachment" of the baby to the breast, is indeed the key to successful breastfeeding. For effective sucking, the baby must form an effective seal around the nipple and areola to eject the milk from lactiferous sinuses. When the baby merely grasps and sucks the nipple, it leads to soreness of the nipple, poor feeding and engorgement of breasts.

How to ensure that baby is having good "attachment" to the breast?

The following features suggests that the baby is having good "attachment" or "latching" for effective feeding.

- Baby's mouth is wide open.
- Chin of the baby touches the breast.

- Nipple and most of the areola is grasped inside the baby's mouth.
- Lower lip is turned outwards.
- Mother feels no pain or discomfort while feeding.

How to delatch the baby from the breast?

When baby is satisfied or falls asleep while feeding, he automatically releases the breast. However, when the baby has stopped sucking but is still maintaining strong suction, do not pull him off the nipple. Instead, mother should slide her index finger into the corner of the baby's mouth to break the suction and delatch the baby.

How frequently the baby should be put to the breast?

There should be no fixed timing for feeding the baby. The baby should be fed on demand, day and night, whenever baby appears to be hungry. The yield of breast milk depends upon the principle of supply and demand. The more a baby sucks on the breast, more milk is produced. Most babies would like to be fed every 2–3 hours. The night feeds are required for initial 6–8 weeks or even longer in healthy normal weight babies.

What should be the duration of each feed?

It is variable but most active and healthy babies take 10–15 minutes to finish a feed. Many babies fall asleep after a few sucks and then demand a feed after half to one hour. Mother should actively interact with her baby while feeding by fondling with his ears or stroking the soles. When baby gets lazy after a few sucks, she should try to partially remove her nipple, the baby will wake up again and start sucking vigorously. While feeding, mother should look at her baby intently and interact with him during the process of feeding. *Breastfeeding is an active process and mother must pay her full attention to the baby while feeding.* She should avoid all distractions like watching the television or talking with the mother-in-law and should enjoy the "moment". During breastfeeding, mother provides warmth, skin-to-skin contact, love, affectionate look, tender touch and music of her heartbeats to the baby thus stimulating all the five special senses of the baby! *Apart from wholesome nutrition, breastfeeding provides global sensory stimulation to the baby.*

The composition of the breast milk is not constant during the process of breastfeeding. The initial or "fore-milk" which flows when a baby starts taking the feed, is thin and rich in protein and lactose while the latter or "hind-milk" is thick and energy-dense due to high content of fat. During each feed, the baby should be allowed to completely empty one breast so that both his thirst and hunger are satisfied by taking both fore-milk as well as hind-milk. Baby should be allowed to feed as long as he wants at one breast before offering the other breast. During the next feed, other breast should be offered first to ensure good milk supply in both breasts. Moreover, when a baby is fed mostly on fore-milk (shifting the baby to the other breast without completely emptying one breast) he is likely to pass greenish semi-loose stools and demand feeds more frequently.

How long to continue breastfeeding?

During initial 6 months, exclusive breastfeeding is given, even water should not be given to the baby during hot summer months. The baby will drink more milk when thirsty and would have better weight gain. Exclusively breastfed babies never develop diarrhea and they have adequate weight gain during first 6 months of life. Breast milk is a complete food for the baby and there is no need to give supplements of vitamins (except vitamin K and vitamin D) and minerals to healthy full term babies of healthy mothers during first 6 months. The quality of breast milk can be improved by giving nutritious diet and supplements of vitamins and minerals to the nursing mother. If mother is malnourished or baby is having intrauterine growth retardation (IUGR), multivitamin and iron drops may be given to the baby. There is no role of giving *janam ghutti, jaiphal* (nutmeg) and gripe water to babies. Semi-solid home-made weaning foods should be offered after 6 months of age but breastfeeding should be continued as long as feasible, at least for a minimum period of 1–2 years. During 6 months to 1 year, milk products (like curd, custard, *dalia, kheer,* cheese) may be given but liquid milk should be introduced after one year and given with a glass or a cup. *In the care of healthy term babies, there is thus no role of bottle feeding which should be avoided because bottles and teats are a potential source of infection.* Breastfeeding may be continued as long as feasible or desired but it is important to ensure that the baby gets adequate nutrition by taking sufficient quantities of home-based supplementary feeds of cereals, pulses, vegetables and fruits.

What is nipple confusion?

Some mothers start 1–2 bottle-feeds along with breasfeeding with the mistaken belief that otherwise it will not be possible to wean the baby off the breast. It is unwise and strongly discouraged because firstly the mechanisms for sucking from the breast and rubber teat of the feeding bottle are different and secondly according to current recommendations there is no place for bottle-feeding in the care of healthy babies. Bottle-feeding is easier for the baby because he can readily get the milk by pressing the soft rubber teat while in case of breastfeeding, the baby has to firmly take a big bite of the breast tissue under the areola and suck with a considerable effort with the help of coordinated movements of lips, gums and tongue. Breastfeeding demands more effort on the part of baby and is usually more tiring compared to bottle-feeding. *Once a baby gets used to the easier option of taking milk from the bottle, he refuses to accept the breast because we are all lazy and so are the babies.* Moreover, the baby may start sucking or biting at the nipples (the way he does to the rubber teat of the bottle) because of "nipple confusion" with unsatisfactory sucking efforts and development of cracked nipples. Unnecessary introduction of bottle-feeding with the mistaken belief that the mother has insufficient lactation is the commonest cause of lactation failure.

How to know that the baby is getting enough milk during breastfeeding?

During breastfeeding when milk drips from the other breast, it suggests that mother has satisfactory lactation. As a safeguard against the mess and embarrassment of leaking breasts, mother can place absorbent breast pad under the bra. When a baby is adequately fed, he is satisfied, happy and playful for 2–3 hours after a feed. Most babies pass urine after every feed. When a baby passes dilute water-like urine at least 6–8 times in a day, it suggests that baby is having enough feed. Some babies enjoy sucking their fingers and it is not suggestive of inadequacy of breast milk. *The best criterion that the baby is getting enough milk is the satisfactory weight gain.* During first 4 months, most babies gain 30 gm weight every day (750–900 gm/month). The baby must be weighed on a reliable weighing scale (and with same clothes) during each visit to the hospital for vaccination and routine check-up. "Test weighing" (weighing the baby just before and after breastfeeding) is unnecessary and not recommended to assess the adequacy of lactation. Excessive crying alone should not be taken as an evidence of poor lactation because babies cry due to a variety of reasons like discomfort of wet napkins, excessive wind or intestinal colic, gastroesophageal reflux, exposure to cold or excessive clothing, insect or mosquito bites, boredom, etc.

What is the usual stool frequency during breastfeeding?

Most healthy breastfed babies pass 4–6 golden-yellow sticky stools. Babies fed on cow's milk or formula feed tend to be constipated but are more vulnerable to develop infective diarrhea. Some babies may pass a stool during or soon after a feed because of an overactive gastrocolic reflex. There is no need to worry about this problem because baby would continue to have satisfactory weight gain. It should not be confused with diarrhea and in any case exclusively breastfed babies are unlikely to develop infective diarrhea.

Diet during Lactation

It must be remembered that the nutritional cost of lactation is higher than the nutritional cost of pregnancy. The nursing mother should take additional 550 kcal/day and 25–30 gm extra proteins, vitamins (especially vitamins A and D) and minerals especially calcium. She should take a well-balanced diet with sufficient quantity of proteins in the form of milk and milk products, pulses, legumes, eggs and poultry. She should consume sufficient quantities of green leafy vegetables and seasonal fruits. It is recommended that a nursing mother should take 2.6 gm of omega-3 fatty acid and 300 mg DHA every day through dietary sources or nutritional supplements. Fish and sea-food are excellent sources of omega-3 fatty acid and DHA. Nursing mother should drink plenty of water and liquids to replenish the fluids lost through breast milk. Intake of balanced nutritious diet by the nursing mother is associated with improved nutritional quality of her breast milk. Healthy breastfed infants of healthy mothers do not need any supplements of vitamins (except vitamin K and vitamin D) and minerals during first six months of exclusive breastfeeding.

Common Problems during Breastfeeding

Regurgitation

Most healthy babies regurgitate some curdled milk after a feed but they continue to gain weight satisfactorily. Regurgitation is more common in bottle fed babies compared to breastfed infants. During feeding, baby swallows some air which causes distension and discomfort till baby is able to eructate. In order to prevent regurgitation of feed, the baby should be burped. After each feed (sometimes even after the intake of one-half of the feed), the baby should be held against the shoulder and abdomen is gently pressed by patting baby's back. Alternatively, mother can make the baby sit in her lap to help him to eructate the swallowed air. After burping, the baby should be put to bed in the right lateral position with head end slightly raised.

Engorgement of breasts

Some mothers develop engorgement of breasts on the second or third day after delivery, if breastfeeding is delayed or given infrequently and baby has not learnt the art of correct "attachment" to the breast. It is more common in a primigravida mother. The breast become heavy, swollen, red, hard and painful. Mother may develop some fever apart from discomfort in the breasts. She should be asked to wear a well-fitting bra round-the-clock. Local application of warm packs and intake of a safe analgesic, like paracetamol, relieve pain and congestion. At times hot fomentation may aggravate engorgement due to increase in blood flow. In such a case, cold compresses (with chilled cabbage leaves with a hole in the center for the nipple) may be more beneficial. At times, alternate cold and warm water compresses in-between feedings provide significant relief. The congestion is best relieved by expressing milk with hand or a breast pump. The baby can be put to breast after expressing some milk when breasts become soft. When a baby is unable to suck directly from the breast, he can be given expressed breast milk (EBM). Early feeding and frequent sucking by the baby prevents development of engorgement of breasts.

Sore or cracked nipples

The most common cause of sore nipples is poor "attachment" to the breast. When a baby merely sucks at the nipple (instead of nipple and areola), hardly any milk comes out. The baby becomes frustrated, tries to suck vigorously or may bite the nipple thus damaging its delicate skin. The nipple may also get damaged by pulling the baby forcefully from the nipple without delatching. Avoid frequent washing of breasts with soap and water which may lead to dryness, cracking and chaffing of nipples. Mother should wear loose clothes and avoid the use of bra to allow the cracks to heal. The plastic breast shields or plastic-lined nursing pads should not be worn because they hold the moisture. Mother can use a nursing bra with a breast shell to avoid direct pressure over the tender nipples. After breastfeeding, mother should express some milk and apply over the nipples. The "hind-milk" contains fats and anti-infective substances which serve as an emollient and promote the process of healing. The breastfeeding should be continued and mother can be asked to apply some emollient cream (ultrapurified medical grade lanolin) over the nipples in-between the feed. If nipples are extremely sore, she can use a nipple shield for feeding.

Retracted or inverted nipples

There are wide variations in the shape and size of breasts and nipples. Nipples may be small (or too large), flat or inverted. Most babies are able to feed effectively from a small or flat nipple. When nipples are inverted or retracted, it can cause serious feeding difficulties leading to engorgement of breasts. Mother can be asked to pull out the flat or inverted nipple with her thumb and index finger. The nipple should be rolled between thumb and index finger and pulled out before putting the baby to the breasts. Syringe method is effective for treatment of inverted nipples if manual pulling is unable to rectify the problem (**Box**). Alternatively, nipple shield can be used for feeding till baby is able to suck directly from the nipple.

B

Syringe method for treatment of retracted nipples

- Take a 10 mL plastic syringe and remove its piston.
- After cutting the barrel half a centimeter from the nozzle, insert the piston from the cut end of the barrel.
- Place the smooth or non-cut end of the bevel of the syringe around the nipple and withdraw the piston gently. The nipple will gradually protrude into the barrel. After 30–60 seconds, release the suction gently by pushing the piston.
- Repeat the procedure 5–6 times before each breastfeeding.
- As soon as the nipple becomes prominent, mother should hold the nipple and areola in her thumb and index finger and offer it to the baby to hold and latch.
- Mother should be asked to wear a breast shell under the bra to avoid compression of nipples.

Frequently Asked Questions (FAQs) about Breastfeeding

Should a sick baby be given breastfeeding

Breastfeeding is an ideal food for a sick baby. Many a times, a baby refuses to accept any other food or drink but continues to take breastfeed. When a sick baby is active and able to suck, he must be given breastfeeding. A critically sick baby can be given expressed breast milk (EBM) with a nasogastric tube.

Should breastfeeding be continued when mother is ill?

Most illnesses in the mother do not contraindicate breastfeeding. Breast milk cannot transmit disease causing germs unless there is infection or abscess in the breast. The sick mother is likely to produce antibodies against the infective organisms and these antibodies cross-over through the breast milk and protect the baby. The baby cannot catch cold through breast milk but baby can get infected by close contact with her mother through hands and droplets thrown by her by talking, laughing, coughing and sneezing. Mother with jaundice can safely breastfeed her baby but she should observe strict aseptic precautions to prevent transmission of hepatitis A and E viruses through hands, feeding utensils and clothes (fomites). When a mother is critically sick or suffering from cancer (and receiving anti-cancer medicines) or AIDS, she is advised to bottle feed her baby. When a mother is critically sick or admitted to the hospital, breast milk should be expressed (and may be given to the baby with a cup and spoon) to prevent engorgement of breasts.

B

What medicines should be avoided by the nursing mother?

In general what is safely tolerated by the nursing mother is safe for her suckling infant. Mother should avoid intake of sedatives or sleeping pills as they can make her baby lazy and inactive. Intake of medicated laxative by a mother can cause diarrhea in her suckling baby. It is safe for a nursing mother to take milk of magnesia, liquid paraffin and glycerin suppository for relief of constipation. Intake of certain antibiotics like cephalosporins and amoxicillin by nursing mother may cause mild diarrhea in her suckling infant. Intake of anticancer, antithyroid drugs, anticoagulants and certain antidepressant drugs contraindicate breastfeeding.

What foods should be avoided during nursing?

Mother who is breastfeeding should take a well-balanced nutritious diet without any chillies or condiments. Excessive indulgence in any particular food, fruit or fruit juices should be avoided. It is well known that intake of lentils with their covering like *urad dal*, kidney beans, Bengal gram and *kabli chana* (chick peas) by the nursing mother may cause wind, discomfort and loose motions in her suckling infant. Cruciferous vegetables like cabbage, cauliflower, broccoli sprouts, turnips, radish, beans, mustard leaves (*sarson ka saag*) may also cause distension and gas both in the mother and her suckling infant. When a mother feels that intake of a particular food item consistently upsets her baby by causing wind, colic or loose motions, she should avoid it or take it in moderation.

Can twins be reared on breastfeeding alone?

Many mothers can rear twins on exclusive breastfeeding without any complementary feeds. Many lower mammals are endowed with several breasts (and nipples) depending upon their average litter size. It would appear that two breasts should be sufficient to effectively suckle two babies before they are able to accept weaning foods. Mother can offer alternate breast for feeding each twin baby. If weight gain is unsatisfactory with exclusive breastfeeding, complementary feeds should be given

B

alternating with breastfeeds. However, mother of twin babies must receive tremendous support, encouragement and assistance by family members because it is an herculean task to simultaneously nurture and look after two babies. She would also need additional calories, proteins and micronutrients to maintain her own health and sustain the growth of two babies.

How can a working mother breastfeed her baby?

Mother should take most of her maternity leave after the delivery of her baby. She should extend her leave as much as she can so that she can ensure exclusive breastfeeding as long as possible. If she has to get back to work, she can follow any one of the following alternatives.

1. Availability of a creche near the vicinity of work place is useful so that she can visit her baby for breastfeeding during office hours and lunch break.

2. When a baby is 4 months old, he can be fed with a pre-cooked cereal, soft *rice-dal* gruel (*khichdi*), curd and mashed banana or *cheeku* (sapodilla). Thus a working mother can introduce weaning foods earlier than the current recommendation of 6 months.

3. Mother can express her milk and store it in a container having a tight fitting lid. The milk can be safely stored for 8 hours in room temperature and up to 24 hours in a refrigerator. She can breastfeed her baby before going to work and on returning back. When she is away, expressed breast milk (EBM) can be fed to the baby with a spoon. *It is desirable not to introduce bottle feeding to avoid nipple confusion and reduce the risk of infective diarrhea.*

Technique for Expression of Breast Milk

It is useful to know the proper technique to express and store the breast milk, which may be required in following situations.

i. To maintain lactation when a sick or premature baby is unable to suck from the breast.

ii. To provide milk for tube feeding of a premature or sick baby.

iii. To relieve engorgement of breasts.

iv. When a mother plans to join her office when her baby is still on exclusive breastfeeding.

B

| Manual expression of breast milk |

- Take a wide-mouthed thoroughly washed container having a tight lid. Wash hands with soap and water.
- Sit comfortably. Soften the breast by gently massaging it with both hand starting from near the chest and moving forwards towards the nipple. Massage the breast several times to transfer milk in the lactiferous sinuses which are located under the areola.
- Hold the areola between thumb and index finger and press it inwards to fill up the lactiferous sinuses.
- Place a wide-mouthed container underneath the nipple. Compress the lactiferous sinuses by pinching the areola between your thumb and fingers to express the milk. Press and release the thumb and fingers several times until milk starts to drip out. Rotate the thumb and fingers around the areola so that all traces of milk is removed from the lactiferous sinuses. Collect milk from one breast for at least 3–5 minutes.
- Repeat the process on the other breast. Store the milk if it is not required immediately.

The milk can be expressed manually or with the help of a mechanical or an electrical breast pump (**Box**).

How to store the expressed breast milk (EBM)?

The milk should be collected in a clean wide-mouthed container having a screw cap or a tight lid. Milk can be safely stored for 8 hours in the cool place of the room or up to 24 hours in a refrigerator. It can be stored up to 3 months in a deep freeze at −20°C. The stored milk should never be boiled or heated in the microwave oven as it will destroy the protective components of milk. It can be thawed or warmed by placing the container in a bowl of warm water. The container should be gently shaken to recombine the separated fat globules before feeding. Give EBM with a spoon or *paladay* and strictly avoid the use of a feeding bottle to avoid "nipple confusion" and risk of infection.

Should breastfeeding be given on demand or every 2 hours by clock?

The baby should be fed on demand (and not by clock) whenever baby is hungry and cries for feed. There is no need to unnecessarily disturb or wake up a sleeping baby to give him a feed. Whenever

B

the baby cries because of hunger (check that he is not crying because of wet diaper or discomfort) he should be offered a feed whether it is day or night and irrespective of your convenience or comfort. Most babies are likely to demand a feed after every 2–3 hours.

Should a baby born by cesarean section be given formula feeds during initial few days of delivery?

In most cases of elective cesarean section, mother can breastfeed her baby as soon as she has recovered from general anesthesia. In case of spinal or subdural anesthesia, she can breastfeed soon after the delivery. Nevertheless, when a mother has undergone cesarean section, she needs more support and encouragement to breastfeed. She needs to identify the posture of comfort and should be provided with assistance for holding or supporting the baby. During initial one or two days, she can breastfeed while lying down in bed.

However, in a case of emergency cesarean section, when a mother is critically sick, the baby may be given expressed breast milk (EBM) with a cup and spoon or *paladay* till she is well enough to breastfeed. Introduction of bottle feed should be avoided because it may lead to "nipple confusion" thus causing difficulties in subsequent breastfeeding. It is important to remember that the ability to breastfeed is dependent upon your will power and keenness or commitment to breastfeed rather than your mode of delivery or comfort level.

Should breast and nipple be washed with soap and water before every feed?

There is no need to wash the breasts and nipples with soap and water before each feed as it may lead to dryness, chaffing and crack-ing of nipples. Daily bath and maintenance of personal hygiene is all that is needed by the nursing mother. She should wear nursing pads to prevent ugly patches on her clothes due to leakage of milk.

Can a mother with small breasts is able to breastfeed her baby effectively?

Just like other attributes, breasts come in different shapes and sizes. Irrespective of the size of breasts, every woman is endowed with enough glandular tissue to effectively breastfeed her baby.

Adequacy of lactation depends more on keenness and confidence of mother, freedom from pain and discomfort, sucking stimulation provided by an active and healthy baby rather than the size and shape of breasts or nipples. Nevertheless, there may be genetic or constitutional factors which may determine that mothers in certain families are better milk producers than in others.

Is it true that formula fed babies are more healthy and "chubby" compared to breastfed babies?

It is true that formula fed babies gain weight faster and look "chubby" but they are "unhealthy" and at an increased risk to develop obesity, diabetes mellitus and coronary artery disease later in adult life. The animal milks and formula milks have higher content of proteins and solutes which leads to excessive weight gain. The composition of human milk is ideal and best suited for optimal physical and mental growth of human babies. Nature has profound biological wisdom and milk of an animal is best suited for serve the biological needs of its own offsprings—and is not meant or suitable to serve the nutritional needs of babies of other species.

Is it true that if a mother was unable to breastfeed her first baby, she will not be able to breastfeed her second baby?

It is untrue because if you have the necessary desire, motivation and will power and if you have the perseverance and positive frame of mind, you can always succeed in every human endevour in life. Never ever have a defeatist attitude in life, you can achieve whatever you believe and crave for. When you start thinking that you cannot successfully breastfeed, it is unlikely that you would succeed.

Is it true that when a baby cries frequently, it is an indication that the breast milk is insufficient?

Apart from hunger, the babies cry due to a variety of other reasons like discomfort because of wet napkins, wind or colic, exposed or overclothed, over stimulated or bored baby, nappy rash, insect bites, etc. When your milk drips on the mere sight of your baby or drips from the other breast while you are feeding the baby, baby is passing urine at least 8 times or more in a day and having satisfactory weight gain, it suggests that you are having satisfactory lactation. Starting one or two complementary bottle feeds on the mistaken belief that mother is having insufficient lactation, is the commonest cause of lactation failure and its consequences.

Is it true that breastfeeding is more troublesome, inconvenient and demanding for the mother as opposed to bottle feeding?

Infact, the truth is otherwise. Bottle feeding demands more efforts on the part of mother for sterilization of feeding bottles, preparation of formula, ensuring right temperature of the milk before feeding, maintenance of strict asepsis—especially when all this needs to be done by mother herself without the help of the husband, other family members or maid. Breastfeeding is certainly more convenient and less bothersome especially during night. Mother is likely to regain her figure faster because fat stores laid during pregnancy are utilized to sustain lactation.

Is breastfeeding likely to make the breasts more saggy and unattractive?

It is not the act of breastfeeding but pregnancy *per se* that affects the shape, size or firmness of the breasts. During pregnancy, structural changes occur in the breasts for promotion of lactation and even if breastfeeding is denied to the baby, the breasts are likely to sag unless strong support is provided with a bra and mother undertakes vigorous exercises of the muscles located under her breasts (pectoralis major). Excessive weight gain during pregnancy, hereditary factors and increasing age are other factors which make the breasts less globular, saggy and soft. Breastfeeding should not be blamed for something which is going to happen sooner or later.

Should breastfeeding be stopped when baby has cut his teeth?

Most babies cut their first tooth around 6–7 months but breastfeeding is continued till at least one year or even longer till all the milk teeth are in place. Most babies are smart and do not bite the nipple because they know it is their life line. However, an angry young fellow may create mischief by biting the nipple either to relieve irritation of the gums or due to frustration of not getting enough milk. Mother should not laugh or approve this prank and she should firmly say "no biting" and calmly delatch the prankster from the breast and divert his attention by talking or playing with the baby. When mother does this several times, the baby gets the message of her disapproval and eventually drops the habit.

B

Should nursing mothers avoid exercise because it may sour the milk due to elevation of lactic acid?

There is no evidence to suggest that exercise leads to souring of milk unless the mother indulges it to the point of exhaustion. Aerobic exercises and yoga are the best. Mother should wear a firm sports bra and do the exercise immediately after having given feed to the baby. She should drink extra glass of water before and after the exercise especially during summer to maintain good hydration status.

Should breastfeeding be stopped when mother becomes pregnant?

It is desirable that parents should adopt family planning measures to prevent next pregnancy till the elder sibling is at least 2 years old. The second child should be born when the elder sibling is about 3 years old and relatively independent and attending a play school. However, when mother gets pregnant early, breastfeeding can be continued till mid-pregnancy. The baby should be started on supplementary feeds, if he is above 4 months of age. In this case, the weaning foods can be introduced at 4 months of age instead of the conventional recommendation of 6 months. Prolonged breastfeeding by the pregnant mother may adversely affect the nutritional status of the infant and imposes profound nutritional demands on the mother which may adversely affect the growth of the fetus.

BREAST MILK JAUNDICE

Most newborn babies (whether bottle or breastfed) develop some degree of jaundice which is called "physiological jaundice" which usually disappears by 2 weeks of age. In some healthy babies who are exclusively breastfed, the "physiological jaundice" becomes more intense and takes longer time to disappear. There are several factors which aggravate jaundice in breastfed babies but there is nothing "bad" about the breast milk of the mother whose baby develops "breast milk jaundice". Infact "breast milk jaundice" may confer some health benefits to the baby because bilirubin is a strong antioxidant. The child remains active, feeds normally and there is no risk of brain damage due to elevated serum bilirubin. *It does not need any treatment.* Some doctors stop breastfeeding for 2–3 days but many others continue breastfeeding and the course of jaundice remains similar with both the options. In babies with breast milk jaundice, urine remains colorless (like water) while stools are normal yellow-colored. Jaundice disappears without any treatment but may take 6–10 weeks to wane off. A similar type of jaundice may occur in babies with hypothyroidism (cretinism) and your doctor may order blood tests to exclude it. However, when prolonged jaundice in a newborn baby is associated with yellow or high-colored urine and white or clay-colored stools, the child must be seen by a pediatrician for further investigations.

BREATH HOLDING SPELLS

In some children, a violent temper tantrum may be followed by a breath holding attack. The child gets angry (due to unfulfilled demand or frustration) or gets hurt, cries loudly (by putting his heart and soul into it) and after a long uninterrupted cry, holds his breath and becomes blue. Rarely the attack may lead to a fit or convulsion. When enough carbon dioxide accumulates in the body by holding the breath, it provides the necessary trigger to the breathing center in the brain and child starts breathing again. After the spell, the child may continue to cry or whimper and start asking for the same demand which triggered the attack. When a crying spell, is triggered by pain due to injury, it may cause reflex cardiac asystole with sudden onset of extreme pallor, loss of posture due to flabbiness of muscles and at times a tonic convulsion or stiffening of the limbs.

The spells usually occur in children between 6 months and 3 years of age but in some babies they may start as early as newborn period. The condition may run in families and affected children may have autonomic dysfunction. Iron deficiency makes children more vulnerable to breath holding spells. The spells occur in over sensitive and over demanding babies of anxious, concerned and apprehensive parents and grandparents. It would appear that breath holding spells are a sort of "blackmailing" tactics on the part of the child to get his demand fulfilled. The episodes are frightening to the family and many a times the parents give-in to the demands of the child. The child learns to use these spells as a tool to get what he wants and makes parents feel helpless and at the mercy of the child. These children are over indulged or pampered, over demanding and lack patience or coping skills to manage their frustration, disappointment and anger.

Treatment

The breath holding spells are harmless and do not pose any danger to the life or brain of the child. The frequency of spells increases, if parents or grandparents show extreme anxiety and panic during the attack and when child is rewarded after the spell. There is no need to panic or sprinkle cold water on the face of the child. Parents should accept the spell coolly and with confidence that no harm will come to the child by holding his breath. If mother or other relatives start shouting or create undue panic and alarm, the child is likely to hold his breath more often and for a longer period. You should try to reduce episodes of frustration by meeting some of his genuine or acceptable demands. Parents should follow a sensible middle-of-the-road approach and should neither deny nor succumb to all the pranks and demands of their child. When a child starts crying loudly due to a temper tantrum and it appears that he is going to hold his breath, he should be pinched and the child will continue to cry and breathe. Administration of iron supplements may reduce the frequency and severity of breath holding spells if child has iron deficiency anemia. The spells usually disappear after the age of 3 years when child learns other ways and means to express his anger and frustration for meeting his demands.

Bronchial Asthma (see Asthma)
BRONCHIOLITIS

Acute bronchiolitis is a viral infection due to respiratory syncytial virus (RSV) involving the bronchioles which are tiny air passages in the lungs. It usually affects infants below one year but toddlers may also get it. It is more common in premature babies and infants who received assisted ventilation during newborn period. After initial symptoms of fever, cough and cold, there is progressive

B

worsening of cough, rapid breathing and wheezing. In severe cases, there is marked breathing difficulty, with indrawing of chest and upper abdomen. There may be feeding difficulty, marked irritability and crying because of oxygen lack. About 40% infants with acute bronchiolitis may develop attacks of recurrent wheezing when there is familial predisposition or atopy or asthmatic bronchitis.

Treatment Ensure adequate intake of fluids and feeds. Fever should be controlled by administration of paracetamol. Provide steam inhalation or cold humidification (with a nebulizer) with water containing common salt, 2–3 times in a day. Avoid use of cough suppressants and sedatives. Whenever child is having breathing or feeding difficulty, consult your doctor without delay. In severe cases, the child may need hospital admission for administration of oxygen and nebulization with epinephrine or hypertonic (3%) saline. Antibiotics are given, if there is superadded bacterial infection. The complete recovery may take several days and weeks.

BROWNISH STAINING OF TEETH

The foundation of teeth is laid in the mother's womb as early as 6 weeks of fetal life. Good health and nutrition of the mother during pregnancy lays a sound foundation for baby's teeth. Intake of tetracyclines should be avoided during pregnancy as they may get deposited in the tooth buds leading to permanent yellowish-brown staining of teeth. Children should not be given tetracyclines during first 8 years of life because of risk of yellow-staining of permanent teeth. Poor oro-dental hygiene and intake of colored medications (especially iron containing syrups) may cause brownish discoloration of teeth. In adolescent children brownish, discoloration of teeth can occur due to cigarette smoking, tobacco chewing or taking *guthka* and *paan* (betel leaves with *katha*, lime and nutmeg). The enamel of teeth may become mottled and brown in color if fluoride content of water is high (>2 parts per million). Severe jaundice during newborn period may cause yellow staining of permanent teeth in association with manifestations of brain damage (kernicterus).

BURNS AND SCALDS

Burns may occur due to fire, fireworks, contact with a hot object and electric shock. Most burn accidents occur in the kitchen or due to fireworks used during various festive occasions. The severity of burns depends upon the extent or surface area of the body burnt, site and depth of burns. In first degree burn, only outer layer of skin is burnt. Skin becomes red and is tender to touch. Second degree burn is more deep leading to formation of blisters, swelling and weeping due to rupture of blisters. In third degree burns, all the layers of skin are involved along with underlying structures, subcutaneous tissues like muscles and nerves. The skin looks dry, pale, swollen and charred.

Treatment Do not panic, keep yourself cool and composed. Wrap the child with a bed cover or blanket and extinguish the flames. The child should not be allowed to run. *Pour tap water or cold water over the burnt area for 10–15 minutes to reduce tissue damage.* Burnt area can be covered with a cool towel. Dab dry the skin with a clean towel and wrap the child in a clean white sheet. Give sips of water and paracetamol or ibuprofen to relieve pain and discomfort. If burnt area is small and superficial, apply silver-sulfadiazine cream (silverix). Avoid use of home remedies like application of turmeric or oil over the burnt site. Do not use cotton to cover the burnt area, as it will get stuck to the damaged skin. When burnt area is larger (more than 10% body), there are second or third degree burns (blisters and charring) and when vital parts of the body like face, hands, feet and genitals are affected, the child must be immediately rushed to the hospital. Even a small area of full thickness burns may cause severe disfigurement unless it is managed with due care and professional competence. During journey to the hospital, the child should be reassured and given sips of water or oral rehydration solution.

Prevention

- Children should not be allowed to enter the kitchen.
- Keep the match box out of reach and out of sight of children.
- Children should play with firecrackers only under the direct supervision of adults.
- They must wear shoes and put on clothes made of non-synthetic material like cotton while playing with firecrackers.
- Never light fireworks inside the house.
- Keep the doors and windows of home closed on Diwali night to prevent entry of firecrackers.

- Do not burst crackers near the vehicles.
- Keep a bucket of water handly while playing with firecrackers.

Scalds

Scalds are more common than burns and occur due to contact with hot water and other hot liquids like milk, tea, coffee, soup, or due to steam. The child may get burnt when you are drinking a hot cup of tea or coffee while holding the child in the lap. Accidents are common during inhalation of steam or spilling of hot water bucket in the bathroom. The child may pull a table cloth, spilling hot tea or milk over himself. You must check the temperature of the hot water meant for his bath or hot drinks before offering to him.

Treatment Pour cold water over the burnt area or place it under the running tap for 5–10 minutes so that skin temperature is brought down immediately. Give paracetamol or ibuprofen to relieve pain. Apply antiseptic cream like silver-sulfadiazine cream over the burnt area. The child should be taken to the hospital if blisters have formed. The blisters are ruptured with a sterile needle while keeping the wrinkled skin on.

Home Remedies

Apply aloe vera gel or calendula cream over the burnt site and cover with dough prepared from wheat flour. Dough remains cool for a long time without dripping and can be easily molded to effectively cover the burnt site. The dough can be covered with an ice cool towel for 1–2 hours. Local application of honey, 2–3 times in a day, is useful to relieve inflammation and disinfect the wound.

Prevention

- Never take the baby in your lap while drinking a hot drink or taking hot soup.
- Do not leave the child alone near a tea pot or hot water bucket.
- Never keep a tray with hot food or hot drink on the dining table with a hanging table cloth.
- Always keep the handles of cooking pots towards the back side of the stove or cooking range so that they are out of reach of the child.

B

- When planning hot water bath, the temperature of water should be brought to a comfortable level before child is taken to the bathroom.
- Be extremely vigilant and careful while giving steam inhalation. It is better to use a facial steamer rather than a pot with boiling water.

Chemical Burns

Burns can occur due to contact with strong acids, alkalis, caustic soda, toilet cleaner, unslaked lime and certain dyes. Fingers are most commonly affected. Wash the burnt area under a constant flow of tap water till all traces of chemical are washed away. At times a child may drink a strong acid or alkaly causing life-threatening burns of the mouth and food pipe. The child can be given a small amount of water or milk to dilute the residual chemical in the mouth. Never give large volume of liquids and never try to induce vomiting as it may cause rupture of the food pipe or stomach. Milk of magnesia and antacids can be given to neutralize strong acids. After the first aid, child must be taken to the hospital because most chemical burns are rather deep.

BURPING

During feeding, most babies swallow some air which causes discomfort till baby is able to belch or eructate the swallowed air. Along with belching, most healthy babies regurgitate some curdled milk after a feed but they continue to gain weight satisfactorily. Burping is the technique to enable the baby to eructate the air swallowed during feeding. After each feed (whether breast or bottle feeding), mother should make the baby sit in her lap or hold the baby upright against her chest to help him eructate the swallowed air. Mother can gently compress the tummy of the baby against her chest and rub or stroke the back of the baby to facilitate belching. In some babies, who are prone to frequent regurgitations, burping may be done twice during a feed, i.e. once when one-half of the feed has been taken and then after completion of the feeding. After burping, the baby should be put to bed in the right lateral position with head end slightly raised. When despite effective burping, the baby continues to have regurgitations and weight gain is slow, the possibility of gastroesophageal reflux disease (GERD) due to lax sphincter at the junction of esophagus and stomach should be ruled out.

CAPUT SUCCEDANEUM

When labor is prolonged and difficult, the head of the baby may look odd-shaped with a diffuse boggy swelling over the presenting part. The swelling is seen at birth (unlike cephalhematoma which appears few hours after birth) and it pits on pressure. The nose and ears of the baby may be compressed and eyes may appear swollen. The baby may look deceptively unwell but there is nothing to worry. These changes subside within few days without any treatment.

CEPHALHEMATOMA

During the process of vaginal delivery especially when vacuum is applied, the blood may leak out and collect under the outer covering of one of the skull bones. When enough blood has leaked out over next few hours, it forms a well-defined soft or cystic lump on one side of head over one of the skull bones. It is called cephalhematoma and usually occurs few hours after birth. It may be associated with underlying linear fracture of skull bone. It is harmless but when swelling is excessively large in size, it may be associated with anemia and jaundice in the baby. The swelling gradually resolves over a period of several days or weeks depending upon its size. No cold or hot fomentation should be done over the swelling.

CEREBRAL PALSY (Spastic child)

There is motor disability which occurs in early life due to disorder of brain development or because of brain damage in fetal life, during delivery or at birth and early infancy. There is stiffness or spasticity of limbs which is more marked in the lower limbs so that the child may keep the legs criss-crossed like scissors. The child would have delay or inability to sit, stand, walk and difficulty in holding objects or performing skills with hands. The child may have convulsions, visual and hearing defects and mental retardation. The degree of mental subnormality may be variable. The speech is after delayed and there is lack of clarity. There may be irregular tremors or movements of limbs. There may be difficulty in swallowing and feeding with drooling of saliva.

Causes The common causes of cerebral palsy include extremely premature babies, delayed crying with lack of oxygen to the brain at birth (birth asphyxia), severe jaundice during first week of life (kernicterus), metabolic disorders (hypoglycemia and inborn error of metabolism) and infection of brain (meningitis).

Treatment Cerebral palsy is a non-progressive disorder and is managed by early stimulation and physiotherapy. Active and passive movements of various limbs and exercise of different groups of muscles are done under the supervision of a trained physiotherapist. *Massage should not be done because it may further increase the muscle tone and spasticity.* The child should be made self-reliant and independent to undertake daily activities of life, like feeding, bathing, and dressing, even if the child may do it slowly or awkwardly. Some children with cerebral palsy may have unique or specialized capabilities like interest in painting and music. Parents should identify any other special attributes and harness them effectively by guiding and inspiring the child. After getting hands-on instructions from a physiotherapist, the parents should continue the exercises and manipulations at home.

There is no role of drugs or "brain tonics" for treatment of cerebral palsy. Muscle relaxants may be tried to relieve spasticity. Botox injections have been used to reduce spasticity but they are expensive and benefit is short lived. You should seek the advice of an orthopedic surgeon for special shoes, braces, splints and surgical procedures to relieve tightening of muscles and tendons. There are special institution or associations (Spastic Society of India) in big cities and their expertize can be effectively utilized. Because of feeding difficulties, these children may have to be fed with a liquid or semi-solid diet. Avoid over feeding because they have a tendency to become overweight because of lack of physical activity. The child must be provided with routine immunizations as per the recommended schedule. Parents should have a positive attitude and should not feel desperate or despondent in facing the challenge of the specially abled child. Parents should join the support group of parents of children with cerebral palsy so that they can harness the moral support to handle the challenge with greater poise and determination.

CESAREAN SECTION

When pregnancy progresses to term, the bag of water (amniotic sac) ruptures followed by spontaneous onset of labor pains. In large majority of pregnancies (>90%), the baby is born through vaginal delivery either spontaneously or with the help of assistance by an obstetrician, like use of forceps, vacuum extraction or widening of the vaginal passage by episiotomy. When a baby cannot be delivered through the vaginal route either because of narrow or deformed pelvis (osteomalacia) or there is development of a life-threatening complication in the fetus or mother, the baby is delivered through the abdomen by a surgical procedure.

Cesarean section may be planned or may be required as an emergency procedure. Elective cesarean section is done when (i) pelvic outlet is narrow, (ii) breech presentation, (iii) multiple pregnancy, (iv) previous delivery by cesarean section and (v) mother wants that baby to be born by C-section to bypass the pain of vaginal delivery. More often, emergency cesarean section is done when there is (i) poor progress of labor despite a fair trial, (ii) severe toxemia of pregnancy, (iii) Rh-isoimmunization, (iv) fetal distress, and (v) antepartum hemorrhage (placenta previa).

Cesarean section may be done under general anesthesia or spinal anesthesia (subdural block) when mother remains conscious during the procedure. Instead of a conventional midline vertical abdominal incision, these days a horizontal incision is made above the pubis to reduce the risk of unsightly scar. Cesarean section is usually a safe procedure and common complications include transient breathing difficulty in the baby (wet lungs), infection, delay or difficulty in breastfeeding and prolonged convalescence. It must be remembered that C-section is an unnatural or unphysiological mode of delivery and should be practised when there is a risk either to the life of the baby or mother.

CHICKENPOX (*Chhoti mata*)

It is a viral infection due to varicella. Infection occurs through droplets from cough or direct contact with a patient with chickenpox. After 2 to 3 weeks of exposure to a patient, child develops mild fever, cough and cold. After 3–4 days of onset of fever, skin rash appears in crops mostly on the trunk and proximal parts of limbs. Skin rash has all types of lesions like flat red spots, papules and fluid-filled vesicles (like dew drops). Itching is usually present. Chickenpox is usually a mild disease in healthy children but can be serious or severe in adolescents and adults. Patient is contagious during the phase of "cough and cold" and remains contagious till all the scabs have formed.

Treatment Patient is given symptomatic treatment with paracetamol and antihistaminic (to relieve itching) and advised to take plenty of liquids and nutritious diet without any chillies. Aspirin should never be given to a child with chikenpox because of potential risk of development of Reye syndrome. Bath is given daily with an antiseptic soap. Local application of a soothing calamine-containing lotion provides relief to itching. The nails should be kept trimmed to prevent scratching and superadded bacterial infection.

Complications The common complications include secondary infection of skin lesions, pneumonia, cerebellar taxia (difficulty in walking due to lack of balance which usually recovers) and rarely encephalitis. After recovery, the virus may remain dormant in the baby and may manifest as herpes zoster or shingles (painful streaks of blisters on one side of the face or trunk) during adulthood.

Prevention Chickenpox vaccine is given anytime after the age of 15 months in children who had not suffered from natural infection. A second dose of vaccine is recommended after the age of 5 years. In children above the age of 12 years, two doses of vaccine are given at an interval of 4 to 6 weeks. The vaccine also provides protection against development of shingles.

CHOCOLATES

There is age old relationship between children and chocolates. Children are crazy to consume chocolates which is the most popular gift given to them on all occasions. Chocolates are loaded with sugar and calories, and they are recognized risk factors for development of obesity and caries teeth. However, cocoa-based dark chocolates are no longer considered as a junk food because they are credited to have several health benefits. Cocoa is nature's richest source of polyphenols (especially flavanol) which stimulates the production of nitric oxide (NO) which vasodilates blood vessels to bring down blood pressure. Cocoa-based flavanols reduce inflammation by reducing levels of 5-lipooxygenase (5-LO), a key enzyme for the synthesis of leukotrienes. Dark chocolates have the highest oxygen radical absorbance capacity (ORAC) compared to any other food. It is credited to reduce aggregation of platelets and raise the level of heart-friendly high density lipo-proteins (HDLs). Chocolates contain tryptophane and phenyl-ethylamine which increase the level of "feel good" neurotransmitter serotonin which gives a feeling of pleasure and well-being. Intake of dark chocolates in moderate amount is both health and heart-friendly and are preferable to other calorie-dense junk foods and snacks, but always keep in mind that excess of everything is bad.

CHOKING (Foreign bodies)

Choking and suffocation due to foreign bodies may occur in toddlers and preschool children. Toddlers are notorious for "mouthing" small objects like coins, buttons, peas, groundnuts and beads. Children between 1 and 2 years should not be offered popcorn, round candies, grapes or roasted Bengal gram and nuts because of potential risk of accidental choking and aspiration into air passages. Children should not be tickled or made to laugh while eating due to potential risk of choking. Children have an uncanny habit of inserting objects into their body holes. They can put a safety pain, splinter, crayon, pencil, etc. into their mouth, nose, ear or vagina.

The aspiration of foreign body may cause a sudden bout of coughing and choking. The child may develop gasping or difficulty in breathing and may become blue. The child is unable to speak or cry. Choking may lead to sudden death or accident may be over-looked and child develops symptoms of persistent or recurrent respiratory infections.

First aid When a rouneded object like a coin, bead or a nut is swallowed into the stomach, it is spontaneously passed out in the stool in next 12–24 hours. When a foreign body is lodged in the esophagus, give mashed potatoes or banana to dislodge it. When an object or insect has lodged in the nostril or ear canal, do not make any attempts to remove it unless it is hanging out of the orifice. Otherwise you may push the foreign body deeper. You should seek the help of an ENT specialist to remove the foreign body from the nose and ears.

When a child is choked or suffocated by a foreign body, do not panic but act immediately. Never try to sweep or recover the foreign body with your fingers because it may get further pushed and impacted in the throat or wind pipe. In case of an infant or toddler, suspend the baby upside down by supporting his chest and abdomen over your left arm. Alternatively, you can sit on a stool or an armless chair and place the child on his tummy across your thighs with his head hanging down while legs and feet are lifted up. Give 4–5 good thumps or blows between his shoulder blades. Most of the time the impacted object may be expelled out and the child may take a sigh of relief.

Heimlich maneuver When the aforementioned procedure to remove the foreign body fails or the child is grown up, Heimlich procedure is more appropriate and effective to remove the foreign body. The child is made to stand and lean forward. The child is held firmly from behind by interlocking your hands over the center of upper abdomen just below the rib cage or breast bone. The locked hands are sharply pulled upwards 4–5 times with thrusting movements to raise the pressure inside the abdomen and chest. The resultant sudden increase in the intrathoracic pressure is likely to dislodge and push out the foreign body. Heimlich maneuver should be conducted quickly with a sense of purpose but without any panic. If breathing stops or child becomes blue and unconscious, start cardiopulmonary resuscitation (CPR) and rush the child to the hospital.

CHORIONIC VILLUS SAMPLING

Chorionic villus sampling (CVS) or biopsy of chorion of the placenta is being increasingly used in advanced centers for antenatal diagnosis of genetic or metabolic defects (by DNA probes and PCR studies) and chromosomal abnormalities. The procedure is useful for antenatal diagnosis of a number of life-threatening genetic diseases, like thalassemia, hemophilia, Duchenne's muscular dystrophy, cystic fibrosis, etc.

The procedure is performed between 10 and 12 weeks of gestation. Under continuous ultrasonographic guidance, a catheter is passed through the cervix into the uterus. The catheter is inserted into the chorion of the placenta and chorionic tissue is sucked with the help of a 20 mL syringe filled with 5 mL of tissue culture medium. It is an outpatient procedure and must be done by an experienced obstetrician. The procedure can also be performed during second trimester of pregnancy (>12 weeks) through transabdominal route under the guidance of ultrasonography. Many centers prefer to undertake transabdominal CVS because of reduced risk of infection, bleeding and abortion. When procedure is performed on an Rh-negative mother, she must be given 50 μg anti-D immunoglobulins intramuscularly before the procedure to prevent Rh-isoimmunization.

CIRCUMCISION

Surgical excision of foreskin has been practiced for over 6000 years as a religious ritual. Circumcision should not be done just because child is having a long foreskin or for relief of enuresis and masturbation. The medical indications for circumcision include scarred opening of prepuce (due to persistent nappy rash), recurrent formation of pus at the tip of penis (balanitis) and recurrent episodes of urinary tract infection due to phimosis (non-retractable prepuce or foreskin). The procedure should be done by a pediatric surgeon under proper anesthetic cover. There is recent evidence to suggest that circumcision is associated with reduced risk of HIV, urinary tract infection, carcinoma of penis, sexually transmitted genital ulcer and carcinoma cervix (among the spouse).

CLEFT LIP (Hare lip)

The baby is born with a cleft or gap in the upper lip. The incidence of anomaly is around 1 in 800 births. There may be a unilateral single cleft or two clefts one on either side, with the central part of lip jutting or protruding out. The nose appears flat and asymmetrical. The defect may be isolated or associated with other anomalies especially cleft palate. These infants have difficulty in sucking from breast or bottle. They are best fed expressed breast milk (EBM) with a spoon or *paladay*. There should not be undue anxiety because the defect can be completely repaired by a pediatric or plastic surgeon. It is desirable to get the lip repaired before the baby leaves the hospital or the repair can be done within the first few weeks of life. Early surgical repair is associated with better cosmetic results.

C CLEFT PALATE

Cleft in the palate (roof of the oral cavity) is usually associated with cleft lip but may occur as an isolated anomaly. Isolated cleft palate may be associated with a hole in the heart or ventricular septal defect. When celft palate is associated with a small and retracted jaw (micrognathia and retrognathia), a large tongue which has a tendency to fall back and block the throat, the condition is called Pierre-Robin syndrome. Cleft palate is cosmetically less frightening but it seriously interferes with feeding in early life and causes speech difficulties (nasal twang and indistinct speech) later in life. The baby is unable to suck from breast or bottle and feeding is associated with risk of regurgitation through the nose and aspiration into the lungs. The baby is at an increased risk to develop ear infection (acute otitis media).

The baby should be fed in a sitting or upright position with a wide flat teat which can close the gap in the palate. Most mothers find it easier to feed expressed breast milk (EBM) with a spoon, *paladay* or a dropper. The surgical repair is recommended at the age of one or one and a half year. The cosmetic results are good and quality of speech is better when repair is done by a plastic surgeon. Most infants do need speech therapy to improve the clarity of speech before they join the play school.

CLUB FEET (Talipes equinovarus)

It is a congenital deformity where the feet are stretched downwards at the ankles and turned and rotated inwards. The upper surface of the foot cannot be made to touch the front of leg or shin. The defect may be limited to one side but usually both feet are affected. The abnormality may be positional due to crooked position of the fetus because of less quantity of the amniotic fluid. It may be associated with other developmental defects or spinal deformity (spina bifida, meningocele) in some babies.

Treatment When deformity is mild and limited to soft tissues, it can be corrected by physiotherapy. The affected foot is pulled outwards and then dorsiflexed to touch the front of foot with the shin. The manipulations are done several times in a day. In severe cases which are associated with bony deformity, application of plaster of Paris cast is recommended under the supervision of an orthopedic surgeon. Correction of complete deformity is achieved by changing the cast every week for a period of 6–10 weeks. At times surgical procedure may be needed to correct the deformity and lengthen Achilles tendon. In most cases, the feet will become entirely normal and child will be able to walk and dance normally, if early and effective treatment is instituted.

COLOR BLINDNESS

Color blindness is an X-linked (sex-linked) disorder which is mostly seen in boys. The girls in general have better color sense and they do not suffer from color blindness. It is estimated that 1 out of 10 men suffer from some degree of color blindness. The color blind person has difficulty in identifying few colors and they see them as shades of gray. Color blind people are disqualified to join certain services where it is important to distinguish between different colors like aviation, merchant navy or shipping, railway drivers, chemical industries, web designing, etc. Color vision is tested with the help of a pseudoisochromatic plate or Ishihara compatible (PIP) 24 color vision test plates. There is no specific treatment for the disorder. Total color blindness with loss of visual acuity and nystagmus is indicative of a serious retinal disorder.

COLOSTRUM

The golden-yellow milk produced during first 2–3 days after delivery is called colostrum. It has a higher protein and vitamin A content and is rich in protective antibodies (secretory immunoglobulins). It is best suited to serve the nutritional needs of the baby and virtually works like the "first vaccine shot" for the baby by blocking the entry of pathogenic bacteria through the gut. *It should never be discarded and is indeed the ideal first feed for the baby.* During first few days, the milk yield is low but it is enough to meet the nutritional needs of the baby. Healthy babies born at term do have enough stores of energy (glycogen in the liver) and do not need any complementary feeds. The practice of introducing bottle feed, during first 1–2 days when lactation is gradually building up, is an important cause of lactation failure. Bottle feeding leads to "nipple confusion" (because baby uses different technique to feed from a rubber teat of a bottle compared to breastfeeding) with reduced hormonal stimulation to the breasts because of reduced sucking efforts.

COMMON COLD (Upper respiratory catarrh)

Common cold is the most common acute respiratory infection in children. It is the commonest cause of absenteeism in school and is caused by over 200 different viruses. The infection occurs throughout the year but is more common during change of weather and in winter. Most children are likely to suffer, on an average, 4–6 episodes of common cold in a year. Infection occurs when child comes in contact with a person suffering from cold, i.e. parents, siblings or maid at home and classmates in the creche, play school or regular school. It is a highly contagious disease and infection is transmitted by the patient directly through air droplets by coughing and sneezing. The infection may also occur through contact with soiled hands and clothes, like towel and handkerchief of the patient. The patient with common cold is most infectious a few hours before the onset of symptoms and 1–2 days after the onset of illness. After contact with an infected person, the symptoms start after 24–48 hours of incubation period. When a child starts attending a day-care center, creche or play school, he is likely to get frequent episodes of cold due to greater risk of exposure from schoolmates. The risk of infection is higher when body defences are low (poor diet), exposure to sudden changes in the environmental temperature (air conditioned room or car to a hot environment), pollution, tiredness or lack of activity, overcrowding (visit to a crowded place like public transport, market, cinema) and lack of exposure to sunlight.

Symptoms It is characterized by sudden onset of fever, cough, sneezing, running of nose (coryza) and watering of eyes. There may be sore throat, headache and body aches. Nasal congestion due to swelling of the inner lining (nasal mucosa) of the nose leads to blockage of the nose. Infants become miserable due to blockage

C

of the nose as it interferes with their sleep and feeding behaviour. When nose is blocked, infant cannot continuously suck from the breast or bottle and has to stop sucking frequently to take a breath through the mouth. The child may be irritable and restless due to fever, headache, body aches and nose block. There is general malaise and loss of appetite. The bout of cough may be followed by vomiting in infants. Some children with common cold may develop associated viral diarrhea.

What conditions can mimic common cold?

Children with allergic rhinitis (hay fever) manifest with persistent watery nasal discharge, marked wheezing and watering of eyes. There may be itching in the eyes and nose. There is no fever and cough is absent or minimal. These children are more prone to develop enlargement of adenoids and features of bronchial allergy, such as asthmatic bronchitis, wheezing or bronchial asthma. Antihistaminics are useful in these children for relief of nasal symptoms but they may worsen the bronchial symptoms by drying the secretions with inability to expectorate or cough out the phlegm.

Streptococcal pharyngitis or "strept throat" must be differentiated from common cold because of its potential risk of causing serious complications, like acute rheumatic fever and post-streptococcal acute glomerulonephritis. It occurs in children above 2 years of age and is characterized by high grade fever, sore throat and enlargement of lymph nodes in the neck. *There is no running of the nose or watering of the eyes and cough is minimal or absent.* Tonsils are enlarged and intensely congested with visible pus points in their follicles. Unlike common cold, "strept throat" must be treated with an oral antibiotic like penicillin or erythromycin or amoxicillin for 10 days to prevent serious damage to the heart and kidneys.

Complications Common cold is a self-limited disease and most cases resolve spontaneously within 3–5 days. It is important to remember that "common cold like symptoms" may precede the onset of several serious childhood diseases like measles, chicken-pox, mumps, whooping cough, acute poliomyelitis, etc. Super-added bacterial infection may occur and spread to sinuses (sinusitis), middle ear (acute otitis media) and lungs (pneumonia).

In some children, common cold constitutes an important trigger for increased bronchial reactivity in children who are predisposed to develop attacks of bronchial asthma.

Treatment There is no specific treatment for common cold which is a self-limiting condition. *It is said that untreated common cold lasts for 7 days and when you treat, it disappears in one week.*

- Give paracetamol or ibuprofen for relief of fever, headache and body aches. Aspirin should be avoided in children with viral infections because of potential risk of causing serious toxicity (Reye syndrome).

- Steam inhalation with a warm-mist humidifier or a steam vaporizer is useful to relieve nasal congestion. Avoid instillation of medicated nose drops because of risk of "rebound congestion" due to chemical rehinitis. Saline (0.6% solution of sodium chloride in water) drops or inhaler is an effective and safe nasal decongestant without any side effects. Refer to "nose block" for detailed guidelines for relief of nasal congestion in infants.

- Cough mixtures containing nasal decongestants, antihistaminics and cough suppressants are no better than home remedies. Antihistamines may worsen both the nose block as well as the cough by drying the secretions. In children who are predisposed to develop asthmatic bronchitis, antihistamines may worsen the wheezing due to drying of bronchial secretions which becomes viscid and thick.

- Give plenty of warm liquids in the form of plain water, milk, herbal tea, chicken soup, vegetable soup, etc. They are soothing to the throat and keep the secretions thin and liquified. The child should be encouraged to take a balanced nutritious diet and avoid food items which are known to cause irritation in the throat like condiments, ketchup, fried items, cold drinks, sour fruits, etc.

- There is no role of antibiotics in an uncomplicated case of common cold. The antibiotic may be required if there is superadded bacterial infection. The indications for use of an antibiotic include thick nasal secretions, pain in the ear (acute otitis media), severe headache (sinusitis), spread of infection to lungs (pneumonia) and persistence of fever beyond 3 days.

Home Remedies

In view of the self-limiting nature of common cold, a number of home remedies are popular.

- Gargles with warm saline water and steam inhalation are useful to relieve irritation of throat and nasal congestion. The efficacy of steam inhalation can be improved by adding carom seeds (*ajwain*), eucalyptus, lavender, holy basil (*tulsi*) leaves, mint (pudina), menthol, etc.
- Give herbal tea made with holy basil leaves (*tulsi*), ginger (*adrak*), cinnamon (*dalcheeni*) and honey.
- Mix juice of 8–10 *tulsi* leaves and 20 g ginger into 10 mL honey. Give 1–2 mL of the mixture at night or whenever there is a bout of cough.
- Chest rub with a liniment containing eucalyptus and menthol are useful to relieve nasal and chest congestion.
- To 50 g jaggery (*gurh*), add one teaspoon of powdered black pepper (*kali mirch*), half teaspoon of cloves (*laung*) and one teaspoon of ginger (*adrak*) juice. Mix the contents thoroughly on a slow fire and make small pellets or round lollies for sucking them to relieve irritation and inflammation of the throat.
- Roast carom seeds (*ajwain*) over a hot dry *tawa* or *karahi* and tie them in a thin muslin cloth. Let the child sniff or place it near the pillow to relieve nasal congestion.
- Take 250 g each of poppy seeds (*khas khas*), almonds, and sugar candy (*mishri*) and 50 g white pepper (*Dakni mirch*). Roast almonds and poppy seeds on a hot *tawa* or frypan. Mix all the ingredients and grind them in a mixer grinder. Give one teaspoon of the mix twice a day with hot water or milk during change of weather or during winter months for prevention of colds.

Prevention

- There is no effective vaccine against common cold because it is caused by a large number of viruses. Flu-cum-H1N1 vaccine is available but it prevents only influenza and H1N1 infections while cold due to other viruses is not prevented.
- Whenever child comes back home from school, shopping spree, play or a party, he must wash his hands and face with soap and water, rinse and blow his nose to prevent the cold virus to take hold.
- Avoidance of visits to over crowded public places and reduced exposure to environmental pollutants may reduce the episodes of respiratory infections. Children should be properly clothed

and effectively covered (cap, mittens or gloves and socks) during winter.

- Common cold is highly contagious and it is difficult to prevent its spread to other family members, if one person is affected. The patient should be asked to cover his mouth and nose while coughing and sneezing. He should frequently wash his hands with soap and water and use a personal towel and handkerchief or disposable paper napkins to reduce the risk of transmission of infection. Isolation of the patient at home is virtually impossible.
- Good nutrition with adequate intake of micronutrients (vitamins and minerals) from food or supplements is useful to maintain adequate body defences to ward off infections.
- Breastfeeding provides protection against a variety of infections including common cold because human milk is replete with a large number of protective factors. It is important to ensure that mother provides exclusive breastfeeding (not even water should be given!) to her baby during first six months of life.

Complementary Feeds (*see* Weaning)

Congenital Hypothyroidism (*see* Cretinism)

CONGENITAL MALFORMATIONS (Developmental defects, birth defects, anomalies)

Congenital malformations refer to developmental defects which are present at birth. The defect or abnormality is present at the time of birth but at times its manifestations may appear later in life either due to complications or because of adverse environmental or dietary factors. The defect may be minor and purely cosmetic or it may be life-threatening or major demanding surgical or medical intervention. The usual incidence of major congenital malformations is about 2% among live born babies. Among these, about 0.5% are caused by chromosomal disorders and 0.6% by single gene disorders or inborn errors of metabolism. In over 50% cases of congenital malformations, no obvious cause is found.

Causes

During first 3 months of pregnancy (phase of embryogenesis), various organs of the baby are being formed. The eyes, ears and nose are taking shape and various body organs, like brain, heart, lungs and kidneys, are being formed. During this critical phase of development of the fetus in the womb, if anything goes wrong in his environment, the baby can develop structural defects. Occurrence of viral fever (especially rubella or German measles) and intake of medicines by the pregnant woman during early pregnancy may lead to development of structural defects or congenital malformations. There is an increased risk of development of birth defects, if fetus is exposed to X-rays during the phase of embryogenesis (first 3 months of pregnancy). Nutritional deficiencies (especially folic acid) may be associated with increased risk of defective development of the brain and spinal cord (neural tube defects).

Birth defects, especially those due to chromosomal abnormalities, are more common, if mother is elderly (above 35 years of age). When there is missed abortion (spotting of blood during early pregnancy) or failed abortion following intake of certain drugs (to abort a fetus of unwanted sex), there is a greater likelihood of having a baby with birth defects. Genetic defects (inborn errors of metabolism) are more common among couples who are close blood relatives or first cousins. Birth effects are more common in babies who are born preterm and low birth weight babies (especially those with intrauterine growth retardation or IUGR).

High-risk Situations

There is an increased risk of congenital malformations or genetic defect in a child in following situations.
1. Elderly mother (>35 years).
2. Consanguinity among parents, i.e. couple being first cousins.
3. Intake of certain drugs, exposure to X-rays or viral infection during first trimester (3 months) of pregnancy.
4. Consumption of alcohol, smoking or drug abuse during pregnancy.
5. Gestational diabetes mellitus.
6. Family history of a birth defect or a genetic disorder.
7. History of congenital malformation or genetic defect in a previous sibling.
8. History of recurrent pregnancy loss due to abortions or stillbirths.

Types of Birth Defects

Birth defects may be limited to a single organ of the baby or it may be present in several organs causing a life-threatening emergency with high chances of producing a serious physical and neuromotor disability. Some infants with serious birth defects are born early or die in the womb. Every parent is thus gravely concerned and worried to have a healthy baby. Most parents heave a sigh of relief when they are told that their newly born baby is normal and without any significant or serious birth defects.

Birth defects may occur in any organ of the baby but they most commonly involve skin, muscles, bones and central nervous system (brain and spinal cord). The common birth defects include birth marks (nevi), musculoskeletal defects (extra or fused fingers and toes, club feet), cleft lip with or without cleft palate, various hernias and neural tube defects (spina bifida, meningocele, meningomyelocele, anencephaly). Infants with birth defects may need multiple surgical procedures and prolonged rehabilitation and follow-up by a large number of specialists.

Prevention of Birth Defects

Premarital genetic counseling and avoidance of marriages among close relatives can reduce the incidence of genetic and hereditary diseases. It should be remembered that the safest age for reproduction in women, is between 20 and 30 years. Girls must be protected against development of German measles and chickenpox by timely administration of MMR and chickenpox vaccines. During pregnancy, self medications should be strictly avoided (especially during first 3 months) and drugs should be taken only on the advice of an obstetrician. Smoking, alcohol and drug abuse are known to cause birth defects and must be avoided during pregnancy. Among married women, X-ray examination (and even medications) should be limited during 2 weeks after menstruation (when it is sure that woman is not pregnant) to avoid inadvertent exposure of the embryo (young fetus) to the harmful effects of X-rays and drugs. When a couple is planning to have a baby, mother should take a balanced and nutritious diet including supplements of folic acid. No attempt should ever be made to abort the fetus of unwanted sex by any over-the-counter or Ayurvedic medicines.

CONGENITAL TEETH

Milk teeth start erupting usually after 6 months of age. Some babies may be born with 1 or 2 teeth, which is considered as a bad omen.

If natal tooth is loose, it should be removed because of risk of aspiration. When congenital tooth is well embedded and fixed, nothing needs to be done.

CONJUNCTIVITIS (Red eye)

Infection of eyes or conjunctivitis may occur soon after birth, or anytime subsequently. In newborn babies, infection is usually caused by pyogenic bacteria including gonococci which cause a serious infection. There is marked redness of eyes with swelling of lids and pus discharge. The baby must be seen by a doctor without delay and gonococcal infection ruled out by taking a swab for smear and culture. Eyes should be gently cleaned with sterile cotton swabs soaked in boiled or sterile water by using one swab for each eye. Gonococcal ophthalmia is treated with both topical and injectable antibiotics, like penicillin or ceftriaxone.

In older children, conjunctivitis may occur due to viral, bacterial infections or due to *Chlamydia trachomatis*. Infection may occur if you are putting *kajal* or *surma* in the eyes or when baby rubs his eyes with dirty hand. When baby's towel is not kept clean or is shared by other family members, it is a potent source of infection. Viral conjunctivitis may occur in certain epidemics of cough and cold. The eyes become red and swollen with watery discharge which later becomes thick like pus. There may be stickiness of eyelids on waking up in the morning. During summer months, some children develop redness and itching in the eyes due to dust or pollen allergy. Keep the eyes clean by washing or rinsing them repeatedly with boiled or sterile water. Your doctor will recommend antibiotic eyedrops and ointment. Eyedrops are convenient and should be put in the eyes every 1–2 hourly on day 1 and 4 hourly subsequently while ointment (single use applicaps) is applied at night for its overnight effect. Avoid use of *surma* and *kajal* to reduce the risk of infection and lead toxicity. Towels and handkerchiefs should not be shared as they are potential source of transmission of viral and bacterial infections.

CONSTIPATION

Passage of infrequent dry and hard stools is called constipation. In Indian culture, constipation is believed to be the root cause of many ills due to accumulation of toxins in the body though there is no scientific basis for it. Infants fed on cow's milk or a formula are often constipated due to formation of hard casein stools. Some breastfed babies may develop constipation especially if mother is taking a decoction of fennel (*saunf*) and carom (*ajwain*) seeds. There is no need to worry or give any medications, if stools are not hard and baby has no difficulty in passing the stools. You can give extra sugar, honey, sweet lime or orange juice to the baby for relief of constipation. Insertion of a lubricated rectal thermometer or a rubber catheter is often followed by evacuation. *The use of laxatives should be avoided in newborn babies.* When constipation is persistent and bothersome to the baby, you should consult your doctor to exclude any developmental defect in the rectum or anal canal and cretinism (hypothyroidism).

In older children, constipation is often due to poor intake of diet or intake of low-fiber diet and not drinking enough fluids. Intake of certain medications (opioids, iron supplements, NSAIDs) and high grade fever may cause constipation due to dehydration and poor intake of food. Severe constipation (obstipation) is common around 2 years of age in fussy children due to dietary and psychological reasons. The passage of dry and hard stools may cause injury to the lining of anal canal leading to slight bleeding and formation of a fissure or ulcer. The condition becomes self-perpetuating as child refuses to sit on potty because evacuation is associated with discomfort and pain. Instead, when there is pressure for evacuation, the child stands in a corner and tries to "withhold" stools and does not relax or let go. In some children, it is a phase of psychological development where the child "refuses to part with anything belonging to him including his stools". During this stage, child is rebellious and refuses to do anything that pleases his parents. The situation may progress from bad to worse and evacuation is achieved only by enema or insertion of a glycerine suppository. At times the semiliquid stools may trickle out spontaneously around the hard stools (encopresis) staining the undergarments and giving the wrong impression that the child has developed diarrhea.

Intractable constipation dating back to birth, may occur due to congenital narrowing of anal canal or lack of proper neural development in the colon and rectum (Hirschsprung's disease). Constipation in association with delayed neuromotor development

C

and general lethargy, poor activity, poor muscle tone and course features of the face is highly suggestive of deficiency of thyroid hormone (cretinism). Alternating diarrhea with constipation may occur due to inflammatory bowel disease, celiac disease and chronic amebiasis. Children with cerebral palsy, psychomotor retardation and neuromuscular disorders are likely to be constipated. In long-standing cases of severe constipation, loaded rectum compresses the urinary bladder causing stasis of urine with recurrent episodes of urinary tract infection.

Treatment

Early treatment of constipation prevents development of self-perpetuating psychological constipation. Constipation is best managed by psychological support and modification of diet. Avoid intake of food items which are known to cause constipation, i.e. cow's milk or formula feed, rice (except parboiled or brown rice), yoghurt, cheese, banana, white bread and junk food. The child should be encouraged to drink plenty of water and take extra sugar or corn syrup, fruit juices, honey, butter, ghee, lentils (*dals* with *chhilka*) and high fiber whole grain cereals. Ensure adequate intake of green leafy vegetables like salads, spinach, *lauki*, *tori*, carrots, beans, peas, sweet potatoes, etc. Intake of fresh seasonal fruits (citrus fruits, papaya, grapes, melon, guavas, pears, peaches, plums, bale fruit) and dry fruits (especially prunes, apricots, dates and figs) are most useful to regulate the bowel movements.

The child should be encouraged to sit on the potty regularly especially after the meals when he is more likely to have a bowel movement. Increase in physical activity and gentle massage of abdomen from above downwards or in a clockwise direction may help by improving the tone of abdominal and intestinal muscles.

In intractable cases, the stools can be softened and impaction relieved by insertion of a glycerine suppository through the anus or by enema. Judicious modification of diet and use of mild laxatives or stool softeners like milk of magnesia, polyethylene glycol, osmotic agents (lactulose which imbibes water into the gut) and prokinetics (drugs which improve the gut motility) are effective. Drugs should be given for a short period of 2–3 weeks and constipation should be managed by and large by modification of the diet. The child should not be scolded and instead provided

Home Remedies

1. Massage of navel (with a tip of finger), abdomen and calves with mustard oil is useful for relief of constipation.
2. Give 1–2 teaspoons of *isabgol chhilka* (psyllium husk) in milk or warm water at night.
3. Soak over night 4–5 dates (*khajoor*) or 1–2 figs (*anjeer*) or 5–6 raisins (*kishmish or monaka*) in one cup of water. Let the child eat the contents and drink the water in the morning.
4. Give one glass of hot water with one teaspoon honey and lemon juice daily first thing in the morning.
5. Ask the child to drink lot of water and suck few sticks of liquorice (*malathi*) every day.

with emotional support and tension-free atmosphere to ensure relaxation of his body, mind and sphincters.

CONTRACEPTION (Family planning methods)

It is true that only girls become pregnant but contraception is the joint responsibility of both the partners. Teenagers should be conversant with the available contraceptive methods so that they can make informed decisions during their sexual explorations. After marriage, the couple should practice two-family norm and there should be an interval of at least 3 years between two children by using a safe, reliable and effective contraceptive method. All the contraceptive methods are user-dependent and if a method is not strictly adhered to, pregnancy may accur.

1. *Rhythm method.* During the menstrual cycle, 10th–18th days of the menses are the most fertile because ovum is released during that time period. Sexual intercourse immediately before or soon after the menstrual period is thus relatively safe but not fool proof.
2. *Withdrawal method (coitus-interreptus).* Removal of penis from the vagina before ejaculation reduces the chances of conception but compromises pleasure and is not fool proof.
3. *Condom.* When a male partner wears a condom over the erect penis before penetration, it is an effective and safe method to prevent occurrence of pregnancy. A contraceptive jelly or vaginal cream can be used concomitantly to enhance

protection. *The use of condom also protects against the risk of sexually transmitted diseases (STDs) like gonorrhea, syphilis, AIDS/HIV, etc.*

4. *Diaphragm or cervical cap.* It is also a barrier technique like condom but is worn by the woman. It is technically more difficult to use and must be inserted in the vagina no more than 6 hours before intercourse and should remain in place for at least 6–8 hours after the sexual act. A contraceptive jelly or cream must also be used to improve protection.

5. *Intrauterine device (IUD).* A copper-T or coil can be inserted into the uterus by an obstetrician and it effectively prevents implantation of the fertilized ovum in the womb. There is increased risk of pelvic inflammatory disease (PID) and chances of infertility later in life. It does not provide any protection against sexually transmitted diseases (STDs). It is not recommended for use in unmarried teenage girls.

6. *Birth control pills.* They regulate the woman's hormonal cycle and prevent the release of ovum. It is an effective contraceptive method but pill has to be taken regularly everday. It must be remembered that pills do not provide any protection against STDs. *A combined use of an oral contraceptive by the woman and a condom by the man is the best option to prevent both pregnancy as well as STDs.*

7. *Depot injection.* A long-acting hormone preparation can be given by injection to prevent ovulation. Depot medroxy progesterone acetate (Depo provera) provides protection for 90 days and is popular worldwide. Norplant is a subdermal implant of a long-acting progesterone (levonorgestrel) which slowly releases the drug in the circulation and provides contraception for up to 5 years.

8. *Post-coital or morning-after pill.* In case of unprotected, unplanned or forced sex, a high dose hormone pill (i-Pill) can be taken as a safeguard against development of pregnancy. They are available, over-the-counter (OTC) without doctor's prescription. Two tablets of Ovral® (0.5 mg levonorgestrel and 0.03 mg ethinyl estradiol) should be taken as early as possible after the sexual act followed by 2 tablets 12 hours later. Alternatively, one tablet of Norleva® should be taken as early

as possible after the coitus (preferably within 72 hours) followed by a repeat dose after 12 hours. The postcoital pills may cause marked nausea, vomiting and mood changes. The safer and more effective option is to take mifepristone 600 mg (progesterone antagonist) as a single dose as early as possible after the sexual intercourse. The frequent and repeated use of "morning-after" pills may lead to development of polycystic ovary disease (PCOD), hormonal imbalance and relative infertility. They do not provide any protection against sexually transmitted diseases (STDs).

CONVULSIONS (Seizures, fits)

Sudden involuntary stiffening, twitching or jerky movements of a limb or whole body is called a convulsion or seizure. It occurs due to paroxysmal electrical discharge from a group of neurons in the brain. There may or may not be loss of consciousness. It may be associated with staring look or uprolling of eyeballs. It may or may not be associated with electroencephalographic (EEG) changes. Common causes of seizures include sudden onset of fever (febrile convulsions), localized (tumor, trauma, scar) or generalized (hypoxia, pyogenic or tubercular meningitis, encephalitis) disease of the brain or metabolic disorder in the body like reduction in blood glucose, calcium, sodium and magnesium levels. A number of drugs are known to lower the threshold for seizures in children. The list includes fluoroquinolones, theophylline, chlorpromazine, metoclopramide, piperazine salts, caffeine, isoniazid, mefenamic acid, local anesthetics (application of xylocaine over the anus) and drugs of abuse. Inhalation or ingestion of camphor during *puja* ceremony is an important cause of convulsions in children.

CORD CARE

Umbilical stump is an important site for entry of bacteria and spores of tetanus. Umbilical cord must be cut with a sterile knife or blade. Even when a new razor blade is used for cutting the cord, it must be sterilized before use by boiling in water for 10 minutes. The cord should be clamped with a rubber band or a disposable clip. Surgical alcohol or betadine lotion can be applied to the tip and base of the stump once daily after the bath. The stump should be left open without any dressing. *Never apply any "home antiseptics" like cow dung or turmeric over the stump.* The umbilical stump usually falls after 5 to 10 days but may take longer, if it is dry and shriveled or when infected. The delayed falling of the cord is also a useful marker of immunodeficiency disorder.

CRACKED NIPPLES (Sore nipples)

Mother may develop sore nipples if there is poor attachment of the baby to the breast. When a baby merely sucks at the nipples (instead of nipple and areola), the baby gets very little milk. The baby is likely to suck vigorously or may bite the nipple in frustration thus damaging the delicate skin of the nipple. Pulling the baby forcefully from the nipple without delatching may also damage the nipple. Frequent washing of breast with soap and water may lead to dryness and cracking of nipples.

When nipples are sore, mother should wear loose clothes and avoid the use of a bra to allow the cracks to heal. She can use a nursing bra with a breast shell to avoid direct pressure over the tender nipples. The plastic breast shields should not be worn because they hold the moisture. After nursing, mother should express a little milk from the breasts and let it dry over the nipples to provide a protective covering which facilitates the process of healing. The "hind-milk" (milk at the end of feeding) contains fats and anti-infective substances which serves as an emollient and soothing agent. The breastfeeding should be continued and you can apply some emollient cream (ultrapurified medical grade lanolin) over the nipples in-between the feeds. If nipples are extremely sore, a nipple shield can be used for feeding till cracks have healed. If a baby has developed white patches in his mouth (thrush), antifungal lotion should be applied inside the baby's mouth and over your nipples.

CRADLE CAP

Some newborn babies develop a brown crusts on the top of their scalp. The crust forms due to collection of natural secretions (sebum) of hair follicles and skin of the scalp. It is a form of dandruff. There is nothing special that needs to be done and it gradually disappears as you gently shampoo and brush the scalp. Do not try to remove it forcibly. You can apply some coconut oil or oily topscum of boiled and cooled milk and shampoo the scalp with savlon or cetrimide after 15 to 30 minutes. The crust will gradually come off with daily shampooing and gentle brushing but it may take several days or weeks to completely resolve.

CRETINISM (Congenital hypothyroidism)

The clinical syndrome due to deficiency of thyroid hormone at birth is called cretinism. It is the commonest hormonal disorder in children and an important cause of preventable mental retardation. Cretinism may occur due to absence or abnormal location of thyroid gland (which is normally located below the Adam's apple infront of the neck) or due to defective production of thyroid hormone (thyroxine). Cretinism may occur due to deficiency of iodine which is widely prevalent in sub-Himalayan regions and hilly terrains in our country. Many people in these areas develop enlargement of thyroid gland (goiter).

Clinical features Cretinism is difficult to diagnose in newborn period because clinical features may become apparent only after a few months. Because early diagnosis and prompt replacement therapy is crucial for prevention of mental retardation, many hospitals routinely screen all newborns at birth. The common symptoms of hypothyroidism include lethargy, inactivity, poor feeding and constipation. Skin may be dry and mottled, and facial features may look coarse. Physiological jaundice may persist beyond 2 weeks of age. The first suspicion of cretinism may arise when baby does not give a smile to the social interactions or overtures of the mother at 4–6 weeks of age.

When treatment is delayed, the clinical features of cretinism become obvious. Skin and hair become rough and dry. Facial features become coarse and puffy, with a large tongue and hoarse cry or voice. Abdomen is distended and there is an umbilical hernia. The child is extremely slow and lazy without any interest in usual play activities. The child looks short and stumpy. The constipation may become worse. The developmental milestones are delayed. Rarely, hypothyroidism may occur in an older child or during adolescence. It is suspected by excessive weight gain or obesity, lethargy, mental dullness, poor academic performance (fall in grades in school), slow linear growth and constipation.

Screening Early diagnosis of hypothyroidism and replacement therapy within 2 weeks of age is mandatory to ensure normal physical and mental development. It is, therefore, desirable to screen all newborns before they are discharged from the hospital. TSH screening can be done at birth (cord blood) or after 3–4 days after birth. TSH level of more than 50 μIU/mL in cord blood or more than 20 μIU/mL after day 3 are suggestive of hypothyroidism. T_4 level may be normal or low (<8 μg/dL) in these infants.

Treatment Early replacement therapy with thyroxine is associated with prompt recovery. Eltroxin or thyronorm is given on empty stomach in a daily single dose of 10–15 μg/kg. The dose is adjusted by maintaining T_4 level between 8 and 12 μg/dL. As the child grows, the dose of thyroxine gradually comes down to 2–5 μg/kg/day in older children and adolescents. It is an extremely cheap medicine but need to be taken throughout life under the supervision of a doctor.

CROUP

Croup occurs most commonly due to viral inflammation of larynx (laryngitis) or wind box. It is characterized by sudden onset of noisy crowing or grunting sound (stridor) while breathing in. It is usually associated with hoarseness of voice and a barking cough. There is associated fever, anxiety, breathing difficulty and air hunger or hypoxia. In children between 1 and 3 years, spasmodic croup may occur during exposure to cold or when child wakes up in the early hours of the morning. There is no preceding cold or associated fever. The condition is benign and may recover spontaneously but may recur on subsequent days.

Treatment The child should be handled calmly and given steam inhalation with a warm-mist humidifier or a steam vaporizer. No sedative should be given to the child. There is no role of antibiotics or cough mixtures. When child is restless, having breathing difficulty or fever, he should be taken to the hospital. Administration of oxygen, nebulization with racemic epinephrine and a single intramuscular shot of dexamethasone (0.3–0.6 mg/kg) provide prompt relief.

CRYING BABY

During the first few weeks, most newborn babies sleep during the day and they are awake, playful and troublesome during the night. This behaviour is probably due to continuation of their *in utero* pattern of activity. The baby has no concept of day and night because there was perpetual darkness in the womb. During pregnancy, when mother is up and about during daytime, the baby is rocked in the pool of amniotic fluid and sleeps. During the night when mother is resting, the fetus is active and playful. This patterns of behaviour gradually disappears but "change over" may take several weeks or months in some babies. To facilitate the "change over", you can interact and play with the baby during the day time so that he sleeps less during the day and sleeps better at night.

Most babies cry when they are either hungry or having discomfort. The cry may be a signal of unpleasant sensation because of a full bladder before passing urine, painful evacuation of hard stools, discomfort of wet napkins or nappy rash. Some babies may cry before passing urine due to discomfort of a full bladder, they become quiet and dazed while passing urine and start crying again after having passed urine due to wet napkins. The experienced or sensitive mother can differentiate between the cry used as a signal for feed and the cry of discomfort. Infant with "wind" or abdominal colic is likely to cry loudly by flexing legs toward abdomen, is likely to have audible gurgling sounds in the abdomen and usually feels comfortable when placed in a prone position with buttocks raised which facilitates the expulsion of gas. The common causes of excessive crying at night are listed in the **Box**.

Most babies cry while falling asleep (as if they are not keen to sleep and want to play). Excessive inconsolable crying may occur

Common causes of night crying

- Hunger
- Wet diaper
- Evening colic
- Nasal congestion
- Over clothing or underclothing
- Insect bites (mosquitoes, bed bugs, mites)
- Teething
- Pin worms
- Diaper rash
- Excessive light or noise
- Gastroesophageal reflux disease (GERD)
- Bone pains (leukemia)

due to a serious disorder like meningitis, inflammatory conditions (abscess, acute otitis media, infection of bone or joint, torsion of testis, obstructed hernia, injury, dislocation of elbow or nursemaid's elbow), milk allergy, anal fissure, open diaper pin, DTwP vaccine (whole cell pertussis vaccine), etc. Brain damaged children are prone to bouts of excessive crying. Crying may occur as a side effect of administration of some drugs.

Treatment The specific treatment depends upon the underlying cause of crying. When a child is having bouts of inconsolable crying, and associated with fever or failure to take feed, he must be promptly taken to a pediatrician. You must respond promptly to a child in discomfort by picking and cuddling him without any fear of spoiling the child. Most cyring infants are comforted when picked up but when an infant becomes more uncomfortable on picking up, it indicates a painful condition in the limbs, joints and bones. Diaper should be checked for soiling and feed given, if child is hungry.

Paracetamol is useful for relief of discomfort due to teething or any inflammatory painful condition or injury to limbs. Application of a soothing cream or bland coconut oil (never apply mustard oil!) is useful for treatment of nappy rash and relief of anal itching. Application of *hing* (asafoetida) dissolved in warm water around the navel and giving a decoction of carom (*ajwain*) and fennel (*saunf*) seeds may provide relief. Gripe mixture can be given if it is formulated without alcohol. Anti-colic drops can be given half an hour before the anticipated time of crying spells on the advice of a doctor.

CYANOSIS

When hemoglobin is not properly oxygenated due to lack of oxygen because of serious diseases of the heart or lungs, the blood becomes blue in color owing to formation of carboxyhemoglobin. It is usually associated with air hunger (because of hypoxia) with blueness of nails, lips and tongue. Children with cyanotic heart disease (blue babies) are blue without any breathing difficulty except when associated with complications or heart failure. Monitoring of arterial oxygen saturation with a pulse oximeter is a useful non-invasive method to assess the severity of hypoxia. Isolated blueness of finger or toe nails (peripheral cyanosis) may occur because of exposure to cold.

DANDRUFF (Seborrhea)

Dandruff (*roosi*) is very common in children who have an oily skin. The follicles of scalp hair secrete an excess of oily material (sebum) which dries up to form whitish flakes on the scalp. There may be associated fungal (*Malassezia furfur*) infection. At times, even eye brows and eye lashes may show white flakes of dandruff. There may be itching over the scalp. In some children, it may be associated with skin rash which may be confused with atopic dermatitis. Rash commonly involves face, neck, areas behind ears, axillae and diaper area.

Treatment

The hair should be washed daily with a shampoo. Coconut oil should be massaged into the scalp and shampoo done after half an hour. *Do not apply any oil after hair wash.* The comb and brush should be washed frequently and should not be shared by other family members. If dandruff persists, a medicated shampoo

Home Remedies

- Rub aloe vera (*kanwaar gandal, kanwaar patha*) gel into the scalp and leave it on for 15 minutes before shampooing the hair.
- Massage the scalp with a mixture of olive oil and almond oil followed by application of juice of one lemon 2–3 times in a week. Leave the oil on for half an hour before shampooing the hair.
- Massage the scalp with warm coconut oil containing juice of one lemon and leave it on for half an hour before doing the shampoo. The best outcome is achieved when procedure is followed daily.
- Add few drops of eucalyptus oil or tea tree oil in your shampoo and massage thoroughly. It is effective in removing the flakes of dandruff.

containing an antifungal agent (ketoconazole, miconazole) should be used on the advice of a doctor. Inflamed scalp lesions respond to local application of corticosteroid cream.

DARK CIRCLES UNDER THE EYES

Discoloration of the skin with bogginess under the eyes is uncommon in children. It is most commonly due to familial or hereditary predisposition. The common causes include inadequate sleep (stress and fatigue), blocked nose, chronic sinusitis, allergic rhinitis (hay fever), food allergy, gluten intolerance and exposure to sunlight. The condition is more common in children with fair skin or deep-set eyes.

Treatment There is no specific treatment except to identify and manage the underlying predisposing condition. The child should be advised to take plenty of water and consume a balanced diet with plenty of green leafy vegetables and seasonal fruits. Stress and fatigue should be avoided and relieved by taking adequate rest and sleep. Sun screen cream with a minimum of SPF 30 protection is a useful preventive measure when going out of doors. When dark circles have developed, skin creams containing vitamin K and retinol can be rubbed over the affected areas 2–3 times in day for several months.

Home Remedies

- Relax, lie down in bed and close your eyes. Apply thick slices of cooled cucumber or raw potato slices over the eyes for 10–15 minutes daily.
- Keep the used tea bags in the refrigerator. Lie down, close your eyes and apply the cool and damp tea bags (standard tea and not green tea) on the eyes for 10–15 minutes daily.
- Massage lids and area below the eyes with almond oil daily at night.
- Pressing the mount on the palm above the index finger and doing *pranayam* daily for at least 5 minutes are useful to remove dark circles.

DEAFNESS

Hearing loss is an important cause of delayed speech and must be ruled out whenever there is isolated delay in speech and language development in an otherwise healthy child. Hearing loss may adversely affect social and emotional development, behaviour, attention and school performance. High-risk children are routinely screened at 3 months by otoacoustic emission (OAE) testing and brainstem evoked response audiometery (BERA) for early diagnosis of deafness. The hearing loss may be *conductive* due to diseases of external ear or middle ear (acute otitis media) or *sensorineural* due to disease in the inner ear, cochlea or central nervous system. It is important to diagnose deafness as early as possible so that hearing aid is provided latest by 6 months of age in order to ensure proper speech development. In sensorineural deafness, it is possible to cure deafness by cochlear transplant surgery.

DEHYDRATION

Deficiency of water in the body is called dehydration. It occurs most commonly due to vomiting and diarrhea. Other causes of dehydration include excessive passage of urine (diabetes mellitus and diabetes insipidus), loss of water due to excessive sweating or rapid breathing (high grade fever, pneumonia, heat stroke) and poor intake of water (severe illness, inability to drink).

The child becomes irritable due to excessive thirst, eyes are sunken, tongue and buccal mucosa become dry. Skin is dry (because of lack of sweating), shrivelled and inelastic. When skin of abdomen or chest is pinched and released, it takes several seconds to assume its normal appearance. When urine output is reduced or no urine is passed for 6 hours in an infant and 12 hours in an older child, it indicates that the dehydration is severe. The child may become drowsy and refuse to drink leading to further aggravation of dehydration.

Treatment The underlying cause of dehydration should be identified and managed appropriately. Excessive crying in a child with vomiting and diarrhea is because of dehydration rather than pain abdomen. Children are at the mercy of parents or caretakers to fullfil their nutritional and fluid needs. The child should be offered plenty of water and oral rehydration solution (ORS). Other home-based fluids, like milk, coconut water, lentil-water (*dal ka pani*), soup, *chhaj*, etc., can be given. When child is passing adequate quantity (same frequency and volume of urine as before the onset of illness) of colorless or light-colored urine, it indicates satisfactory hydration status. When a dehydrated child (i) refuses to drink, (ii) vomiting is intractable or (iii) diarrheal losses are profound, or (iv) child develops abdominal distension, he must be taken to the hospital for intravenous rehydration.

DENGUE FEVER

Dengue fever is an acute viral infection due to any one of the four serotypes of flaviviruses which is transmitted through the bite of *Aedes aegypti* mosquitoes (which have characteristic black and white stripes). Most epidemics occur during or soon after rainy season and disappear after onset of winter. The first or primary dengue infection is a self-limiting viral fever but when it is due to reinfection (especially with DEN 2) in a subject who had primary infection in the past, it may lead to development of life-threatening severe dengue disease.

Common Features

Fever occurs 5–8 days after the bite by an infected mosquito. There is sudden onset of high grade fever with chills, flushed face, headache, pain in the eyes (especially on movements of eyes), body aches especially severe backache (break bone fever). Fever may be camel hump type, i.e. fever drops after 2–3 days with marked sweating followed by rebound fever of lower severity which lasts another 2–3 days. There may be faint pink skin rash 2–3 days after the onset of fever. *Cough and running nose, which are hallmarks of common cold and flu, are not seen in dengue fever.* Rarely, bleeding from nose may occur during acute phase of primary dengue infection. In most cases of primary infection, fever settles in 5–6 days without any complications.

In severe cases of dengue fever (especially when it is reinfection), there is development of petechiae (bleeding spots under the skin) over the face and extremities after 2–3 days of onset of fever. Pain in upper abdomen (due to enlargement of liver) and vomiting are also suggestive of severe disease. Bleeding from nose, mouth and gastrointestinal tract in the form of blood-stained vomitings and blood in the stools are ominous. *Most complications of dengue fever occur when fever is settling down.* During this period, some patients may develop profound leakages from capillaries which leads to puffiness of face, swelling of hands and feet and accumulation of fluid in the chest and abdominal cavities. Due to profound leakage of plasma through the capillaries, the blood volume falls leading to shock-related symptoms in the form of restlessness, cold extremities, fainting, rapid pulse, low blood pressure and reduced production of urine.

Laboratory Investigations

During an epidemic, every episode of fever (especially without running of nose and cough) should be considered as dengue fever unless proved otherwise by investigations. The diagnosis of dengue hemorrhagic fever (DHF) is suspected when there is fever with body aches, pain in the eyes, low platelet count (less than $100,000/mm^3$) and rise in hemoglobin or hematocrit (because of leakage of plasma from the capillaries). Accumulation of fluid in the abdomen and chest can be diagnosed early by an ultrasound examination. The presence of dengue-specific NS1 antigen and IgM antibodies are useful early markers of definitive diagnosis. The elevation of dengue-specific IgG antibodies usually appears later during second week of illness but if they are elevated early, it is suggestive of reinfection with a likelihood of having a severe disease.

Treatment

Dengue fever due to primary infection is a self-limiting condition and recovery occurs spontaneously in 5–6 days. *There is no specific treatment or any role of antibiotics and antiviral agents.* Fever and body aches should be controlled by administration of a safe antipyretic and analgesic agent like paracetamol. The temperature should be kept below 101°F by using paracetamol and tepid water sponging of the body and extremities. The use of NSAIDs (like ibuprofen and mefenamic acid) and aspirin should be avoided due to their potential risk of causing and aggravating bleeding manifestations. The child should be encouraged to drink plenty of fluids (water, soups, juices, coconut water) and take balanced nutritious diet.

During an epidemic of dengue fever, all patients with fever, should be evaluated by a doctor and investigated for baseline hemoglobin or hematocrit, platelet count and tourniquet test. These parameters should preferably be checked at least once daily for 4 to 5 days. *The period when fever is settling down (usually 5 days after the onset of fever) is indeed the most critical phase for development of complications.* Patients who develop bleeding manifestations, upper abdominal pain with vomitings, low blood pressure, elevation in hematocrit or hemoglobin level (due to leakage of plasma from capillaries) and low platelet count ($<50,000/mm^3$) should be admitted to the hospital. These patients need intensive medical management with intravenous fluids and high quality supportive care by trained nurses. Recovery is heralded by improvement in appetite and sense of well-being. During recovery, some patients demonstrate marked exfoliation of skin with itching of extremities, palms and soles. Most patients complain of profound weakness and lethargy or depression after recovery.

D

Prevention

The detailed preventive measures for control of mosquitoes are listed under mosquito-borne diseases. *Aedes aegypti* mosquitoes breed in and around dwellings and flourish in fresh water. They are likely to bite the human victims during daytime. During an epidermic, the school authorities should liberalize the dress code and allow children to wear long sleeved shirts and full pants or *pyjamas*. The mosquito-repellent skin cream or spray should be applied to the exposed areas of skin (except face) at least 3 times in a day. It is hoped that an effective quadrivalent (incorporating all the four dengue viruses) dengue vaccine is likely to be available in the near future.

Home Remedies

Dengue fever is a life-threatening disease and patient should be under the close supervision of a physician. Home remedies should be used under strict medical advice. The following remedies are credited to increase the platelet count.

1. Pomegranate juice and black grape juice are useful.
2. Crush or grind one fresh papaya leaf, strain the juice, add honey and give it to the patient twice daily till platelet count is stabilized. Juice contains enzymes, chymopapain and papain, which prevent destruction of platelets.
3. Grind 10 *tulsi* leaves with one black pepper and make a peasized pill and give it with water.
4. Prepare herbal tea of fenugreek leaves and give it frequently to the patient.

DHA (Docosahexaenoic acid)

Polyunsaturated fatty acids (PUFAs), i.e. omega-3 and omega-6 fatty acids, are essential for health and well-being. Docosahexaenoic acid (DHA), a long chain metabolite of omega-3 fatty acids, is the predominant structural fatty acid in the brain and retina. During pregnancy, fetus is completely dependent on the maternal dietary intake of omega-3 fatty acids and DHA and after birth breast milk is a rich source of DHA. The DHA content of breast milk is 30 times more than cow's milk. The pregnant and nursing mothers should take 2.6 gm omega-3 fatty acids and 300 mg DHA daily to sustain the rapid growth and maturation of brain and retina during fetal life and infancy. When the child is weaned off the breast, his requirements of omega-3 fatty acids and DHA must be met from dietary sources like vegetable oils (flaxseed, linseed, soy, peanut), green leafy vegetables, kidney beans (*Rajmah*), nuts (walnuts, almonds, peanuts) and above all fish oil, fish, seafood and seaweed (algae). Unfortunately, an average vegetarian diet does not provide adequate quantities of omega-3 fatty acids and DHA during preschool years. Apart from nutritious balanced diet, nutritional supplements fortified with DHA should be provided to preschool children.

DIABETES MELLITUS

Diabetes mellitus in children (type-1) is uncommon compared to adult-onset diabetes mellitus (type-2). Diabetes mellitus in children is a serious disease and is treated by administration of insulin (insulin-dependent). The exact cause of diabetes mellitus in children is not known. It may occur following a viral infection of pancreas, a gland which produces insulin and is located deep in the center of abdomen. There is no genetic predisposition (unlike adult-onset diabetes mellitus) but it is more common in bottle fed babies. Due to increasing incidence of obesity in adolescent children, type-2 diabetes mellitus may occur in childhood. Girls with polycystic ovarian disease (PCOD) also more vulnerable to develop type-2 diabetes mellitus.

Clinical Features

The onset of disease may occur at any age but it is more common in school going children. There is marked elevation of blood glucose level (due to lack of insulin) which leads to excessive urination (polyuria), marked thirst (polydypsia) and increased appetite (polyphagia). Despite excessive intake of food, the child remains lean and thin. At times, the disease may manifest as an emergency (without any prior warning symptoms) due to diabetic ketoacidosis or diabetic coma. It is characterized by sudden onset persistent vomitings, abdominal pain, fever, severe dehydration, drowsiness or coma.

Treatment

Diagnosis is confirmed by elevation of blood glucose level and glycosylated hemoglobin (HBA1C). The child would need life long specialized care under the supervision of a pediatric endocrinologist. The child would need specialized care with insulin injections with the help of relatively painless insulin penjet or constant infusion pump. A nasal spray of insulin is being marketed which is likely to greatly simplify the management of diabetes mellitus. The child would need carefully regulated diet and physical activity. The blood glucose should be monitored regularly at home with glucose strips with the help of an electronic device (Accu-chek®). Glycosylated hemoglobin (HBA1C) should be checked every 3 months to assess the adequacy of blood sugar control. Most children with diabetes mellitus can lead a normal life under the expert guidance, supervision and emotional support provided by the doctor and family members.

DIAPER RASH (Nappy rash)

Diaper rash is common because of soakage of bottom with urine and stools. Babies cared with non-soakable cotton nappies are unlikely to develop the rash. The use of tight fitting plastic panties and soakable diapers is the main culprit. The rash affects the areas of skin covered by the diaper and often spares the creases of the groin. The affected skin becomes red and macerated due to prolonged contact with a wet and soiled napkin. The rash is more likely to develop following an episode of acute diarrhea. When nappy rash persists for more than 3–4 days, superinfection with a yeast, like *Candida albicans* commonly occurs. Candidal infection is usually associated with discrete spots in the form of red pimples or vesicles at the margins of the rash. In girls with persistent soakage of napkins, ascending urinary infection may occur. In boys, the foreskin (prepuce) of the penis may be severely affected leading to scarring or phimosis which may lead to difficulty in passing urine.

Treatment The soakable diaper or plastic nappies should not be worn at home except at night. The baby must be cleaned and dried immediately after passage of each urine and stool. The bottom should be kept dry as far as possible. You must have liberal supply of nappies so that you can change a wet nappy immediately after each voiding. The nappies should be thoroughly rinsed in water to get rid of all traces of detergent and soap. They should be sun dried and ironed to kill the germs. Nappy rash is best treated by keeping the baby naked and exposing the buttocks to air and sunlight. Local application of a bland oil (coconut) or soothing cream containing aloe vera, calamine and zinc oxide facilitates recovery. Avoid local application of an irritant oil like mustard oil. When candidal superinfection is suspected, local application of a cream containing nystatin or miconazole is followed by prompt resolution.

DOG BITE

Dog bite either due to a pet or a stray dog is common in children. Dog bite is associated with a high risk of transmission of rabies which is invariably a fatal disease. Rabies can also be transmitted through the bites of cats, bats, monkeys, mongoose, jackals and cattle. In India, rats, mice, bandicoots, squirrel and rabbits have not been shown to transmit rabies. Children are more likely to have dangerous dog bites on the head, face and neck. Pet animals must be effectively immunized against rabies and other diseases on the advice of a veterinary doctor.

First-aid Wash the wound thoroughly for several minutes with soap and running water. No home antiseptics, like turmeric, chilly powder or oil, should be applied over the wound. You can apply tincture iodine or betadine lotion. The child should be immediately taken to the doctor for further management.

Tissue-culture antirabies vaccines are safe (unlike sheep brain vaccine) and must be administered as early as possible. The standard schedule consists of giving 4 doses by intramuscular route on days 0, 3, 7 and 14. In case of bite by a domestic dog, the animal should be watched. If the dog is alive after 10 days of bite, the 4th dose of vaccine on day 14 may be omitted. When a fully immunized person is bitten by a potentially rabid animal, it is recommended to give him only 2 doses (days 0 and 3) of vaccine, if the prior vaccination was done within 2 years. In case of wound on the face and neck, multiple bites or bites associated with oozing of blood, rabies immunoglobulins (RIG 20 iu/kg) should also be given along with the first dose of vaccine. RIG should be infiltrated around the wound within 24 hours of bite. Tetanus toxoid is given if the last shot was taken 10 years ago. Antibiotics are indicated, if wound is contaminated.

Prevention of Dog Bite

Children should be sensitized to develop a humane and compassionate attitude toward animals and provided with basic safety tips to safeguard against bites by domestic and stray animals.

- Do not disturb any animal that is sleeping, eating or feeding her puppies.
- Do not approach, stare and touch an unfamiliar animal.
- Never leave the young child with a dog unsupervised.
- Always allow the pet dog to see and sniff you before touching it.
- Children should be taught not to run or cycle past the stray dog.
- When a stray dog approaches you, never stare or run, but be calm and stoic, and look away and ignore the animal.

DOWN SYNDROME (Mongolism)

It is the commonest chromosomal defect (1:800 live births) wherein there is an extra chromosome 21 (Trisomy 21). The defect is more common in babies of elderly mothers (>35 years). In about 5% cases, Down syndrome occurs in young mother due to translocation (a portion of chromosome-21 is dislocated and get attached to another chromosome). In such as child, the chromosome count shall be 46 and not 47 as in a classical case of trisomy-21.

The child with Down syndrome has a flat face with a flat nasal bridge and a small and flat head with a wide gap between the skull bones at top of the head (anterior fontanel). The eyes are placed wide apart and slanted upward and outward. The mouth is small and usually open with protrusion of tongue which is fissured. Neck is short, ears are small and placed at a lower level. Instead of two horizontal creases in the palm (heart and head lines), there may be a single palmar crease (simian crease). Hands are small, little finger is short and incurved. There is a wide gap between 1st and 2nd toes (sandal gap) with deep furrows over the soles. The muscles are flabby and child's limbs can be placed in any position. The developmental milestones are delayed and child has mental subnormality of varying grade. There may be other associated defects especially structural defects of the heart (hole in the heart or endocardial cushion defect) and intestines (duodenal atresia and Hirschsprung's disease). Dental problems, poor eye sight, defective hearing and thyroid dysfunction may be associated and should be looked for. These children are prone to develop frequent respiratory infections. Girls with Down syndrome are usually fertile while boys are invariably infertile. The diagnosis can be easily made by looking at the child and is confirmed by analysis of chromosomes (karyotyping).

Treatment

There is no specific treatment for Down syndrome. Mongol babies are pleasant, lovable and docile. They have great liking for music and dance. They are prone to develop frequent episodes of cough and cold, chest and ear infections (otitis media) due to poor immunity. They should be protected against exposure to viral infections which should be identified early and treated promptly. When hypothyroidism is associated, it is treated with replacement therapy with thyroxin (thyronorm, eltroxin). The associated defects in the heart and intestines may need surgical correction. They can be sent to a mainstream inclusive school having facilities for special or challenged children. The parents should join and interact with the members of the Down Syndrome Association for emotional support and guidance. Parents should seek genetic counseling for prospects of having a normal child. It is extremely rare to have two children with Down syndrome in a family.

It is possible to make antenatal diagnosis of Down syndrome during early pregnancy by triple and quadruple test, ultrasound examination of fetus and chromosomal studies on chorionic villus sampling. The normal pregnancy can be allowed to continue while medical termination of pregnancy can be advised when mother is carrying a baby with Down syndrome.

DROOLING

Saliva is produced to keep the inner lining of mouth wet and it contains anti-infective agents and digestive enzyme ptyalin. It aids in swallowing, digestion and maintenance of oral hygiene. Drooling of saliva occurs either due to excessive production of saliva or inability to swallow the saliva as a result of obstruction in the throat or food pipe (esophagus) or neuromotor incoordination. Some normal children continue to drool without any obvious cause. Teething is associated with irritation of gums, putting fingers in the mouth and drooling. Drooling is common in children who keep their mouth open to breathe because of blockage of nose and enlargement of adenoids. Stomatitis and mouth ulcers (aphthous ulcers) are associated with drooling of saliva. Children with mental retardation and cerebral palsy cannot swallow their saliva and may have persistent drooling throughout childhood. The condition is managed by treating the underlying cause.

DROWNING

Drowning is a leading cause of accidental deaths in children. Drowning accidents may occur in a bath tub, swimming pool, lake, rivulet and tube well. Drowning may occur during natural calamities like floods. During the monsoon, the roads and streets may get flooded with rain water. The open sewers pose a hazard to unsuspecting children playing or wading through rain water. The drowning victim is likely become cold, blue, apneic (gasping or no breathing), drowsy or comatosed depending upon the duration of submersion in water.

First-aid Place the child on his tummy (face down) and clean the mouth of any secretions and debris with a handkerchief. Chest and abdomen are gently pressed to expel water from air passages, stomach and lungs. If child is gasping or not having any breathing, cardiopulmonary resuscitation (CPR) should be started. The child should be dried and effectively covered with woollens to prevent hypothermia (fall in body temperature). The child should be taken to the hospital while CPR is continued during the journey.

Prevention

Drowning accidents are preventable, if following guidelines are followed.

- Infants should never be left alone, even for a moment, in the bath tub, water bucket or inflatable pool.
- Never run to attend the door bell or a telephone call by leaving the child alone in the bathroom.
- Keep the bathroom door latched and always keep the commode covered with the lid.
- Children with history of seizures (epilepsy) should not be permitted to swim.
- Swimming pools should be equipped with safety measures, adequate fencing and well-trained life-guards.
- Children above 4 years of age should be taught to swim under the supervision of parents and a trainer.

DUCHENNE MUSCULAR DYSTROPHY

Duchenne muscular dystrophy (DMD) or pseudohypertrophic muscular dystrophy is an X-linked or sex-linked recessive disorder affecting male children. The symptoms usually start after the age of 2 years with unsteady gait and frequent falls. The child has difficulty in climbing upstairs and develops waddling gait (like a duck). Gower's sign is a characteristic feature of DMD and is elicited by asking the child to rise from a squatting position. The child makes efforts to lift up the trunk by supporting his weight on the arms by placing his hands on the floor. He slowly tries to stand up by making a great effort as if climbing up on his body by taking support with his hands which are placed on the ankles, knees and finally thighs. The enlargement (hypertrophy) of calf muscles is usually seen after the age of 4 to 5 years. These children are likely to have cardiac dysfunction, frequent respiratory infections and mental retardation.

Treatment The child should be encouraged to remain active by walking, climbing stairs and cycling. Physiotherapy and graded physical exercises are useful to maintain muscle strength.

Corticosteroids, antioxidants and vitamin E have been used with variable results. There is a hope that in the near future, the disease may be cured by newer technologies like stem cell or myoblast transplantation and gene therapy.

DYSENTERY

When there is passage of blood and mucus or pus in the diarrheal (loose) stools, the condition is called dysentery. Bacillary or bacterial dysentery is more common than amebic and it is usually associated with fever, abdominal colic and tenesmus (frequent urge to pass stools). In amebic dysentery, there is no fever or toxemia, stools mostly comprise of blood or mucus with little fecal matter. Amebic dysentery may run a protracted course over several months with episodes of loose motions, constipation and abdominal pain simulating irritable bowel syndrome. In severe constipation, the hard stool may be coated with streaks of blood and it should not be confused with dysentery. In children with polyp in the rectum, there is passage of fresh blood (without any fecal matter) through the anus.

Treatment Bacillary dysentery is treated by administration of paracetamol, antispasmodic and oral rehydration solution (ORS). Fluoroquinolones (norfloxacin, ciprofloxacin) are useful to eradicate infection. Amebic dysentery is treated by administration of tissue (metronidazole, tinidazole) and gut (diloxanide furoate, diodoquinol) amebicides. When bleeding per rectum persists or recurs frequently, the child should be examined by a pediatric surgeon to exclude rectal polyp.

DYSLEXIA

Dyslexia is the commonest cause of learning disability and is characterized by difficulties in reading, writing and learning the spellings. Around 8–10% children are affected who may have either normal or above normal intelligence. Boys and girls are equally affected. The exact cause is unknown and it appears there may be defective neurological wiring or processing of information in the brain due to genetic or acquired factors. The functional MRI studies of brain have shown that left angular gyrus is not used when a dyslexic child reads. Dyslexics are more rooted to use the right side of their brain, instead of the left to read and spell. Early recognition of dyslexia is important because slow learning may adversely affect the confidence and self-esteem of the child. These children may be taunted by their classmates and ignored by teachers leading to isolation, anxiety and depression. The child may be labelled as lazy, careless, stupid, indisciplined or mentally slow. The child with dyslexia has following learning disabilities and associated problems.

The child has poor skills of reading, writing and learning spellings. The child has poor handwriting, tends to write slowly and hesitatingly, at times contorting the face and protruding the tongue while writing. These children can process 3D information better because they have excellent visuo-spatial ability and can solve puzzles, make designs with blocks and play video games better.

- These children are confused between right and left direction of alphabets which appear as mirror image of each other like 'b', 'd', 'p', 'q'. The child may read 'was' as 'saw', 'pit' as 'tip', 'pan' as 'nap', 'car park' as 'park car', etc. Instead of writing from left to right, some children tend to write from right to left.
- They are unable to follow and perform actions in a sequential order, such as describing the days of the week or months of the year. The child may have difficulty in reciting nursery rhyme or remembering the exact sequence of a story.
- The child may be clumsy and may have difficulty in dressing, buttoning, tying shoe laces and often gets confused between right and left.

Treatment

Early recognition of the problem is important so that confidence and self-esteem of the child are not adversely affected. The child should be assessed by an educational psychologist for diagnosis and management of the condition. The child should be examined for any visual and hearing defect. The commonest cause of learing disability is poor concentration and low level of intelligence which should be excluded by assessing IQ. The dyslexic child should remain in the mainstream school and encouraged to pursue other activities and hobbies of his interest. The child must be encouraged and protected against the embarrassment and teasing by other classmates. They should be given coaching in phonetics by special educators. They can be provided help by computer-based reading programs. The good software that promote phonemic or phonic fluency include Read, Write and Type, Learning System and Read Naturally and Read it. Mother should educate herself in the concept of phonemes (breaking every word or sound into several parts) and phonetics to provide training to her child at home.

Famous Dyslexics

Many dyslexics are gifted with special attributes like ability to solve complex problems by providing novel or creative answers. Some dyslexics have the special ability to see things in 3D format or multidimensional manner. They may have special visual, spatial and lateral or novel thinking abilities. No wonder a number of politicians, scientists, inventors, artists and thinkers were dyslexics. Famous people who had reading and spelling difficulty in school but became legendary include Akbar the Great, Albert Einstein, Leonardo da Vinci, Pablo Picasso, Galileo, Thomas Edison, Graham Bell, Henry Ford, Benjamin Franklins, Agatha Christie, Steven Hawkins, Bill Clinton, Tony Blair, etc. They all created history. Therefore, one should never feel despondent in life, every challenge has a blessing in disguise.

DYSMENORRHEA

When menstrual periods are associated with marked discomfort and pain, it is called dysmenorrhea. Dysmenorrhea is common in teenage girls especially during their initial menstrual periods which are likely to be irregular. It may be associated with nausea, loose motions, fatigue and headache. Pain and discomfort can be relieved by giving paracetamol or ibuprofen. Local fomentation with a hot water bottle kept over the lower abdomen and perineum is useful. A combination of antispasmodic and an analgesic, like dicyclomine hydrochloride and mefenamic acid, is useful to relieve the painful contractions of the uterus. Dysmenorrhea usually disappears after pregnancy and with the use of oral contraceptives. Most adolescent girls are anemic, they must be given an hematinic containing iron, folic acid, B complex vitamins and magnesium. When dysmenorrhea is severe and intractable, the child should

Home Remedies

- Reduce salt intake 1–2 days before the onset of periods, which is likely to reduce pelvic congestion.
- Eat a bowlful of papaya during the periods as it facilitates menstrual flow and relieves constipation.
- Intake of one cup of carrot juice daily during the periods is beneficial.
- Take a long leaf of aloe vera, wash it thoroughly and put it into a mixer to extract the juice. Strain and filter the juice. Drink one tablespoon of juice with honey daily during the menstrual periods. Fresh juice should be prepared every day.
- Carrot and parsley soup is also useful to relieve uterine cramps during menstrual period.
- Intake of flaxseeds or flaxseed oil (salad dressing) is useful to reduce uterine cramps. Flaxseeds are rich in omega-3 fatty acid which is credited to suppress production of prostaglandins. Other foods which are rich in omega-3 fatty acid (fish, walnuts) are also beneficial.

be assessed by an obstetrician to rule out endometriosis and pelvic inflammatory disease (PID).

EARACHE

Ear pulling or earache is common in children and usually occurs due to middle ear infection (acute otitis media), infection of the ear canal (otitis externa), wax, insertion of a foreign body and trapping of an insect or a fly in the ear canal. Infants may pull at their ears when they are tired, sleepy, bored, hungry or during teething. At times, toothache may be referred to the ear. Infants with dandruff may have identical scales in the ear canal leading to constant itching and pulling of ears. Wax is formed by normal secretions produced by the gland in the outer part of the ear canal. It helps to trap dust and other small particles and provides protection to the eardrum. No attempt should be made to remove normal wax from the ears. During air travel, ear pain may occur during take off and landing because of pressure changes. The baby should be put to breast or bottle, or given a pacifier or dummy nipple during take off and landing. Older child can be given a candy or chewing gum and ears kept plugged with a cotton bud.

Treatment Pain and discomfort can be relieved by administration of paracetamol and a sedative like chloral hydrate or promethazine hydrochloride (phenergan). Warm fomentation with a heated napkin or lowel provides comfort. Wax and foreign body visible at the opening of ear canal may be removed with tweezers. Never push a hair pin, matchstick, toothpick or cotton bud to remove the wax or insect. Focussing bright light into the ear canal may at times attract the mosquito to fly out. Impacted wax in the ear can be softened by instillation of wax softener drops followed by removal of wax by syringing by an ENT specialist. It is dangerous to put oil into the ears (fungal infections) or nostrils (lipoid pneumonia) in children. When there are dry scales in the ear canals, it can be moistened with the help of cotton buds soaked with olive oil or coconut oil.

ELECTRIC SHOCK

Electric shocks are uncommon but are usually life-threatening. Toddlers love to put their fingers into small holes including electrical sockets (power points). They can get an electric shock by biting and chewing an electric cord or by poking metal objects, like a steel rod, fork and knife into an unprotected electrical outlet. Electrical accidents are common in bathroom when electric current makes contact with water. Accidents can also occur when electrical tools and toys are used incorrectly without supervision of an adult.

First-aid Switch off the current immediately or remove the plug from the socket. If that is not possible, push the child away from the source of current with a wooden rod or rolled-up magazine or newspaper. *Never touch the child with your bare hands if he is attached to the source of current.* All victims of electric shock must be rushed to the hospital immediately. Even when electric shock does not appear to be severe, it may cause deep burns and damage to the internal organs especially heart and brain.

Prevention

- When constructing a new house, instal safety circuits in the wiring so that fuse blows off automatically when there is electric shock.
- The electric sockets should be kept "child proof" by covering them with dummy plugs or made inaccessible to the child by installing them at a height or blocking them with heavy furniture.
- Do not amuse the child by repeatedly switching the light or fan on and off.
- The electrical appliances should be always kept unplugged so that child cannot put them on or off.
- Avoid using electrical tools and toys near bathtub and kiddy pool.
- Do not buy toys for young children which operate on main electrical supply.

ENCEPHALITIS

Encephalitis refers to inflammation of the brain parenchyma (encephalon) and is an important cause of death and neuromotor disability. The common viruses causing encephalitis include Japanese encephalitis virus, herpes viruses, measles, mumps and enteroviruses.

There is abrupt onset of high-grade fever, vomiting and progressive alteration of consciousness. Seizures and neurological deficits are common. There is progressive increase in intracranial pressure with marked irritability, confusion, delirium, drowsiness and coma. Unlike meningitis, the meningeal signs (neck stiffness, photophobia) are absent or minimal.

Treatment The child is admitted to pediatric intensive care unit and provided symptomatic and supportive treatment for control of fever, seizures, raised intracranial tension and electrolyte disturbances. Specific therapy is provided when child is diagnosed to have cerebral malaria and herpes simplex encephalitis. The disease carries high mortality and marked risk of neuromotor sequelae among the survivors. The common neurological sequelae include epilepsy, paralysis of one or several limbs, learning disability and mental retardation.

Prevention Japanese encephalitis vaccine (*JEEV*) can be given to children living in endemic areas. Two doses of vaccine, 4 weeks apart are administered through intramuscular route (0.25 mL in children between 1 and 3 years and 0.5 mL in children above 3 years). Measles and mumps can be prevented by routine administration of measles and MMR vaccines at 9 months and 15 months respectively.

EPILEPSY

When episodes of seizures are recurrent and there is no associated fever or underlying metabolic cause, it is called as epilepsy. Children are more prone to develop seizures compared to adults. Epilepsy may be generalized (twitchings of both upper and lower limbs with loss of consciousness) or partial and localized (twitchings of one side of the body or one limb without loss of consciousness). Most cases of generalized (grandmal, petitmal, myoclonic) epilepsy are familial in nature while partial epilepsy occurs due to a localized disease process in the brain like birth asphyxia, injury, infection, infarction, tumor, granuloma (tuberculoma, cysticercosis), vascular malformation or developmental defect of the brain. Epilepsy may or may not be associated with neurological deficits, delayed neuromotor development, mental retardation and behaviour disorder. Epilepsy is a disease and not a curse by nature or possession by an evil spirit.

First-aid During an episode of convulsion, clothes should be loosened and child protected against injury. The child should be placed on a bed with head kept low and face turned to one side to prevent choking due to secretions or vomitus. No attempt should be made to force open the mouth with a teaspoon. Never pour any water over the face or make the child smell a shoe. The child can be administered a dose of diazepam through rectum (Direc-2 rectal diazepam 2 mg/mL or Rec-DZ rectal solution 2 mg/2.5 mL and 5 mg/5 mL) or midazolam through a nasal spray (Insed nasal spray provides 0.5 mg midazolam per metered dose) and taken to the hospital.

Treatment

The child should be investigated and managed by a pediatric neurologist. A large number of effective anticonvulsant drugs are available. The dose of anticonvulsant drugs should be gradually increased and least number of drugs should be used in the lowest dose to control the seizures. Anticonvulsant drugs must be taken regularly and their administration should never be delayed or stopped suddenly because it may lead to intractable seizures. Over 80% of epileptic children can be effectively treated with one or more medications. In a select group of children who do not respond to drugs, surgical treatment has been used with success for control of intractable seizures. Children with epilepsy should be advised to avoid potentially hazardous activities like swimming and driving unless fits are well controlled. When seizures are controlled for 2 years, the patient can be gradually weaned off the drugs during a period of 3 months.

A large majority of children can attend a regular school and grow up to have normal or even above normal intelligence. Many great intellectuals and leaders, like Sir Isaac Newton, Socrates,

Alexander the Great, Julius Caesar and Napoleon Bonaparte, made outstanding contributions in life despite having epilepsy.

EVENING COLIC

It is the most common cause of unexplained crying in infants between 2 and 8 weeks of age. The crying spells occur every day at the same time in the evening or night in a clockwise regularity. The infant cries loudly, pulls up the legs over the abdomen and face becomes flushed. The gurgling sounds may be felt by placing the hand over the abdomen and child may pass wind to get temporary relief. Excessive crying may lead to further swallowing of air thus initiating a vicious cycle of colic-crying-colic. The spell of crying may last for 2–3 hours until baby is tired and falls asleep. The condition is seen in equal frequency in both breast and bottle fed babies. The crying spells usually disappear by 12 weeks of age.

The exact cause of evening colic is unknown but may occur due to intestinal colic ("blocked" wind), milk allergy, over sensitive and over reactive infant, excessive stimulation by the parents/grandparents, parental anxiety, abnormal emotional tension at home, etc. Babies are very sensitive and easily affected by the mother's tension and nervousness. When a mother is over reactive and upset by baby's crying, a vicious cycle is set up, with the baby crying more and mother becoming more jittery, as she is unable to handle the situation.

Treatment

Nothing seems to provide a consistent or fool proof relief to a baby with evening colic. The child usually cries with his "heart" and full vigor and the whole family is extremely upset and demoralized by unexplained inconsolable spells of crying. Holding the baby upright against the shoulder, rocking, cuddling, patting, kissing, prone positioning, taking him for a drive, etc. usually provide temporary relief. Local application of asafoetida (*Hing*) dissolved in warm water around the navel area usually provides relief. Placing the baby in a prone position with raised buttocks (knee-chest position) provides relief by expulsion of wind. Administration of antispasmodic drops, or decoction of carom (*ajwain*) and fennel (*saunf*) seeds, or gripe water are useful. The nursing mother should avoid intake of cruciferous vegetables (cabbage, cauliflower, turnips, radish, broccoli sprouts, kale, mustard leaves, etc.), lentils (especially kidney beans, Bengal gram, *urad dal*, etc.) and fruit juices to reduce the chances of development of excessive wind in the baby. There is some evidence that administration of probiotics may provide some relief to the baby with evening colic. When the family and physician are exhausted by trying various remedies and maneuvers, suddenly one day the condition resolves spontaneously after 6–8 weeks of nightmare!

EXANTHEMATOUS ILLNESS

Many infective illnesses especially viral in origin are associated with a skin rash (exanthem). They are preceded by symptoms akin to common cold (prodrome) which is followed by development of a characteristic skin rash, such as diffuse redness (macules), pin-head sized elevated lesions (papules), blisters (vesicles), pustules (pus-containing blisters) and petechiae or purpura (bleeding in the skin). There may be associated enanthem, i.e. internal eruption over the mucous membranes of the oral cavity. During recovery, there may be peeling or desquamation and pigmentation of the skin. The common viral exanthemata include measles, German measles (rubella), chickenpox and mumps and are described at their appropriate places in the text. They can be prevented by timely and effective immunization.

EXCESSIVE SWEATING (Hyperhidrosis)

Many children have excessive sweating which is usually limited to the head and palms. It is most commonly due to constitutional or genetic predisposition. It is of no significance although most parents are unnecessarily worried that it may cause weakness. Sweating of palms with nail biting is suggestive of anxiety. Excessive sweating is common during hot and humid climate, physical activity or exercise, and when fever is brought down by use of an antipyretic medicine (paracetamol or ibuprofen). Cold sweating may occur in pulmonary tuberculosis, congestive heart failure, sudden fall in blood glucose (hypoglycemia) and blood pressure (shock) and excessive secretion of thyroxine (hyperthyroidism or thyrotoxicosis).

EYE INJURY

Children are more prone to accidents and injuries. Injury to eye/s may occur due to a sharp object, cricket ball, stone, pellet, arrow or a firecracker. When there is a serious injury to the eye, it should be covered with a sterile gauze pad and child should be rushed to the emergency department of a specialized eye hospital.

Foreign object When you can see the grain of dust or sand, or a hair in the eye, you can attempt to remove it. Wash your hands with soap and water and take a moist sterile wick to remove the foreign body while some one else holds the baby and keeps the eye open. You can attempt to remove the foreign body if it is located beneath the upper or lower eyelid or over the white portion (sclera) of the eye. When foreign body is lying over the central brown part of the eye (cornea), never try to remove it because of potential risk of causing injury to the cornea. You can flush the eye by pouring water as described below.

E

Chemical injury Accidental entry of corrosive agent like lye, detergent or chemical spray are most damaging to the eyes and should be handled with ulmost urgency. Flush the eye immediately and thoroughly by pouring plain luke warm water from a jug or kettle for at least 15 minutes. Keep the head turned towards the side of affected eye, keep the eye open with your thumb and index finger, and pour the water over the inner side of affected eye so that it drains away from the normal eye. *You must ensure that the chemical run off during flushing does not enter the normal eye.* There is no need to put any eyedrops or ointment in the eye and child should not be allowed to rub his eye/s. After 15 minutes of thorough flushing, the child should be rushed to an ophthalmologist.

FAILURE TO THRIVE

The basic aim of child care is to ensure that every child is assisted to achieve his or her optimal genetic potential for physical growth and mental development. Physical growth of children depends upon an interaction between nature (genetic potential, constitution, developmental defect and chronic systemic illness) on one hand and nurture (nutrition, health care, safe and stimulating environment, love and affection) on the other. When a child fails to have satisfactory weight gain and linear growth (slow or poor gain in height), he is diagnosed to have failure to thrive (FTT). It is not possible to make the diagnosis of FTT on the basis of one or two isolated measurements of weight and length or height. Instead the weight and length or height of the child should be taken on a periodic basis during visits to the health clinic for immunizations and recorded on a road-to-health card. In a healthy child, the growth curve should run along the 50th percentile. *When the growth curve is flat or it gradually drops down, the child needs urgent attention to reverse the trend.* Failure to thrive should not be confused with food fussiness in children belonging to well-to-do families when "the child is not eating to the satisfaction of parents" but is otherwise active and playful though not chubby as per their expectations.

Causes

The common causes of failure to thrive include poor or unsatisfactory feeding (bottle feeding with diluted milk or formula, delay in the introduction of weaning or complementary foods) and recurrent or chronic infections. The child may be born small (premature, intrauterine growth retardation) and may have a developmental defect (congenital malformation, chromosomal or genetic defect). The child may have a chronic systemic disorder affecting any organ or system of the body. Psychosocial deprivation (lack of love, tender loving care), neglect and child abuse is an important cause of FTT. A detailed assessment and investigations by a pediatrician are mandatory to identify the underlying cause of FTT.

Treatment

The management depends upon the underlying cause of FTT. The faulty child rearing and feeding practices should be identified and corrected. The underlying chronic infections or infestations should be identified and appropriately treated. Wheat-free or gluten-free diet (celiac disease), lactose-free milk (lactose intolerance) and exclusion of milk protein (cow's milk allergy), when indicated, provide prompt symptomatic relief and resumption of normal growth. The presence of a systemic chronic or recurrent disease should be identified and appropriately managed. The child should be encouraged to take energy-dense high-protein balanced nutritious diet like full-fat milk, cheese, lentils, eggs, dry fruits and nuts. Nutritional supplements containing micronutrients (vitamins and minerals) and high biological value protein can be provided as an interim measure.

FAMILY LIFE EDUCATION (Sex education)

Family life education is not merely knowledge about the anatomy of sexual organs and how reproduction occurs but includes information on dynamics and principles of family life. Children learn about the facts of life by watching their parents and asking innocent and spontaneous questions. Sex is not merely passion, it must be sublimated to compassion by integrating it with love, tenderness, consideration and feelings of respect for each other. Parents should set a good example for their children by showing attributes of helpfulness, thoughtfulness, kindness and mutual respect for each other even when they disagree. A child who sees love, affection and mutual respect among parents is likely to imbibe and practice these qualities during courtship and married life.

Children around 3 years of age understand the differences between a boy and a girl. At this stage, they start asking several innocent and embarrassing questions to their parents. It is important to answer their questions in a matter-of-fact manner in a simple language depending upon their level of understanding to satisfy their curiosity.

Reproductive Health Education

There is a wrong belief in our society that children should not be taught about sex as if sex is immoral or bad. There is a need to accept and appreciate that sex indeed is a vibrant and divine energy because it creates new life. Apart from basic anatomy and physiology of sexual organs, children should be taught about the spiritual dimensions of sex. They should be taught as to how passion or lust should be allowed to flower into love and how love can be sublimated to evolve into compassion for all human beings.

Adolescent children (5th grade onward) should be taught about the biology of reproduction and risks of unprotected sex. This must include broad aspects of family life education and moral and spiritual aspects of sex. The sex should never be associated with fear, guilt, anxiety or aggression. It is not possible to impose a particular attitude towards sexual morality but we should be able to prepare and motivate the youth to take informed decisions in matters of their sex life. Adolescent children need guidance from their parents regarding day-to-day issues pertaining to sexual organs like menstruation in girls and "wet dreams" in boys. Girls often confide these issues with there mothers, while boys are a bit wary of their fathers and both are reluctant to talk about sex issues openly.

Sexual Hygiene

Children should be explained about the need for personal and sexual hygiene during adolescence and adult life. Boys should be told to retract the foreskin during bath to wash off the dried secretions (smegma) that collects over the glans of the penis. Girls should be told to wash the bottom thoroughly with soap and water during the bath and after attending every call of nature. *Care must be taken to wash the vulva from front backwards, so that there is no risk of fecal bacteria entering the vagina or urethral orifice.* Girls must be explained about the importance of using clean pad or sanitary napkins during menstruations. Health education should provide detailed information for prevention of sexually transmitted diseases (STDs) and method of contraception for prevention of unwanted pregnancies. It is true that only girls become pregnant but contraception is the joint responsibility of both the partners.

FEBRILE CONVULSIONS

Sudden onset of high-grade fever in some children may lead to development of convulsions. They are most common during 6 months to 3 years of age. The exact cause of febrile convulsions is not known but immaturity of the brain in children and hereditary predisposition are believed to be common predisposing causes. There is some evidence that children with iron deficiency anemia are more likely to have febrile convulsions. Even before the mother realizes that the child has fever, he becomes stiff and develops jerky movements or twitchings of upper and lower limbs. There may be uprolling of eyes, clenching of teeth and loss of consciousness. Most episodes are brief in duration and usually last between 2 and 5 minutes. Convulsions usually stop by the time mother contacts the doctor and they do not recur during the subsequent course of the fever. However, they can occur again when child gets another episode of fever after a few weeks or months. Febrile convulsions do not occur in children below the age of 6 months or after the age of 5 years.

F

Treatment

There is no need to panic or get alarmed because convulsions stop automatically within a few minutes. The child should be placed on a bed and head kept turned to one side so that secretions in the mouth are drained out without any risk of aspiration and tongue does not fall back and block the wind pipe. Efforts should be made to bring down the body temperature by switching on the fan and sponging the body with tap water. In a convulsing or unconscious child, rectal paracetamol (Anamol rectal suppository 125 mg and 250 mg and Paracetanal suppository 80 mg and 170 mg) and diazepam or nasal midazolam can be administered as an emergency measure. When child is conscious, the medications can be administered orally. When convulsions are prolonged for more than 10 minutes or child is getting repeated convulsions during a bout of fever, he must be taken to the nearest hospital.

Prevention

When your preschool child is known to get episodes of febrile convulsions, you should be vigilant but not worried because febrile convulsions do not cause any brain damage or impose any threat to life. Iron supplements should be given if child is anemic. The onset of fever should be identified early and promptly managed by administration of paracetamol or ibuprofen and hydrotherapy. Child can be administered clobazam (0.5 mg/kg/dose twice a day) during first 2 days of fever to reduce the risk of febrile seizures. Febrile seizures are benign and there is no role of long-term anti-convulsant therapy which is practiced as a standard protocol for treatment of epilepsy.

FEVER

Fever is the commonest signal or symptom of disease in children. It provides a warning that something is wrong with the child. Fever and pain often coexist because fever is usually associated with headache and body aches. There are diurnal variations in body temperature, it is lowest in the morning and highest in the afternoon (maximum oral temperature of 99.9°F or 37.7°C). The body temperature is more unstable in children and diurnal or daily variations are more marked especially during summer months. *Fever is defined as an elevation of oral temperature to >100°F or 37.8°C.* Fever is a protective response on the part of the body to fight an infection. However, during fever the requirements of fluids, food and oxygen go up because of rise in the metabolic rate of the body. And in young children (6 month–3 years), fever may cause convulsions or fits in susceptible families.

Is fever a friend or a foe?

Fever is not an "illness" but response on the part of body that it is fighting an infection. Most fevers serve to heal, rather than harm. It inhibits the growth and virulence of disease producing microbes. Fever enhances the disease fighting capabilities of the body to kill the microbes. It is well known that septic patients with fever have a better chance to survive as compared to septic patients with hypothermia (fall in body temperature) which occurs in malnourished children, cancer patients and newborn babies (especially prematurely born and low birth weight babies). In preantibiotic era, artificial fever was produced by injecting malarial parasites to treat tertiary syphilis. Therefore, unnecessary reduction of mild to moderate fever (<101°F or 38.5°C) may be likened to "disarming the body which is trying to fight an infection".

Causes of Fever

Fever occurs due to a variety of causes but the commonest cause of fever in children is acute viral infection like common cold. Sore throat due to tonsillitis (strep throat) is common in school going children. Other common causes of fever include gastro-intestinal infection, ear infection (acute otitis media), pneumonia, malaria, typhoid fever, tuberculosis and urinary tract infection. Fever may occur following administration of some vaccines in children. During hot summer months, fever may occur due to exposure to high environmental temperature. Drug fever may occur following administration of certain drugs or when multiple antibiotics are given for a prolonged period of time. Fever may occur in children with autoimmune disorders (rheumatic fever, rheumatoid arthritis) and cancer. Teething should never be blamed as a cause of fever.

Common Symptoms

The child with fever becomes inactive, less playful, irritable and cranky due to headache and body aches. There is loss of appetite but he may crave for water. The urine output may decrease and it may become high colored due to concentration. The face may be flushed, head and trunk are warm to touch while hand and feet may be cold especially when fever is shooting up. Most fevers are associated with feeling of cold but when chills and shivering (rigors) are marked, it is suggestive of blood-borne infection, like viremia, septicemia and malaria. Depending upon the cause of fever, there may be associated specific symptoms which help the physician to make the diagnosis.

What are the hazards of fever?

Fever makes the child uncomfortable due to associated headache and body aches, and elevation of heart rate and breathing rate. The metabolic rate of the body is increased leading to greater demand for fluids, food and oxygen. In children with pneumonia and heart disease, fever may lead to fall in oxygen tension (hypoxia) and elevation in carbon dioxide (hypercarbia). High grade fever may lead to delirium and confusion. Fever often leads to loss of appetite, negative nitrogen balance and weight loss. In certain families, young children (6 months–3 years) may develop febrile convulsions when their body temperature shoots up suddenly.

General and Supportive Care

Most viral fevers are self-limiting and child only needs good supportive care. The child should be kept in a cool, well-ventilated room with light and comfortable clothes. The extra layer of covers and clothing should be removed to allow the body to lose temperature. The cultural belief that keeping the child with fever under a fan leads to pneumonia does not have any scientific basis. The child should be encouraged to take extra fluids and nutritious diet. Food should never be denied to children with fever because they already have loss of appetite and their metabolic needs are higher. No dietary restrictions should be imposed and the child should be encouraged to eat foods and fruits of his liking and choice. The cultural practice of denying certain foods to children with fever, does not have any scientific basis in the modern system of medicine.

> Fever is a friend and not a foe—never try to give it a knocking blow.
>
> —Meharban Singh

Avoid use of aggressive antipyretic therapy because fever is a protective response on the part of the body to fight infection. Paracetamol (15 mg/kg/dose every 4–6 hr) and/or ibuprofen (10 mg/kg/dose every 4–6 hr) can be given when oral temperature goes above 101°F (>38.5°C) or even at a lower temperature if there is associated discomfort, headache and body aches. Early antipyretic therapy is recommended, if there is associated breathing difficulty or past history of febrile convulsions and epilepsy. Paracetamol is a safe and effective antipyretic with minimal side effects. It can be given safely to children with bronchial asthma. Ibuprofen can be co-administered with paracetamol or given alternately. In general, medications should be administered in a precise dose with the help of a plastic syringe or a graduated plastic measure provided by the manufacturer. The use of household teaspoons should be avoided because they are variable and not of a standard size. When child refuses to take oral medications (drowsy, persistent vomiting) paracetamol can be given through rectum.

When fever goes beyond 42°C (104°F) despite adequate antipyretic therapy, effective sponging of the body with tap water is recommended. Place the child on a thick towel or plastic sheet and soak 3 small towels or sheets of flannel in a basin containing tap water for sponging. You can add few drops of eua de cologne in the water. *Cold water should never be used for sponging, it will cause shivering and discomfort with further rise in body temperature.* In winter, even tap water may be too cold, it should be warmed up to body temperature (37°C or 98.4°F) for sponging the body. The child should be completely exposed and sponging done over the forehead, trunk and extremities. The child should be placed

F

Some do's and dont's for children with fever

Do's
- Keep the child in a well-ventilated cool room. Remove unnecessary or extra clothes.
- Give plenty of liquids to drink.
- Give a good nutritious diet of child's liking without any restrictions.
- Give a safe antipyretic like paracetamol and/or ibuprofen. Administer the correct dose.
- Do sponging of the body with tap water by placing the child under a fan if fever is high or unresponsive to an antipyretic.
- Consult your doctor as early as possible for institution of a specific treatment.

Dont's
- Do not panic because most fevers are viral in origin and are self-limiting.
- Do not over clothe or cover the child with a blanket.
- Do not starve the child or impose unnecessary food restrictions.
- Do not give an antipyretic to a child with mild fever.
- Sponging of the body should not be done with ice cold water.
- Avoid misuse of antibiotics which are dangerous both for the patient and society.

under the fan to assist cooling by evaporation. Antipyretic must be given before starting hydrotherapy except in a child with heat stroke where there is no role of fever relieving drug/s. Hydrotherapy should be stopped as soon as body temperature drops to 100°F (38°C) to prevent risk of over cooling. The child with fever must be seen by a family doctor or a pediatrician as early as possible. The site of infection and likely pathogens causing the disease should be ascertained or identified. "Shot gun" antibiotic therapy with multiple drugs should be avoided and a specific antibiotic should be used depending upon the likely diagnosis. *Antibiotics should not be indiscriminately misused as antipyretics.* Efforts should be made to treat the child and not the thermometer! The common do's and dont's in the management of a child with fever are summarized in the **Box**.

The Child with Low Grade Fever

Many children are wrongly diagnosed to have low grade fever and subjected to unnecessary investigations. The usual story is that the child had high grade fever (viral or some other infection like typhoid fever) but parents continue to record the body temperature (either on their own or on the advice of physician) even when initial illness has settled. They find that child is running "low grade fever" (oral temperature 99–99.8°F or 37.2–37.8°C) especially in the afternoon and evening. A number of consultations are sought and investigations are done to identify the cause of fever without realizing that it is a normal pattern of body temperature of the child. The child is otherwise well, active and without any discomfort. He is playful and his appetite is good. Infact, there is nothing wrong with the child if his "temperature" is ignored. The child wants to go to school but parents think he needs rest. All investigations including erythrocyte sedimentation rate (ESR) are normal. No further investigations should be done and parents need to be reassured that there is nothing wrong with the child. Further recording of body temperature should be stopped and child sent to school.

A number of diseases, however, are known to start with a low grade fever. They are often associated with other symptoms of an underlying disease process like loss of appetite, lack of vigour and enthusiasm, weakness, inability or lack of interest to play, easy fatigability, pallor (due to fall in hemoglobin), poor weight gain or loss of body weight, etc. Depending upon the site and nature of the disease process, additional symptoms like cough, dysuria (discomfort in passing urine) or frequency of urination, bowel disturbances (constipation or loose motions), body aches, bone or joint pains, etc. may be noticed. ESR which is a non-specific marker of a large number of diseases, is often elevated. These children do need expert medical advice and a battery of investigations to identify the cause of underlying disease process. A number of diseases, like tuberculosis, chronic infections, cancer (leukemia, lymphomas) and autoimmune diseases, may have this symptoms complex.

FINICKY OR FUSSY EATER

There are different types of feeding and nutritional problems among the economically deprived and illiterate families compared to the affluent and educated ones. Children belonging to poor families are keen to eat but are starving and are undernourished because of lack of food and poverty or ignorance of the parents. These children never refuse to eat, instead they fight with their siblings to get a share of their family food. When you offer to them a dry piece of bread or *chapati*, they will grab and eat it without any fuss. As opposed to this, there are fussy "blackmailers" of well-to-do families who have abundant food but children refuse to eat in accordance with the expectations or to the satisfaction of their parents.

The parents bring their child to the physician with the usual story that "our child eats nothing" or "our child eats like a bird" and "we have tried virtually everything to make him eat but it has been of no use". The meal times are virtual mini-wars. The battle lines are drawn. On one side is the valiant, adamant and determined lone fighter the child, and on the other side of the fence is the whole family with mother and grandparents indulging in all sorts of pranks and gimmicks to make him eat. The child is coaxed, cajoled, forced and bribed to eat. He is distracted by telling a story, showing a picture book, his favourite ad on TV or a cartoon clip. The child is often running around and mother is chasing him with his food plate in her hand. The whole family is worried and concerned about the child with a fond hope that he will eat something. The mealtimes become unpleasant, emotionally surcharged and stressful both for the child and family. The morale of the child is high while the whole family is gloomy and despondent. The worst scenario is that father is physically restraining the child and mother is literally forcing and pushing the food into his mouth. No wonder that the child often spits or vomits the food after the feeding brawl.

Food fussiness is common due to over indulgence or over-concern because of the "only child" or "only male child". The child is not having loss of appetite but it is a behaviour problem. The child is literally "blackmailing" the family. The more he is forced, the less he eats. The child is rebellious and wants his way to exercise his individuality. He has a good appetite for the foods of his liking but they are often denied by the family. The child usually eats well at the neighbour's house or at a birthday party. The child may not be chubby but he is otherwise active, playful and wiry. The parents are worried because he is not gaining weight at a rate he did during the first year of life. It must be remembered that weight gain velocity slows as the child grows. During 3–10 years of age, children gain merely 2 kg body weight during one year as compared to weight gain of 750–1000 gm per month during the first 4–6 months of life.

How to handle the picky eater?

- The development of food fussiness should be prevented by avoiding over indulgence and not paying excessive concern and attention to the child's food.
- No distractions (like showing a cartoon movie or TV ad, picture book) should be used while feeding the child.
- You should honor the individual likes and dislikes of your child and offer a variety of food items to break the monotony. Give him a choice between 2 and 3 food items but not an open-ended or unlimited choice.
- *The best way to make the child eat is "not to try"*. Adopt a relaxed attitude at meal times and let the child enjoy what he likes to eat. Give more attention and show pleasure when child eats well and ignore him when he refuses to eat or fiddles with food.
- You should encourage the child to self-feed even if he creates mess. Most children would like to eat when other family members are eating.

- After giving a reasonable time to finish the food, the plate should be quietly removed even if the child has not finished, without showing any concern and anxiety.
- Children do have a rebellious attitude and many a times a negative statement that "Kabir will not get his food today", many evoke a positive response.
- The whole family including grandparents must participate in the mission approach to change the "blackmailing" tactics of the child. You must appreciate that food fussiness is a behaviour disorder and the child does not have loss of appetite or "sluggish liver".
- There is no role of tonics and appetisers to make the child eat. You must understand the aforementioned family dynamics of food fussiness and emphasis should be placed on changing your attitude and approach in feeding the child.
- Nevertheless, tonics may be given to gain confidence of the mother and to provide supplements of vitamins and minerals. But the reliance should be placed on behaviour management by adopting a relaxed and common sense approach without any anxiety or sense of frustration.

FIRST-AID KIT

Parents should have the know how to provide first-aid to common day-to-day illnesses and accidents in children. The following first-aid items should be stocked in a first-aid box and replenished from time to time.

- Digital thermometer
- *Antiseptic solutions* like isopropyl alcohol, cetrimide (savlon), chloroxylenol (dettol), povidone-iodine or betadine.
- *Antiseptic cream or ointment* silver-sulfadiazine (silverix), povidone-iodine or betadine, polybacterial ointment (T-bact, neosporin)
- *Soothing lotion and skin cream* calamine, caladryl, prucal, calchill, calak-A, counter-irritant ointment or spray (moov, volini), anesthetic cream or gel (lignocaine 5%)
- *Dressing material* cotton bandages, water proof band aid strips, surgical adhesive tape, elastic or crepe bandage, sling for arm, roll of cotton ball, sterilized gauze pads, scissors, bulb syringe or nasal aspirator, tweezer and forceps.

- Commonly used medications
  - Relief of pain and/or fever: Paracetamol, ibuprofen, mefenamic acid
  - Anti-vomiting or anti-emetics: Domperidone and ondansetron
  - Anticolic drops and syrup: Colicaid, meftal spas, cyclopam
  - *Antihistamines:* Promethazine hydrochloride (phenergan), diphenhydramine hydrochloride (benadryl), cetirizine dihydrochloride (cetzine), hydroxyzine hydrochloride (atarax).
  - Oral rehydration salt. ORS sachets
  - Ice pack in the refrigerator and hot water bottle
  - List of important telephone numbers in case of an emergency and poisoning.

Fits (*see* convulsions)

FLAT FEET (Pes planus)

In infants, flat feet are normal because bones are soft and the arch of the feet is filled with a fatty pad. This obscures the normal curve on the inner side of feet giving a flat appearance to the feet. When infant walks with wet feet, it leaves behind a complete impression of the feet on the ground. The physiological appearance of flat feet disappears by the age of 2 years. After this age, flat feet are diagnosed when the inner side of the heel of shoes wear off and arch of the feet is poor when child is asked to stand on his toes. Ask the child to sit and raise the foot off the ground and observe for the arch on the inner side of the foot. When child is asked to walk barefeet, the whole foot touches the ground instead of the inner side of the feet being raised a little bit off the ground. It is more easily brought out by observing the complete impression of the feet when child with wet feet is asked to walk. It may be associated with shortening or contracture of Achilles tendon. Flat feet are less common in societies where young children walk barefeet. Children with flat feet may complain of pain in the feet, ankle or calf and difficulty in running and easy fatigability.

Treatment The child should be encouraged to walk barefeet. Walking barefeet on a pebbled surface or a rough floor is useful. Ask the child to walk or run on toes and try to spread out the toes as widely as possible. Child can be asked to make full range active movements of the feet in all directions. Child can be asked to pick the marbles or pebbles between the toes and sole. Stretching exercises of tendo-Achilles by forcibly trying to touch the dorsum of the foot to the shin are useful when Achilles tendon is short. Special shoes with insoles or inserts (orthoses) may be advised by an orthopedic surgeon, podiatrist (foot specialist) and physical medicine specialist.

FLUOROSIS

Fluorine deficiency is a recognized risk factor for development of caries but in areas where fluoride content of drinking water is in excess of 2 parts per million (>2 mg/liter), the population is at risk to develop fluorosis. It is, therefore, desirable to avoid the use of fluoride-containing tooth paste or fluoridation of water in such regions. The enamel of the teeth gets mottled and discolored brown. Fluorosis may produce crippling deformities of long bones, spine and joints. Knock knees is the most common deformity observed in regions with fluorosis. The bones may look thick and dense on X-rays. There may be damage to peripheral nerves and muscles causing severe deformities and disability.

FOOD FUNDAS FOR A FLAT BELLY

Obesity is becoming a public health issue among adolescents belonging to well-to-do families. It is an outcome of intake of calorie-dense junk food and sedentary lifestyle. There is no easy *mantra* to maintain a fat belly. Lifestyle changes like maintenance of active life (regular exercise, swimming, sports, walking, jogging, aerobics, dancing and yoga) and eating the right type of food without any fasting and bingeing are crucial to prevent obesity and risk of metabolic syndrome X (precursor of type 2 diabetes mellitus). A number of foods are non-fattening and health-friendly and they can be remembered by an acronym. ABS DIET POWER (*see* **Box** on next page).

FOOD POISONING

Food poisoning may be caused by germs or their toxins or by intake of some poisonous foods like wild variety of mushrooms. Intake

Abs diet power			
A	**B**	**S**	**D**
Almonds (and other non-salted nuts and seeds)	Beans (and other legumes)	Spinach (and other green leafy vegetables and salads)	Dairy products (double-toned milk products)
I	**E**	**T**	**P**
Instant oat meal	Egg whites	Turkey (and other lean meat and fish without skin)	Peanut butter
O	**W**	**E**	**R**
Olive oil (and omega-3 fatty acids)	Whole grains cereals (and water)	Extra protein powder	Raspberries (and other berries)

Offer at least six helpings of these foods to your child daily and his body will become a fat-burning machine.

Adapted from Men's Health June 2008.

of stale food especially in summer and consumption of cut and exposed fruits or fruit juices from road-side *dhabas* and hawkers may lead to food poisoning. Food poisoning epidemics are known to occur during community meal programs or religious festivals and marriage parties.

All the members of the family or community who had taken the offending food would manifest symptoms of food poisoning. The symptoms may occur within a few hours if they are due to toxins or may take 2 to 3 days if food is contaminated with pathogenic bacteria. There is colicky pain in abdomen with severe bouts of vomiting and watery diarrhea. The symptoms may be severe leading to development of cold extremities with circulatory collapse and shock. The principles of management are the same as in children with diarrhea, cholera or acute gastroenteritis. The emphasis should be placed on early administration of home-available liquids and oral rehydration solution (ORS). Due to explosive nature of illness, many patients may need referral to a hospital for administration of intravenous fluids.

Home Remedies

- Massage lemon juice over the freckles with your fingers daily. Lemon juice is good for bleaching the skin.
- Mix equal quantity of parsley juice, lemon juice and orange juice and massage over the freckles.
- Mix little quantity of germ wheat in warm honey and apply over the freckles. Rinse it off with warm water after 15 minutes.
- Grind equal quantity of turmeric and sesame seed and make a paste in water. Apply over the freckles and rinse it off after 15 minutes.
- Application of butter milk (milk left after removing butter from curd) over the freckles is useful to reduce the intensity of pigmentation.

FRECKLES

These are light or dark brown spots that occur over sun-exposed areas of skin, such as face, upper chest or back, arms and hand. They are induced by exposure to sun, particularly during the summer and may fade or disappear during the winter. They are more common in individuals with fair skin and golden hair. They appear during pre-school years and increase in number over the years. They can be prevented by reducing exposure to sun and using sun protection cream while going outdoors.

F

GALACTAGOGUES (Lactagogues)

The substances which are credited to enhance milk production are called galactagogues. A large number of Ayurvedic preparations or home remedies are credited to promote lactation. The list includes fenugreek (*methi*) seeds, *tulsi* seeds, fennel (*saunf*), cumin seeds (*jeera*), cinnamon (*daal cheeni*), poppy seeds (*khas khas*), *peepali* (*mug*), garlic, drum sticks (*saijan*), omum (*ajwain*), ginger, asafoetida (*hing*), gum, coriander seeds (*dhania*), alfa alfa, unripe papaya, oats, etc. virtually anything in the kitchen. The very fact that the list of galactagogues is so large, it suggests that there is no fool proof remedy to improve lactation—they are all based on rituals, folklore, faith and figment of imagination. The aforementioned food items are consumed in the form of *laddoos, kheer* or porridge, *burfi, halwa, mukhwas,* sprinklers or decoction like herbal tea. In modern system of medicine, there is no potent or effective galactagogue. Metoclopramide (a drug used for treatment of vomiting) is recommended for promotion of lactation but its efficacy is variable.

GASTROESOPHAGEAL REFLUX DISEASE (GERD)

There is laxity or relaxation of the sphincter between the lower end of the esophagus and stomach. There is regurgitation of stomach contents which is aggravated by straining, excitement, over feeding, conghing and during sleep (with further relaxation of gastroesophageal sphincter).

GERD is common during early infancy and condition improves as the child grows. There are frequent episodes of regurgitation of feeds despite adequate burping. The associated symptoms include irritability, unexplained crying and poor weight gain.

There may be episodes of crying at night with arching of the body due to esophagitis because of reflux of acidic contents of stomach into the esophagus. The regurgitation of stomach contents may be aspirated causing choking and gagging, hoarseness, ear infection (otitis media), lung function or episodes of wheezing. The condition may be confused with intolerance or allergy to cow's milk, pylorospasm or pyloric stenosis.

Treatment The symptoms improve if baby is kept in a semi-upright position at 45° especially after feeds and during sleep. When infant is bottle fed, the feed can be thickened with a rice-based cereal. Prokinetic drugs like domperidone and H_2 blockers (ranitidine), or proton pump inhibitors (omeprazole, lansoprazole) are useful to provide relief. The condition improves as the child grows (assumes upright posture and takes semisolid food) and usually disappears by 2 years of age.

GENETIC DISORDERS (Inborn errors of metabolism)

Every disease and human behaviour is genetically determined and it is codified in the genes which are located in the nuclei and mitochondria of cells. There are 23 pairs (total of 46 chromosomes) in each human cell, 22 pairs of autosomes (with identical or homologous genetic material in each pair) and one pair of sex chromosomes (XX in females and XY in males). Human genome project has identified 100,000 genes and about 3 billion DNA-base pairs have been decoded by DNA probes. *Each gene is credited to control the production of a specific enzyme which is essential for a specific metabolic process in the body.* Single gene disorders are called inborn errors of metabolism or disorders of enzymes. The defective gene may be located in the autosome (autosomal disorder) or sex chromosome (sex-linked disorder). In sex-linked disorders, disease is manifest in boys while girls serve as carriers without suffering from the disease. The common sex-linked disorders include hemophilia, Duchenne muscular dystrophy and G6PD deficiency.

Most inborn errors of metabolism are either life-threatening or produce lifelong disability. Their treatment is unsatisfactory and therapeutic modalities include replacement of a specific enzyme or metabolic end product, reducing the production or increasing the excretion of toxic metabolites, gene therapy (replacing the "bad" gene with the "normal" gene) and organ transplantation

G

(liver, bone marrow or stem cell transplant). The risk of genetic or hereditary disorders is reduced by avoiding marriages among first cousins. In certain genetic disorders, it is possible to make prenatal diagnosis during early pregnancy when option of abortion can be offered to the parents when fetus is affected.

GEOGRAPHIC TONGUE

There is bizarre shapes and patterns of gray-white areas on the surface of the tongue with advancing and slightly elevated and irregular margins resembling like a map. The shape and pattern of the map may change from time to time. It does not cause any discomfort or symptoms to the child and no treatment is required. No attempt should be made to forcibly clean-off the white-gray areas.

GERMAN MEASLES (Rubella)

It is a viral infection which is spread through oronasal droplets. The incubation period varies between 14 and 21 days. There may be fever with symptoms of cough and cold for 1–2 days followed by skin rash on the trunk with enlarged and painful lymph nodes in the neck. The disease is usually mild and resolves within 3 days without any treatment. However, German measles during first 8–10 weeks of pregnancy may cause serious congenital malformations in the fetus (Rubella syndrome). Infants with congenital rubella syndrome (CRS) are usually small in size at birth and may have microcephaly (small head size), cataracts, sensorineural deafness, heart defects (especially patent ductus arteriosus) and neuromotor retardation. These infants may excrete virus in their nasal and throat secretions and urine for as long as one year. They pose a serious risk of infection to pregnant women.

Treatment Rubella is a mild self-limited disease and does not need any treatment. When a pregnant woman is exposed to a patient with rubella or infant with congenital rubella syndrome, she is at grave risk of contracting the viral infection with drastic consequences to her fetus. Mother should be tested for rubella-specific IgM and IgG antibodies in her blood. If the rubella IgM is negative and IgG antibodies are positive, the mother is likely to be immune and nothing further needs to be done. When antibodies are negative, repeat blood samples of the mother should be tested after 2 weeks of the exposure. If second sample of blood shows IgM antibodies, it suggests that she has been infected by rubella virus. In view of the high risk of development of congenital rubella syndrome, mother can be recommended medical termination of pregnancy.

Prevention Rubella can be effectively prevented by administration of MMR (combined measles, mumps and rubella vaccine) vaccine at 9 months followed by a booster at 15 months of age.

GHUTTI

It is a common cultural practice to offer *ghutti* (like glucose water, honey, tea) before putting the baby to the breast. It is believed that the child takes on the personality characteristics of the person who offers *ghutti* to the child. Administration of *ghutti* is a harmful cultural practice because of potential risk of infection and delay in establishing lactation. It is important that colostrum or initial milk which is full of nutritional virtues, should not delayed or denied to the child. There is also a practice of giving a herbal preparation (*Janam ghutti, Baal ghutti, Mughli ghutti*) to the child for treatment of number of ailments like wind, colic, indigestion, acidity, constipation, loose motions, teething, etc. There is no scientific evidence for any health benefits of *Janam ghutti* and it should preferably be avoided.

GIARDIASIS

Giardiasis is a common infestation in children and is caused by *Giardia lamblia*. The infection occurs by drinking contaminated water. The common symptoms include semiloose stool which are usually large, bulky and frothy. There is abdominal discomfort, flatulence, loss of appetite and failure to thrive. The diagnosis is confirmed by examination of stools for cysts and vegetative forms of *G. lamblia*.

Treatment A number of drugs are available to treat giardiasis but cure rates are not satisfactory and reinfection or persistence of infection is common. The commonly used drugs include metronidazole (15 mg/kg/day in 3 divided doses for 10 days) and tinidazole (50 mg/kg single dose) or secnidazole (30 mg/kg single dose). In order to eradicate the infection, all the family members should be investigated and appropriately treated.

G

GIFTED CHILD

The exceptional capabilities of a gifted child may be in the field of intellection or cognition (computer wizard, math genius) or in communication and fine arts like music, dance, painting and acting. The child who is smarter than most of his classmates may get bored because the class work may appear too easy, repetitive or mundane to him. There is no need to have special classes for a gifted child or advance him to a higher class. A well-trained teacher can satisfy and hone the special capabilities of the extra-bright students so that they continue to interact socially with their age-mates in a regular class.

The parents should spend more time with their gifted child to satisfy his curiosity and hunger for learning. They should be provided greater exposure to the bounties of nature by traveling, trekking, visiting zoos and museums. The capabilities of a gifted child can be further enhanced by a special tutor to unravel his full inherent potential. However, the parents should not be over ambitious and the child should be encouraged to develop a well-balanced personality with emotional stability because arrogance may seriously compromise their contribution to the society.

The world love child prodigies, the classical examples include Mozart, Beethoven, Albert Einstein, Ramanujan, Lata Mangeshkar, Zakir Hussain, Budhia Singh (who ran marathon from Puri to Bhubaneshwar at the age of 5 years). The exceptional children do need special attention, encouragement, better apportunities and facilities for flowering of their full potential but they must be protected against exploitation by their parents, trainers and teachers.

GOITER

The enlargement of thyroid gland (located below the Adam's apple) is called goiter. Goiter is more common in people living in hilly areas due to prevalence of iodine deficiency. Physiological goiter is common during adolescence because of increased demand for thyroxine or relative iodine deficiency. Other causes of goiter include infection (thyroiditis), defective thyroxine production (dyshormonogenesis), adenoma and rarely cancer.

Goiter may be associated with diminished, normal or increased production of thyroid secretions (thyrotoxicosis or Graves', disease). The child should be evaluated and managed by a pediatric endocrinologist. The incidence of goiter has considerably reduced because of universal iodization of common salt.

GREEN STOOLS

Many mothers are worried when their baby passes green stools. It may occur at the onset of diarrhea or during teething when stool frequency increases and bile is passed out unchanged. When a baby is taking vegetable soup or iron supplements, he may pass green or greenish-black stools. Stools (and even urine) may develop unusual red color, if a child takes excess of beetroots. When mother is breastfeeding, her diet may influence the color and consistency of the stools of her baby. When infant is mostly fed on foremilk, i.e. during each feed, the baby is fed from both the breasts without completely emptying any breast, he is likely to pass green stools. The foremilk (initial milk) is dilute with higher content of lactose which leads to rapid passage of stools which are likely to be green in color. Hindmilk (later milk) is rich in energy due to high fat content and when there is a balance between the intake of foremilk and hindmilk, the baby is likely to pass usual colored stools.

G

The passage of green-colored stools should not be a cause for concern because the condition usually settles spontaneously. Check whether diet of the baby (or nursing mother) and iron supplements may be discoloring the stools. During breastfeeding, mother should completely empty one breast before baby is moved on to the other breast. Apart from maintaining normal color of the stools, it is likely to be associated with better weight gain of the baby because hindmilk is rich in fat. Administration of probiotics is often associated with normalization of the color of stools.

GREY HAIR

Most mothers are worried to find one or two strands of grey hair with a lurking fear of premature greying of hair. Melanocytes in the root of hair produce a pigment called melanin which keeps the hair dark black in color. Depletion in production of melanin leads to greying of hair which usually starts at old age. There may be familial predisposition to develop premature grey hair. It may occur due to chronic illness (recurrent colds and sinusitis) or undernutrition. Anxiety, tension, stress and fear may trigger the development of grey hair. Exposure to sunrays is an important cause of early greying of hair. The use of unsuitable or poor quality soap and shampoo may cause premature greying of hair. Isolated grey hair should be ignored and they may not progress. A forelock of grey hair may be seen in vitiligo (leukoderma) and certain developmental disorders (partial albinism).

Treatment Associated scalp conditions like dandruff, alopecia (baldness) and nutritional deficiencies should be treated. Administration of high protein diet with multivitamins including vitamin B_{12}, iron, copper, iodine, calcium pantothenate may provide some benefit. If parents and child are worried by excessive grey hair, they can be masked by using a hair dye or herbal *mehndi* (henna) powder.

Home Remedies

- Mix Indian gooseberry (*Amla*) powder with coconut oil (or almond oil) and lime juice and massage the scalp with it. Leave it on for one hour before washing it off.
- Boil dried pieces of *Amla* in coconut oil and massage it on the scalp and keep it on overnight. Soak *Amla* in water overnight and use the water for washing the hair in the morning.
- Fry some curry leaves in coconut oil till they turn dark. Cool them, and massage them on the scalp and leave overnight.
- Massage scalp with margosa (*neem*) oil and leave it on overnight followed by hair wash with a herbal shampoo.
- Prepare strong black tea and add a teaspoon of common salt in a half cup. Massage the scalp with it and leave it on for at least one hour before washing it off.

GROWING PAINS

Children between 2 and 10 years of age often complain of pain in the legs (usually calf muscles) especially during the evening or night. The child is healthy, active and playful. Pain is usually due to fatigue because of excessive play activity throughout the day. Because children are actively growing during this period and pain is benign, the condition is often labeled as "growing pains". Hot water bath and massage are useful to provide relief. When discomfort is marked, a safe analgesic, like paracetamol, provides prompt relief. The presence of associated nutritional anemia and vitamin deficiencies should be treated. When aches and pains are present at multiple body sites, e.g. legs, arms, chest, abdomen and head, it is usually suggestive of a psychological or emotional disorder. When pain is localized to the joints or bones, it should be evaluated by a doctor and investigated to identify the cause.

Halitosis (*see* Bad breath)

HANDEDNESS

Most individuals are right-handed (dominant brain being on the left side) but around 10% of individuals are left-handed. The exact cause of left-handedness is not known but there is some genetic predisposition. When one of the parents is left handed, there is 17% chance of their child being left-handed and when both parents are left-handed, the probability increases to 50%. Left-handedness is more common in boys than girls. Most left-handers are intellectually bright (with greater mathematical capabilities) though the incidence of stuttering and learning difficulties is higher. Majority of left-handed children are also able to use right hand with fair dexterity (mixed handers or ambidextrous).

Handedness is usually established by the age of 4 years. No coercive or punitive methods should be used to force the child to use right hand, if biologically he is destined to be left-handed. The parental tactics would never succeed but may lead to emotional disturbances. The child should be allowed to evolve and express himself the way nature has designed or destined him. Some eminent scientists, artists, and statesmen of the world including Albert Einstein, Alexander the Great, Napolean Bonaparte, Leonardo da Vinci, Hellen Keller, Beethoven, Bill Clinton, cine megastar Amitabh Bachchan and legendary cricketer Sachin Tendulkar (ambidextrous) have been lefties. But the world caters to the needs of the majority, i.e. right-handers, while the left-handers are allowed to fend for themselves by adapting and adjusting to use the daily utility goods that are created for the convenience of right-handers. A store in London has taken up the cause of lefties and sells a variety of articles which are convenient to use by the southpaws.

HEAD BANGING

Some children may start banging their head to the floor after they learn sitting or crawling. They may rock their body or roll their head on the cot from side-to-side leading to loss of hair. These may be symptoms of boredom, stress, anxiety, headache, discomfort of teething, irritation in the ears or a symptom of visual or hearing loss. It may be a feature of low intelligence or an early symptom of autism spectrum disorder. Rocking of the body from forward to backward and rolling of head from side-to-side may be a symptom of self-stimulation akin to thumb sucking or fiddling with genitals. Many a times it is difficult to identify the underlying cause of rocking of the body and banging of the head and both may co-exist.

Body rocking and head banging is usually transient and disappears in due course of time. The child should be provided with greater interaction and play activities to reduce boredom and stress. When condition is severe and persistent, the child should be assessed by a developmental psychologist to exclude mental subnormality and autism spectrum disorder. Hearing and vision of the child should be checked.

HEADACHE

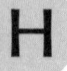

Headache is a common complaint in school going children. It occurs most commonly as a non-specific symptom in association of fever due to any cause (viral fever, tonsillitis, malaria, typhoid, etc.). Exposure to sun or hot 'environment' may cause headache. Headache may occur due to diseases of the organs of the head and face, i.e. brain, eyes, ear–nose–throat (ENT), and teeth. When headache occurs in school, after completing homework or watching TV, it may be due to defective vision or fatigue of muscles of the eyes due to their malalignment (squint). Headache in association with frequent cough and colds with persistent purulent nasal discharge is usually due to sinusitis. Caries teeth may be diagnosed because of headache. Episodes of early morning headache with vomiting is suggestive of raised intracranial pressure due to any cause. Triad of fever, headache and vomiting of acute or sudden onset is suggestive of meningitis. Migraine typically causes episodes of one-sided headache which runs in certain families (refer to migraine for details). Headache due to stress, tension and high blood pressure is less likely in children.

Treatment Most headaches in association with fever are self-limited and disappear when fever resolves. Paracetamol and ibuprofen are safe and effective analgesics for providing symptomatic relief. Headache with aches and pains at multiple body sites is usually psychological or attention seeking behaviour. When headache is frequent and severe or persistent, the child must be taken to the pediatrician. Depending upon the associated symptoms and likely cause, a further consultation is often required with an ophthalmologist, ENT specialist, dentist, and neurologist.

Home Remedies

- Head massage with a soothing oil is useful to relieve headache. In general, mustard or sesame oil or *til* oil is best in winter while coconut or olive oil is recommended in summer. Massage should be done with firm fingers and hand by using rhythmic motions for 10–15 minutes.
- In a child with fever, cold compresses on forehead with water containing eau de cologne promptly relieves headache.
- Holy basil (*tulsi*) leaves pounded with sandalwood powder and made into a paste with water, can be applied on the forehead.
- A paste of 10–12 cloves (*laung*) can be made with milk containing little salt and applied on the forehead and temples.
- Massage of the feet with kneading strokes over the toes and the adjacent sole area, exerts pressure on some pressure points, which is often followed by relief of headache.

HEAD INJURY

Most head injuries at home are minor. The infant may fall from a cot or from the lap of the mother or a maid. *The common practice of tossing an infant in the air or shaking his head vigorously, are dangerous and should be avoided.* The brain of the infant is smaller than the volume of his head cavity and it may get bruised against skull bones when baby is tossed or shaken. Toddlers and older children may get injured by using a walker, falling from the stairs or while flying kites, on the roof top.

First-aid When head injury is associated with bleeding from the nose or ear, vomiting, temporary loss of consciousness or convulsions, he must be taken to a hospital for observation and management. When none of the above mentioned symptoms of serious level injury are present, the child can be given paracetamol for relief of pain. A cold pack can be applied over the site of injury to reduce leakage of blood and bruising. Avoid use of any sedative, as it would interfere with evaluation of consciousness of the child.

Sometimes the effects of head injury become apparent after a few hours or days. When a child is not feeling his normal self and has become drowsy or refuses to eat, or is having headache and/or vomiting on the next day, he should be taken to a pediatrician. The presence of a bump or swelling over the head (without other symptoms) should not be a cause for concern. The swelling is likely to disappear spontaneously in due course of time and there is no need to do hot fomentation.

HEAD LICE

Head lice are common in children especially those living in crowded or unhygienic conditions. These parasites are transmitted from one child to the other or from an adult (maid or caretaker) infested with lice. They can occur due to sharing of combs or hair brushes. Lice do not thrive on pets and do not infest the furniture. The common symptoms include itching of scalp and formation of red bumps on the scalp and neck. The presence of live lice, which can be seen in good day light, confirms the diagnosis. The lice may be seen sticking on the comb or they may fall on the ground during combing. The eggs of lice or nits may be seen as tiny white oval-shaped specks that are attached to the sides of hair.

Treatment Shampoo and comb hair daily and maintain a good standard of personal hygiene. Many preparations containing DDT, lorexane and permethrin or pyrethrins are available which can be used as advised by your doctor. After shampooing when hair are still wet, apply the antilice lotion thoroughly in the scalp the way you apply oil in the hair. Leave it on for 15–20 minutes by covering the scalp with a shower cap and rinse the hair thoroughly taking care that the effluent does not enter into the eyes of the child. When hair are still wet, do combing with a fine bristled comb to remove dead lice and nits. Two treatment protocols at an interval of 7–10 days are adequate to provide cure. It is essential to comb the hair with a fine bristled comb for several days to remove all the nits, otherwise they will hatch the lice again. Daily shampooing and coombing of hair is mandatory to prevent reinfestation. Clothing, towels and bed linen should be washed in hot water and dried under bright sun. Adult member/s of the family or caretaker who is harbouring lice should be treated simultaneously to eradicate the menace.

HEALTHY LIFESTYLE

Parents should encourage children to consume whole grains, green leafy vegetables, fresh seasonable fruits, nuts, seeds and fat-free milk and dairy products. Intake of junk food, cola drinks and tetra-pack juices should be avoided. Water is the best drink and should be consumed in plenty. When a processed snack is unavoidable, you should check the nutrition fact label and follow the "0–2–10 rule" before buying it. The "rule" states that a healthy food choice should contain 0 g trans fat, 2 g or less saturated fat and 10 g or less of sugar. In addition, the child should be encouraged to have daily one hour of outdoor physical activity and limit "screen time" on video games, iPhone, iPad, television or computer to a maximum of two hours in a day.

HEARING

Hearing can be assessed by carefully watching the child for his responses to various sounds. Sudden loud sound may produce a "startle" response, blinking of eyes or change in the activity of the neonate. As the child grows, he will respond to banging of the door, sound of music (showing alertness or dancing movements) noise of an aeroplane, roar of a car or scooter engine, etc. Around 4 months of age, the child would turn towards the sound of a rattle, temple bell, alarm clock or beating of a metallic plate with a spoon. After one year, the child responds to his name when called from a distance or from a different room. Children with autism and mental subnormality may not show normal response to sound even when their hearing is normal.

In high-risk children (premature or sick newborn, severe jaundice during first week of life, family history of deafness), hearing is routinely tested at 3 months of age. The various tests used for assessment of hearing in infants include brainstem evoked response audiometry (BERA), otoacoustic emissions (OAE) and behavioural audiometry. It is important to remember that adequate hearing capability is essential for development of normal speech. Early detection of hearing defect and provision of a hearing aid by 6 months of age is crucial for development of normal speech.

HEART DEFECTS

Congenital heart disease is defined as the structural defect of the heart which is present at the time of birth. About 6–8 per 1000 neonates are born with a cardiac malformation. The cardiac defect may be isolated or it may be associated with other extracardiac defects. There is greater risk to develop a congenital malformation when pregnant woman suffers from an infection or is exposed to certain drugs and X-rays during first 3 months (trimester) of pregnancy. Deficiency of folic acid during early gestation is associated with increased risk of neural tube defects, cleft lip and cardiac abnormalities. Cardiac defects are commonly present in children with chromosomal abnormalities specially Down syndrome. In a large majority of cases, no cause is found.

Children with congenital heart defect are broadly classified into 3 groups: (i) acyanotic (without cyanosis) due to left-to-right shunt, (ii) cyanotic (blueness of lips, tongue and nails) because of right-to-left shunt, and (iii) obstructive lesions which may be cyanotic or acyanotic and usually manifests with shock. The manifestations of cardiac defect may occur during fetal life, at birth or later in life, or it may not have any symptoms for several years. The outcome of cardiac malformations has significantly improved by virtue of an early and correct diagnosis with the help of 2D echocardiography and blood flow or Doppler studies.

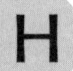

Treatment The child should be given calorie-dense feeds to reduce the physical strain of feeding and promote growth. Iron supplements are given to maintain hemoglobin. Infection should be identified early and managed promptly. Heart failure is managed with furosemide, digoxin and ACE inhibitor like captopril. In some cardiac malformations, prostaglandins are life-saving to maintain the patency of ductus arteriosus. In some cases of small to moderate ventricular saptal defect (VSD), the muscular defect may close spontaneously by 2–3 years of age. In preterm babies with patent ductus arteriosus (PDA), the defect can be closed by administration of indomethacin or ibuprofen. A number of congenital cardiac malformations can be managed with non-invasive percutaneous cardiac interventions. Due to advances in the open heart surgery, a large umber of cardiac defects can be corrected surgically. Stem cell therapy is being tried in children with cardiac ischemia or cardiomyopathy. In end-stage heart disease, heart transplantation has been used in selected advanced cardiac centers.

HEAT EXHAUSTION

Heat exhaustion occurs due to depletion of water and electrolytes during hot and humid summer months. There is mild to moderate elevation of body temperature (up to 100.5°F), with nausea, weakness, fatigue, muscle cramps and headache. The low-grade fever may continue for several days. The sweating mechanism remains intact and child does not develop hyperthermia.

Treatment The patient should be kept indoors in a cool air conditioned room. The child should be given plenty of cold drinks (water with fresh lime and salt, coconut water, *lassi*, butter-milk or *chhaj*, and ORS). Avoid intake of caffeine-containing drinks like coke, tea and coffee, which are likely to cause excessive urination.

HEAT STROKE

When body temperature goes up (hyperthermia) due to elevated environmental temperature in summer, it is called heat stroke. The body temperature goes above 105°F (hyperpyrexia) because of exhaustion or failure of sweating mechanism of the body. Reduced intake of fluids compromises sweating mechanism and predisposes to development of hyperthermia.

There is hyperpyrexia with virtual lack of sweating and dry skin. Headache, dizziness, drowsiness, confusion, disorientation and delirium are common. In advanced cases, convulsions and coma may occur. All the vital organs of the body may be affected. There may be laboratory evidences of renal dysfunction and gross elevation of hepatic transaminases.

Treatment Heat stroke is a medical emergency and child should be taken to the hospital while instituting cooling measures during the journey. All the clothes should be removed and the victim should be given plenty of cold fluids, if he is able to drink. The patient should be kept in an air-conditioned room. The body temperature should be brought down promptly by hydrotherapy with ice cold water, cooling blanket or by placing the child in a tub containing ice cold water. *There is no role of antipyretic agents because there is no alteration in the thermo-regulatory set point in hypothalamus.* Dehydration should be promptly corrected by intravenous administration of glucose-saline solution.

Prevention During hot summer months, the clothes should be loose and light-colored and made of cotton. Children should be kept indoors and play activity should be restricted to early morning or late evening when environmental temperature is comfortable. *Infants should never be kept locked in a car during shopping sprees.* During summer, adequate intake of fluids, and electrolytes should be ensured to promote perspiration and cooling of the body.

HEMATEMESIS

When vomitus is tinged or mixed with blood, the condition is called as hematemesis. The blood-tinged vomiting most commonly occurs after an episode of nasal bleeding (epistaxis) because of swallowing of blood. Gastritis due to intake of certain drugs (aspirin, NSAIDs, theophylline) is an important cause of hematemesis. Massive hematemesis most commonly occurs due to portal hypertension which is associated with marked enlargement of spleen. Rarely, hematemesis in a child may occur from peptic ulcer (*Helicobacter pylori* infection). The child with hematemesis should be taken to the hospital unless it is merely a blood-tinged vomiting because of preceding episode of epistaxis.

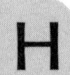

HEMATOMA

A localized collection of blood under the skin or in an internal organ either spontaneously or following an injury (trauma) is called hematoma. There is development of soft swelling with bluish discoloration of skin. In children with a bleeding disorder (like hemophilia or low platelet count), hematoma may occur spontaneously or following a minor injury. Whenever there is a blunt injury or a bump, immediate application of a cold pack and gentle pressure reduces the risk of development of hematoma. When hematoma has formed, it will resolve spontaneously during a few days or weeks when extravasated blood will get reabsorbed back into the circulation. There is no role of alternating hot and cold fomentation for early resolution of hematoma.

HEMATURIA

The passage of blood in urine is called hematuria. It is uncommon in children. The commonest cause of hematuria is acute glomerulonephritis (AGN) after an episode of streptococcal throat infection which has been ignored or ineffectively treated. Other causes include stone in the urinary system (kidneys, ureter, bladder or urethra), urinary tract infection (especially cystitis), vascular malformation, trauma and tumor. Hematuria may occur as a symptom of generalized coagulation or bleeding disorder.

The sudden onset of swelling (puffiness of face, swelling of feet), passage of reduced quantity of pink or tea-colored urine and elevation of blood pressure are suggestive of AGN. Renal stone is characterized by severe colicky pain (which starts from kidney region or loin and radiates towards genitals) with pain and discomfort in passing urine. The child with hematuria must be taken to a pediatric nephrologist for evaluation and management. Treatment is symptomatic and supportive depending upon the underlying cause. Antibiotics are given for treatment of cystitis. Surgery is required for removal of tumor and renal stones.

HEMOPHILIA

Hemophilia is a sex-linked or X-linked genetic disorder wherein boys suffer with bleeding manifestations while girls are carriers of defective gene and do not manifest any symptoms. There is deficiency of clotting factors, such as factor VIII (Hemophilia A or classic hemophilia) or factor IX (Hemophilia B or Christmas disease).

In severe cases, bleeding manifestations may occur at birth due to birth trauma, bleeding from umbilical stump or during circumcision. The bleeding may occur spontaneously or because of minor injury. There may be subcutaneous collection of blood (blue patches on the skin) or hematoma in the muscles. Bleeding into the joint/s (hemarthrosis) is the characteristic feature of hemophilia and commonly involves knees, elbows and ankles. Bleeding may occur from gums, teeth or nose (epistaxis) and rarely from internal organs of the body. The child with a bleeding disorder must be examined and investigated by a pediatric hematologist.

Treatment The child with hemophilia needs constant supervision at home and school to prevent injuries. He should be advised to wear helmets and protective padding gears over the knees and elbows during sports and play activities. He should not participate in contact sports, like football, hockey, boxing and wrestling. He can participate in individual sports, like swimming, cycling, golf, squash, table tennis and badminton. Intramuscular injections should be avoided and all vaccines should be administered subcutaneously. Administration of aspirin and NSAIDs may aggravate bleeding by adversely affecting functioning of platelets and should be avoided. The child must be protected against hepatitis B infection by effective vaccination before administration of any blood or blood products. When injury occurs, subcutaneous hematoma and hemarthrosis should be controlled by rest, application of ice pack, compression and elevation of limb. Early administration of factor VIII concentrate can reduce the severity of bleeding. Surgical procedure should be undertaken only after correction of factor VIII deficiency.

Prevention When mother is a carrier of hemophilia gene, 50% of her sons are likely to suffer from hemophilia while 50% daughters would be carriers. When father is suffering from hemophilia, all daughters will be carriers while all sons will be normal. It is possible to make antenatal diagnosis of hemophilia by chorionic villus sampling if mother is a carrier of hemophilia gene. When fetus is found to be hemophiliac, medical termination of pregnancy can be offered to the family.

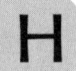

HEMOPTYSIS

When sputum or phlegm is blood-tinged, the condition is called as hemoptysis. The symptom is rare in children because they usually swallow the phlegm which is passed out in the stools. In older children or adolescents, when low grade fever and loss of appetite are associated with bouts of coughing with passage of blood-tinged sputum, it is highly suggestive of tuberculosis of lungs. The diagnosis is confirmed by examination of two specimens of sputum for acid-fast bacilli by Ziehl-Neelsen stain. Rarely, children with bronchiectasis, pneumonia, lung abscess and severe mitral stenosis may have hemoptysis.

HERNIA

The protrusion of intestines through a gap in the abdominal wall is called hernia. There is a boggy soft swelling which becomes small or may disappear on lying down and by gentle pressure. There is no pain or discomfort except when it becomes irreducible or obstructed because of excessive size or narrowing of the abdominal gap. Rarely hernia may get strangulated when intestinal loops get twisted. Obstructed hernia is characterized by severe colicky pain, persistent vomiting and constipation. Strangulated hernia is a medical emergency, apart from symptoms of obstruction, there is risk of development of gangrene of the gut because of obstruction of the blood supply.

Umbilical Hernia

It is a common condition in neonates and infants. The intestines protrude through the navel or umbilicus like a tinny balloon when baby cries or strains. The presence of cough or constipation may increase the size of swelling. The swelling can be reduced by gentle pressure. Umbilical hernia is more common in infants with poor tone of muscles, like protein-energy malnutrition, congenital hypothyroidism (cretinism) and rickets.

Umbilical hernia closes spontaneously in a few months time as the baby's abdominal muscles grow. There is no risk of obstruction or strangulation in umbilical hernia. The associated cough and constipation or any underlying disease should be treated. The cultural practice of placing a coin over it and strapping or bandaging it, is condemned as it may further weaken the abdominal wall and increase the risk of strangulation of the protruding loops of intestines. Surgical correction is rarely indicated except when hernia is extremely large in size and it persists beyond 2 years of age.

Inguinal Hernia

Herniation of intestines into the scrotal sac through the inguinal canal in the groin is called inguinal hernia. There is a soft boggy swelling in the groin which appears on crying and straining and disappears during sleep or lying down. The intestines can be pushed back into the abdomen by gentle pressure. The hernia may be on one side or both sides. It may be associated with undescended testis. Inguinal hernia is associated with a serious risk of obstruction and strangulation and should be operated by a pediatric surgeon as early as possible. The inguinal canal is repaired on both sides to reduce the risk of recurrence of hernia.

HICCUPS

Hiccups are produced by spasmodic contractions of diaphragm (muscular partition that separates chest from abdomen). There are sudden noisy and jerky retractions of the upper abdomen and notches at the upper and lower ends of chest bone (sternum) with audible sounds or hiccups. Hiccups may occur in the womb before baby is born. Among neonates, hiccups usually occur immediately after a feed due to distension of stomach and irritation of the diaphragm. Most grandmothers will tell you that hiccups are good and they indicate that the "baby is growing". Nothing needs to be done and hiccups disappear spontaneously after a few minutes.

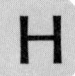

Hiccups are more common in children than adults. They are usually benign and self-limiting. According to old wives' tales, when you develop hiccups, someone in your family is talking or thinking about you. In children, hiccups may occur by eating too fast (gulping air while eating) or by over eating. Intake of hot, spicy and acidic foods may trigger hiccups by causing irritation of food pipe (esophagus) and stomach. Excessive intake of tea, coffee, cola or carbonated drinks are common triggers for hiccups. Emotional stress and excitement may initiate and aggravate hiccups. Children with gastroesophageal reflux disease (GERD) are more prone to get episodes of hiccups. Intractable or persistent hiccups may occur due to intake of certain drugs, irritation of diaphragm due to pneumonia, liver abscess or a surgical procedure and accumulation of toxins because of renal failure. Disoders of central nervous system with involvement of brainstem and vagus nerve may cause intractable hiccups.

Most hiccups are benign and disappear spontaneously or can be aborted by simple home remedies. In intractable causes, the underlying cause should be identified and treated appropriately. Antacids, omeprazole, chlorpromazine and haloperidol are useful for treatment of persistent hiccups. Ketamine is useful for control of intractable hiccups.

Home Remedies

1. Most home remedies are based on distraction and holding the breath. Ask the child to take a deep breath and hold it as long as possible.
2. Drink a glass of cold water quickly or sip water slowly or count slowly without taking any breath.
3. Ask someone to tickle you or frighten you.
4. Put a teaspoon of sugar on the back of your tongue or suck a candy.
5. Put your fingers in the ears and gently wiggle them.
6. Pull out or tug your tongue by holding its tip with your thumb and index finger.
7. Ask the child to breathe into a paper bag (not a plastic bag which can stick against your face and cause choking).

Hives (*see* Urticaria)

HYDROCELE

The collection of fluid around one or both testes is called hydrocele. The scrotal sac may appear tense and boggy, and testis may not be palpable on the affected side. Unlike hernia, the swelling cannot be reduced by pressure or on lying down. Hydrocele is common in healthy newborns (especially premature babies) and usually disappears spontaneously by 3 months of age. Rarely, hydrocele may occur in an older child due to trauma, torsion of testis, inflammation of the epididymis and testis (epididymo-orchitis) and filariasis. In these conditions, hydrocele resolves on treatment of the underlying condition. When hydrocele is persistent, it is drained and surgically repaired as in the case of hernia.

HYDROCEPHALUS

There is excessive accumulation of cerebrospinal fluid (CSF) in the ventricles of the brain leading to excessive increase in the size of head. This may occur either because of excessive production or poor drainage of CSF. The child may be born with hydrocephalus due to block in the ventricles of the brain or it may be acquired later in life as a consequence of infection of the central nervous system (pyogenic or tubercular meningitis).

The head size is large with over hanging or prominent forehead and skull bones are widely separated. The anterior fontanel is large

H

in size and bulging. Veins may be prominent over the forehead and face. The eyes are often rolled downward so that the white part (sclera) of the eye is visible below the upper eyelid (sun-setting appearance). Depending upon the underlying cause, hydrocephalus may be associated with neuromotor retardation, defective vision, seizures and mental subnormality. Several surgical procedures are available to "shunt off" extra CSF into the abdominal cavity or venous system. Early operation gives good results, if it is done before occurrence of brain damage. The procedure may have to be revised as the child grows.

Hyperhidrosis (*see* Excessive sweating)

HYPOTHERMIA

Hypothermia or fall in body temperature is common in premature, low birth weight and sick newborns. These infants have a large surface area with excessive heat loss, poor muscular activity and poor capability to generate body heat. When a baby is born in winter, there is a risk of development of hypothermia unless due precautions are taken to keep the baby warm. The baby should be effectively clothed and covered with woolens from top to toes. The head size of the baby is relatively large and must be covered with a cap to reduce heat loss. Socks and mittens should be worn. The room should be kept warm with the use of a heater, hot air blower or a oil-filled radiator. The windows should be kept closed so that there is no draught of cold air in the room. Body massage should be delayed till baby is at least 3.0 kg in weight. The room temperature (>28°C) that feels slightly warm or uncomfortable to an adult, is best suited to serve the biological needs of the baby. Mother can assess the temperature of her baby by touching the skin of trunk, hands and feet. In a healthy and effectively protected baby, the trunk should feel warm, hands and feet should be reasonably warm and pink in color. When trunk is cold to touch, the infant has serious hypothermia and needs urgent medical attention. When trunk is relatively warm to touch but hands and feet are cold, the baby has cold stress and must be effectively covered and provided warmth. The baby in cold stress may develop intercurrent infection and will not have satisfactory weight gain because energy is being wasted for metabolic heat production and denied for physical and mental growth.

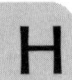

IMMUNIZATIONS

A large number of infectious diseases that can cause disability or death can be prevented by timely administration of safe and effective vaccines. Vaccines are the greatest boon of modern medicine and one of the most effective public health investments. It is a moral obligation on the part of all parents to cooperate with public health authorities to ensure that their children receive all the vaccines in accordance with the recommended national schedule under the guidance and supervision of their pediatrician or family physician.

When a vaccine is administered, it stimulates the immunological system of the body to produce protective antibodies and sensitize the protective cells of the body to mount a fight when the body is invaded by disease-causing microbes. The subsequent or booster doses of vaccines provide an enhanced antibody response because of excellent memory of the immunological system. When a child who has been effectively protected by a vaccine is exposed to the wild microbes through natural infection, he or she is able to fight the assault with complete success or may manifest mild or modified disease without any serious illness or disability.

The vaccines should be taken as per the recommended immunization schedule (see **Box**). However, when a shot is missed, the previously administered dose(s) of vaccine remain valid and there is no need to restart the vaccination schedule. In infants and preschool children, vaccines are administered into the outer side of mid-thigh region while in school going children, they can be given into the outer side of upper arm (deltoid region). The vaccines should never be injected into the buttocks or gluteal region because of poor absorption of vaccine due to thick pad of fat and the potential risk of causing damage to the sciatic nerve. It is important that the parents must keep the vaccination record of their child in safe custody. It is an important document for the doctor and school health authorities.

Side effects By and large most vaccines are safe and they do not produce any side effects. The side effects seen with some of the common vaccines are listed in the **Box**. The common side effects of fever, pain and discomfort can be controlled by administration of paracetamol. Whenever there is an adverse reaction to the administration of the first dose of a vaccine, this fact must be brought to the notice of the doctor or nurse before second dose is administered. The vaccines are highly cost-effective and baby-friendly and no child should be denied the benefits of available vaccines. It must be remembered that exclusive breastfeeding during first 6 months of life and timely administration of all vaccines are crucial to protect children against a variety of life-threatening infectious diseases.

Recommended vaccination schedule		
Age	Vaccine	Dose
	Essential vaccines	
Birth to 2 wk	BCG	Single dose
	OPV[a]	1st dose
	HBV	1st dose
6 – 8 wk	DTwP or DTaP + Hib + IPV	1st dose
	OPV	2nd dose
	HBV	2nd dose
10 – 12 wk	DTwP or DTaP + Hib + IPV	2nd dose
	OPV	3rd dose
14 – 16 wk	DTwP or DTaP + Hib + IPV	3rd dose
	OPV	4th dose
6 mo	HBV	3rd dose (may be given along with 3rd dose of DTP)
9 mo	MMR vaccine	1st dose

(Contd.)

Recommended vaccination schedule (*Contd.*)

Age	Vaccine	Dose
	Essential vaccines	
15 – 18 mo	MMR	2nd dose
	DTwP or DTaP + Hib + IPV	1st booster
	OPV	5th dose
After 2 y	Typhoid vaccine[b]	Boosters every 3 y
4.5 – 5 y	DTwP or DTaP	2nd booster
	OPV	7th dose[a]
	Chickenpox booster	
	HBV booster	
10 y	Tdap or Td or TT booster[c]	Every 10 y
Optional vaccines after one-to-one discussion with parents who can afford		
6 – 8 wk	Rotavirus vaccine + pneumococcal vaccine	1st dose
10 – 12 wk	Rotavirus vaccine + pneumococcal vaccine	2nd dose
14 – 16 wk	Pneumococcal vaccine	3rd dose
12 mo	HAV	Two doses at an interval of 6 mo – 1 y. Attenuated live vaccine (Biovac A) is available which is given in a single dose
15 mo	Pneumococcal vaccine	Booster
	Chickenpox vaccine	Single dose up to 12 y, subsequently two doses 4 – 8 wk apart. A booster dose is being recommended after the age of 5 y
10 – 12 y	HPV	Two doses at 0, and 6 mo during 9–14 years. After 14 years, three doses are given at 0, 1 or 2 and 6 mo.

(Contd.)

Vaccines during special situations (*Contd.*)

- IPV (injectable or inactivated polio vaccine) is given to immuno-compromised or HIV-positive children. It is being administered routinely as a part of post-polio-eradication policy.
- Meningococcal vaccine during an epidemic, Haj pilgrims, sickle cell disease and CSF rhinorrhea. Polysaccharide vaccine is given in a single dose after 2 y followed by boosters every 3 y.
- Pneumococcal polysaccharide vaccine, that is, PPV 23 (chronic lung and heart disease, sickle cell disease, splenectomy, nephrotic syndrome, and immunocompromised child) is given as a single dose or maximum of 2 doses.
- Influenza vaccine is given to children with bronchial asthma, congestive heart failure and immunocompromised child. Initially two doses (single dose is given in children >9 y) are given 4 wk apart after the age of 6 mo, followed by yearly boosters at the onset of rainy season.
- Antirabies vaccine (high-risk individuals, following animal bites).
- Cholera vaccine to control epidemics, visitors to *kumbh mela*, Haj pilgrims.
- Japanese B encephalitis vaccine (endemic areas, during epidemics) is administered (0.5 mL 1 – 3 y, 1.0 mL 3 – 10 y SC) in three primary doses 0, 7, 30 d, booster at 1 y followed by boosters every 3 y.
- Yellow fever is mandatory for travelers to South Africa. It is given as a single dose (>6 mo age) followed by boosters every 10 y. Avoid during pregnancy.

Abbreviations: BCG, Bacillus Calmette-Guérin; CSF, cerebrospinal fluid; d, day(s); DTaP, diphtheria, tetanus and acellular pertussis; DTP, diphtheria tetanus and pertussis (whooping cough); DTwP, diphtheria-tetanus-whole cell pertussis; HAV, hepatitis A vaccine; HBV, hepatitis B vaccine; Hib *Haemophilus influenzae* type B; HPV, human papillomavirus; IPV, inactivated polio vaccine; MMR, measles, mumps and rubella; mo, month(s); OPV, oral polio vaccine; PCV 13, 13-valent pneumococcal conjugated vaccine; PPV 23, 23-valent pneumococcal polysaccharide vaccine; TT, tetanus toxoid; DT, diphtheria toxoid; Tdap, tetanus toxoid with low-dose diphtheria and pertussis; wk, week(s); y, year(s).

[a]Additional doses of oral polio vaccine given under pulse immunization program must be taken by all children below the age of 5 years.

[b]Vi capsular polysaccharide *S. typhi* type 2 conjugated to tetanus toxoid (Typbar TCV) can be given during 9–12 months followed by a single booster at 2 years of age for lifelong protection.

[c]Pregnant woman must receive two doses of TT or Td at 4 weeks interval. The second dose should be taken at least 4 weeks before delivery.

Common side effects of vaccines

Vaccine	Side effects[a]
BCG	A nodule appears 3–4 wk after BCG vaccination. It may soften or ulcerate during next 2–4 wk. No local application or fomentation is necessary. It heals by formation of a thin scar, indicating good "take" for effective vaccination.
DTwP or DTaP	There may be fever with pain, redness and swelling at the site of injection. A small painless nodule may remain for a few days. Sterile abscess may rarely develop. No local application or fomentation is required. DTaP is safer and produces fewer side effects but is less immunogenic. Paracetamol is useful for relief of fever and pain, but it may reduce the immunological response.
Oral polio and rotavirus vaccine	No side effects**
Hib vaccine	Fever, local pain and redness
Pneumococcal vaccine	Fever, local pain, redness, and swelling
Measles/MMR	Some children may develop fever and mild skin rash 7–10 d after the vaccination. A child with egg allergy may show an adverse reaction to MMR vaccine.
Hepatitis B vaccine	Pain and redness at the site of injection. Some children with yeast allergy may show adverse reaction.
Typhoid vaccine	Local pain, fever, malaise and headache may occur. Oral typhoid vaccine may cause vomiting, diarrhea and abdominal pain in some children.
Chickenpox vaccine	Fever and mild papulovesicular skin eruption may occur rarely.
Human papillomavirus vaccine	Local pain, redness, swelling, fever and syncope

Abbreviations: BCG, Bacillus Calmette-Guérin; d, days; DTaP, diphtheria, tetanus, and acellular pertussis; DTwP, diphtheria-tetanus-whole cell pertussis; Hib, *Haemophilus influenzae* type B; MMR, mumps, measles, rubella; wk, weeks.

(Contd.)

Common side effects of vaccines *(Contd.)*

[a]Before giving the next dose of vaccine, ask the mother if the child had any significant reaction to the last dose of vaccine. Allergic reactions may occur with any vaccine but are most common with Japanese encephalitis and yellow fever vaccines.

[b]Oral polio vaccine-related paralytic poliomyelitis is being increasingly reported from developed countries. These countries have changed their strategy and are giving inactivated polio vaccine. Rotavirus vaccine has a potential risk of causing intussusception in susceptible children or when vaccine is administered after the age of 6 months.

IMPERFORATE ANUS

Some infants are born with a flat perineum without any anal opening because of maldevelopment of anorectal canal. In male infants, the anomaly is usually "high" while in girls it is usually "low" in location. In "high" anomaly, there is no dimple or anal impulse when baby cries. "High" anomaly may be associated with a fistula with urinary bladder or urethra, so that meconium (stool of neonate) is passed through urethra along with urine. About one-third infants with imperforate anus have additional congenital defects in the urinary system, heart and sacrum. Lateral invertogram or cross-table X-ray of the infant with elevated buttocks (knee-chest position) is useful to find whether the anomaly is "high" or "low".

Perineum should be carefully examined for the site and size of anal opening in all newborns at birth. In a case of "low" anomaly, modified cut-back operation is done as soon as possible. In "high" anomaly, emergency colostomy is done to provide a conduit for the passage of stools. After 6–8 weeks, definitive corrective surgery is done and colostomy is closed. After 2 weeks of definitive surgery, daily dilatation of the newly created anorectal canal is advised. Efforts should be made to prevent both constipation as well as diarrhea and provide early toilet training to the infant.

INFECTIOUS DISEASES

Infectious diseases are a leading cause of morbidity (illness), disability and death in children. Infections may occur due to viruses, bacteria, spirochetes, fungi and parasites. Children are more prone to develop infectious illness because it is their first or nascent contact with the microbe, they lack protective antibodies and have suboptimal immune defence mechanisms. In most developed countries, the load of infectious diseases has been decreased by improving environmental sanitation, providing health education, safe drinking water, adequate living conditions with lack of overcrowding, enhancing host defences by improved nutrition and better practices in the hospitals to prevent patient-to-patient (nosocomial) or fomites to patients hospital-acquired infections (HAI). A large number of vaccine preventable infectious diseases have been controlled or virtually eliminated (smallpox, poliomyelitis) by universal immunization.

Modes of Spread of Infections

Infectious diseases are transmitted from an infected person to a susceptible host either directly or through an intermediate living host or vector (mosquitoes, rodents, animals) and non-living objects (fomites). The common modes of transmission of infections are listed below:

1. **Direct contact** Infected person transmits infection by close contact, i.e. skin infection and sexually transmitted diseases.
2. **Air-borne or droplet infection** Air-borne transmission of infection occurs by infected droplets or particles that remain suspended in the air following bouts of coughing, sneezing and talking. It is a common mode of infection in cases of cough and cold, viral infection, throat infection, exanthematous diseases and tuberculosis.
3. **Food and water-borne diseases** Contaminated water and food are important sources of infection causing episodes of food poisoning, diarrhea, dysentery, cholera, typhoid fever, viral hepatitis (HAV and HEV) and worm infestations.
4. **Living objects as intermediate hosts and vectors** A number of diseases are transmitted through intermediate hosts or vectors like mosquitoes (malaria, dengue fever, chikungunya, filaria, yellow fever, Japanese encephalitis), sandflies (Kala-azar), dogs (rabies, hydatid disease, leptospirosis), cats (toxoplasmosis, visceral larva migrans), chicken (bird flu, SARs), pigs (Japanese encephalitis, swine flu), cattle (anthrax) and rats (rat bite fever).
5. **Non-living objects or fomites** Direct contact with clothes (handkerchief, towel, sheet, bedding, etc.), medical and surgical instruments, injection needles, books, toys and utensils.

6. **Blood-borne infections** Infection may be transmitted through contaminated needles (abscess, HBV, HIV) and transfussion of infected blood or blood products (malaria, HBV, HCV, HIV, CMV).
7. **Placenta** Maternal infection may be transmitted to the fetus (mother-to-fetus vertical transmission) during pregnancy, labor and delivery (TORCH infections, HBV, HIV).

Duration of Infectivity of Exanthematous Illnesses of Children

Most exanthematous illnesses are highly contagious with an increased risk of infection to close contacts in the family or in a

Average duration of infectivity of common childhood infectious diseases

Disease	Period of infectivity
Chickenpox	One day before onset of skin rash, until 6 days after the rash or when scabs have formed. The scabs of chickenpox are not infective.
Measles	Five to six days before the onset of skin rash, until 5 d after the rash.
Mumps	Two days before onset of swelling of parotids, until swelling subsides (usually about 7 d).
Rubella[a]	One day before onset of skin rash, until 7 d after the onset of rash.
Diphtheria[b]	Two days before the onset of symptoms, until 2–4 wk after treatment.
Whooping cough	Two days before onset of symptoms, until 5 wk after the onset of cough.
Poliomyelitis	Three days before onset of symptoms, until 2 wk after paralysis.

Abbreviations: d, day(s); wk, week(s).

[a]Infant with congenital rubella syndrome can excrete virus for several months. School-going children should be encouraged to come in contact with a patient having rubella to develop natural infection (which is usually mild) and develop lifelong protection. However, it poses a potential risk to unvaccinated or susceptible married women because rubella infection during early pregnancy can lead to development of congenital rubella syndrome.

[b]Three consecutive throat cultures taken 24 hours apart should be negative before the patient is declared free of infection.

public place, like creche, play school, regular school, cinema hall, and public transport. The patient is most contagious before the actual onset of skin rash or symptoms. The risk of infection or exposure during this stage is thus unavoidable. After the onset of symptoms or appearance of skin rash, the period of infectivity varies depending upon the nature of the exanthematous illness (see **Box**). During the period of infectivity of the illness, the child should stay at home and should not go to school or any public place to reduce the risk of transmission of the disease to close contacts.

INSECT BITES

Mosquito bites may cause localized allergic reaction with itching and carry the risk of transmission of life-threatening diseases, like malaria, dengue fever, chikungunya and Japanese encephalitis. In some children with allergic background, mosquito bites may lead to development of generalized skin reaction (papular urticaria). Localized allergic reaction may occur due to bites because of ants and bed bugs. Wasp and hornet stings usually cause local pain, itching, stinging sensation and swelling. In allergic children, a severe hypersensitivity reaction or anaphylaxis, generalized urticaria and breathing difficulty may occur.

Treatment Local application of soothing lotion (containing calamine and camphor), or anesthetic cream and ice pack reduces irritation and itching. When sting is visible, it should be removed with a tweezer, blunt knife or a stiff plastic card. In case of multiple bites or severe reaction, paracetamol and an antihistaminic (phenergan, benadryl, atarax) can be given for relief of pain and itching. In a rare instance of generalized hypersensitivity reaction, the child should be rushed to the hospital. Anaphylaxis is treated by administration of epinephrine through intramuscular route.

Home Remedies

Application of baking powder or common salt dissolved in a few drops of water or vinegar, clarified butter (*desi ghee*), onion juice and honey provide prompt relief against irritation and itching.

INTELLIGENCE QUOTIENT (IQ)

Intelligence or cognition includes several parameters, like comprehension, analytical ability, reasoning, memory and attention span.

Several intelligence tests (like Stanford-Binet, Wechsler) have been devised to assess a wide range of abilities like language development, drawing capability, spatial concepts, numbers, non-verbal skills, reasoning, and memory. In India, culture-specific tests for intelligence have been devised by the Central Institute of Education, Research and Training. On the basis of results of the standardized intelligence test, the examiner can calculate the mental age of the child. The mental age of the child, when compared with his chronological age (actual age in years) and expressed as a percentage gives his intelligence quotient.

$$IQ = \frac{\text{Mental age}}{\text{Chronological age}} \times 100$$

When a child has neuromotor developmental delay or he is not doing well at school, the child should be examined by a developmental psychologist to assess his IQ. The child with an average mental ability has an IQ between 85 and 115. Children with an IQ of above 150 are exceptional or gifted children while an IQ of less than 50 is suggestive of mental retardation.

Apart from IQ, it is important to have a balanced outgoing personality, confidence, courage, self-esteem, enthusiasm, determination, easy adaptability, etc. which are expressed in terms of social, emotional and confidence quotients (SQ, EQ, CQ). Above all, there is a need to look for spiritual quotient (Sp. Q) by assessing qualities like mental peace, poise, balance of mind, compassion and human qualities of heart (rather than head alone) as a barometer of real success in life.

IN-TOEING (Pigeon-toed)

When a child walks or runs, the feet turn inwards (like a pigeon) instead of pointing straight forward. The child may stumble or trip by striking the toes of one foot against the heel of other. There is no discomfort but child may have an awkward gait. The condition affects both limbs but one side is affected more than the other. The condition usually runs in families and has hereditary basis. The condition occurs due to rotational problems of the bones of the lower extremities. Depending upon the site of bone affected, there are 3 variants of pigeon-toeing.

(i) *Inward bending of foot or curved foot* (*metatarsus adductus*). The child's feet bend inward from the middle part of foot like an incomplete club feet. In this variant, when defect is severe, physiotherapy, special shoes and corrective casts provide some relief.

(ii) *Inward twisting of shin bone* (*internal torsion of tibia*). In most cases, the condition self corrects as the child grows.

(iii) *Inward rotation of thigh bones* (*anteversion of thigh bone or femur*). There is some degree of overlapping of thighs and knock knees. Children with this condition often sit in the "W" position with their knees bent and their feet flared out behind their bums.

Treatment Most cases of intoeing resolve spontaneously as the child grows. There is no role of exercises, special shoes and braces. When there is severe bending of feet inward due to metatarsus adductus (akin to club foot), physiotherapy, special shoes and casts may help. When intoeing due to twisting of the thigh and leg bones is severe and persists beyond the age of 10 years and is causing difficulty in walking, surgical correction by an experienced orthopedic surgeon may be considered.

INTRAUTERINE GROWTH RETARDATION (IUGR)

When birth weight of a newborn is less than 10th percentile for the period of gestation, he is called as small-for-dates or small-for-gestational age. When a baby is small at birth, either he is born early (premature) or he is born at term but has suffered from intrauterine growth retardation or fetal malnutrition.

Causes The cause of IUGR may rest with the mother, placenta or fetus. The common causes of IUGR include poor health, nutrition (short and light mother), socioeconomic status of the mother and teenage pregnancy. It is important to remember that growth and well-being of the fetus depend upon the health and nutrition of the mother (not the father!) because she is both the seed as well as the soil where the baby is nurtured for 9 months. In developing countries, a large number of women are malnourished, light in weight and stunted and they are likely to produce small babies because of maternal ill health, frequent pregnancies and malnutrition. The other causes of IUGR include placental dysfunction (due to pregnancy-induced high blood pressure, toxemia of pregnancy), chronic systemic disease of the mother and maternal infections during pregnancy (like malaria, urinary tract infection and tuberculosis) and drug abuse, smoking and chewing tobacco. In about 10% cases, fetal malformations, developmental defects and intrauterine infections (TORCH infections) account for IUGR.

Clinical problems IUGR babies are more vulnerable to have birth asphyxia, passage of meconium *in utero* (respiratory distress due to aspiration of meconium), hypothermia and hypoglycemia. There is recent evidence to suggest that IUGR babies due to fetal malnutrition are at an increased risk to develop type 2 diabetes mellitus, high blood pressure and coronary artery disease later in adult life.

Prevention Adolescent girls should be given a balanced diet, and supplements of iron and calcium so that they are healthy and well-equipped to meet the nutritional demands of the fetus during pregnancy. The best strategy to improve the health and well-being of a nation is to provide education and balanced nutrition throughout the lifecycle (infancy, childhood, adolescence, pregnancy and lactation) of girls.

Management The fetus with IUGR is closely monitored by Doppler ultrasound for any evidence of fetal distress. Timely delivery is crucial to prevent fetal death and ensure intact survival of the baby. Optimal facilities for resuscitation should be available to manage meconium-stained and asphyxiated baby. Early and adequate feeding should be ensured to prevent hypoglycemia. The blood glucose should be monitored for early diagnosis and management of hypoglycemia. The baby should be dried promptly, covered effectively and kept under a radiant warmer to prevent hypothermia. These babies should be screened to identify any congenital malformation. They should be monitored for their physical growth and neuromotor development. Their initial weight gain is rapid but subsequently it slows down and they may not catch-up with normal babies.

INTRAUTERINE INFECTIONS (Fetal or TORCH infections)

During pregnancy, fetus is well protected in the womb against changes in the environmental temperature, light, sound, touch and various infections. Rarely when mother is infected, the pathogens may pass from maternal circulation to the placenta and enter fetal circulation. Intrauterine infections may occur due to viruses, *Toxoplasma gondii* a protozoan, spirochetes and occasionally by bacteria including *Mycobacterium tuberculosis*. They are popularly described with an acronym TORCH wherein T stands for toxoplasmosis, O for others (syphilis, gonococcal ophthalmia, tuberculosis, malaria, varicella, hepatitis B virus, coxsackie-B, Echo, parvovirus, HIV, etc.), R for rubella, C for cytomegalovirus and H for herpes simplex. The incidence of intrauterine infections is low and range between 0.5 and 2.0% of all births. Cytomegalovirus infection and rubella appear to be the most common intrauterine infections though incidence of HIV (AIDS) is gradually increasing.

Intrauterine infections may cause abortion or miscarriage, poor growth of the fetus (intrauterine growth retardation), bleeding manifestations, jaundice, enlargement of liver and spleen, congenital malformations, neuromotor disability due to involvement of the brain. Their treatment is unsatisfactory because most of the damage has already occurred before the baby is born.

JAUNDICE

Yellowness of eyes (due to elevation of serum bilirubin) and passage of high-colored or turmeric-colored urine is called jaundice. Jaundice usually occurs due to dysfunction of liver or hemolysis (breakdown) of red bed cells. Jaundice in the newborns has distinctive causes, different treatment modalities and outcome compared to older children.

Jaundice in Newborns

Almost two-thirds of healthy newborn babies develop yellow discoloration of skin and eyes on the second or third day of life. The jaundice increases during next 2–3 days and gradually subsides without any treatment between 10 and 14 days of life. It is called as "physiological jaundice" and it is harmless and it has nothing to do with infection or viral hepatitis. There is no role of exposing the baby to sunlight because it is ineffective and may cause damage to the delicate skin of the baby.

In some babies, severe and persistent jaundice may occur. The common causes of severe jaundice (serum bilirubin level >15 mg/dL or yellow staining of palms and soles) include blood group incompatibility between the mother and her baby (mother being Rh-negative and baby Rh-positive or mother having O group and baby either A or B group), G6PD deficiency and septicemia. In these cases, the jaundice may occur on the first day of life, there is marked elevation of serum bilirubin (>15 mg/dL) causing yellow staining of trunk, palms and soles and it persists beyond 2 weeks of age. Severe jaundice in the newborn has a potential risk of causing brain damage (kernicterus). These infants should be investigated in a hospital under the close supervision of a specialist dealing with newborns (neonatologist). Severe jaundice in a newborn baby is a medical emergency and is treated by placing the naked baby under special lights (phototherapy) and at times by completely changing baby's blood (exchange blood transfusion).

In some babies who are exclusively breastfed, the "physiological jaundice" becomes more intense and takes longer time to disappear (breast milk jaundice). In these babies, urine remains colorless like water and stools are normal yellow-colored. Jaundice disappears without any treatment but may take 6–10 weeks to wane off. In these babies, congenital hypothyroidism (cretinism) should be rulled out by doing proper investigations. When severe and persistent jaundice in the newborn and early infancy is associated with high-colored urine and clay-colored or pale white stools, it is suggestive of hepatitis or malformation of bile ducts and is associated with poor outcome.

Jaundice in Older Children

The common causes of jaundice in a child are listed below:

1. *Hepatic causes* The commonest cause of jaundice in a school going child is viral hepatitis, which may occur due to intake of contaminated water or food (Hepatitis A and E) or less commonly as blood-borne infection (Hepatitis B and C). Other hepatic causes of jaundice include intake of certain drugs (antitubercular drugs, paracetamol, anti-epilepsy medications, hormones, anabolic steroids), non-viral infections (amebic or pyogenic liver abscess, typhoid fever, tuberculosis, malaria, leptospirosis) and cirrhosis of liver.

2. *Hemolytic jaundice* Jaundice may occur due to acute hemolysis because of G6PD deficiency or chronic hemolysis due to hereditary spherocytosis and sickle cell disease.

3. *Obstructive jaundice* It is uncommon in children and is usually associated with itching, pale or clay-colored stools and elevation of direct-reacting or conjugated bilirubin in the blood. Obstructive jaundice may occur due to HEV-hepatitis, choledochal cyst, gallstones (due to chronic hemolysis) and cholangitis.

4. *Metabolic causes* It is a rare cause of jaundice and need specialized investigations.

Treatment Treatment of viral hepatitis is supportive and symptomatic. Physical activity should be restricted according to the capability of the patient but there is no need for strict bed rest. Diet should be palatable and balanced and in accordance with the liking of the child. Offer carbohydrate rich diet with plenty of fruits, fruit juices and sugar-rich food. There is no scientific basis for elimination of fat from the diet. A number of hepatoprotective drugs are available in Allopathic and Ayurvedic systems but they are of doubtful therapeutic utility. Vitamin B complex is useful to provide non-specific protection to the liver. Ursodeoxycholic acid, cholestyramine and antihistamines are useful to relieve itching due to stasis of bile in the liver.

JITTERY BABY

Some healthy newborn babies are jittery or tremulous on touch or handling. When baby is exposed for a bath, he may show tremulousness of limbs and quivering of chin. They are easily startled by loud noise, bright light or rough handling. Jitteriness usually becomes less when baby is in the mother's lap and during breastfeeding. Jitteriness is self-limiting and generally disappears after 2–3 days. Excessive jitteriness may occurs in babies with low levels of blood glucose (hypoglycemia) and calcium (hypocalcemia) which is more likely to occur in babies of mothers who had diabetes mellitus during pregnancy (gestational diabetes mellitus).

JUNK FOOD

There is growing craze to eat junk food from ever growing self-service jaunts by children belonging to well-to-do families. Children crave for junk food because it is tasty and a status symbol. The excessive intake of unbalanced starchy and fatty junk food (without green leafy vegetables and fruits) is associated with the risk of development of obesity, deficiency of micronutrients and its consequences. Excessive intake of soft drinks, tinned juices, potato chips/crisps, French fries, pizzas, burghers, hot dogs, munching of unhealthy snacks in-between meals, puddings, ice cream, chocolates and sweets should be avoided or their intake restricted especially by children who have a familial tendency to become overweight. There are a number of Indian junk foods which are loaded with calories and unhealthy trans-fats, such as *samosas, kachories, pakoras, poories, bhathuras, muthies, namkeens*, etc.

which should be avoided or taken in moderation. Soft drinks provide empty calories without any essential nutrients and their excessive intake is associated with loss of appetite, restlessness and irritability (due to caffein) and dental decay and caries (due to sugar and acidity). Even canned juices are loaded with empty calories and should be avoided or taken after dilution. Plain water (which is filtered or purified by RO system) is the best drink!

What are trans-fats and their health hazards?

Trans-fats are produced when hydrogen atoms get added to the vegetable oils at high temperatures. Vanaspati is the most common source of trans-fats especially when it is recycled for frying again and again. Vanaspati is commonly used by street food vendors because it is cheap, less greasy, resistant to rancidity and provides flavor and crispness to the fried food items. However, trans-fats are injurious to health because they raise the level of "bad" cholesterol (LDL), lower the level of "good" cholesterol (HDL), cause clumping of platelets and clogging of arteries in the heart and brain. According to WHO, daily intake of trans-fats should not exceed 5 gm. The average content of transfats in common junk foods is shown the **Box**.

Average content of trans-fats per adult serving*	
■ *Bathuras, puries, paranthas, aloo tikkies, samosas, kachoris, pakoras, mathies, dosas, namkeen,* etc.	6.0–9.5 gm
■ French fries, burghers, hot dogs, potato chips, crisps, cookies, doughnuts, cakes, muffins, biscuits, etc.	6.0 gm
■ Pizza, Indian sweets like *jalebis, gulab jamun.*	3.6 gm

*Avoid intake of these "risky foods" more than once a week.
Vanaspati should not be used for frying purposes at home and in general fried foods should be avoided.

The health department of government of India has made it mandatory for the producers of processed foods to indicate the content of the trans-fats on the package. However, 80% of trans-fats that we consume comes from street food vendors, fast food outlets and restaurants which do not serve packaged food. Therefore, public awareness is more important than any governmental guidelines and policies.

KANGAROO-MOTHER CARE

Mother can provide skin-to-skin contact or kangaroo-mother care to her premature and low birth weight babies. It ensures better temperature control, facilitates mother-infant bonding, promotes breastfeeding with better weight gain and reduces the risk of apneic attacks by transmitting healing electromagnetic vibrations of love and compassion from mother to her baby.

Baby is undressed completely except for a soakable diaper, cap, socks and mittens. Mother wears a loose blouse or a gown and places the naked baby upright between her breasts with face turned on one side. The back of the baby is covered with mother's gown or a shawl. Mother can walk with the baby which is properly secured with a sling and she can sleep with her baby having close skin-to-skin contact. When baby can suckle, breastfeeding should be given as often as the baby wants but at least after every 2 hours. During effective kangaroo-mother care, baby's trunk is warm to touch and his palms and soles are warm and pink. It is a useful and cost-effective strategy for care of preterm and low birth weight babies in developing countries who have constraints of technology and trained personnel to manage them.

KAWASAKI DISEASE

The cause of Kawasaki disease is unknown, it is either an infective or an autoimmune disorder. The disease is most common in preschool children. There is high grade fever, marked irritability, skin rash and congestion or redness of eyes. Oral cavity is congested with strawberry appearance of tongue and markedly red and cracked lips. There is swelling, redness and desquamation of hands and feet. Coronary artery abnormalities develop in 25% of untreated patients during 2nd and 3rd weeks of illness.

There is excellent therapeutic response to administration of intravenous immunoglobulins (IVIG) and aspirin. Children who develop coronary artery abnormalities are given low dose aspirin for a prolonged period. The administration of live vaccines should be delayed for at least 3 months after the administration of IVIG.

KEGEL EXERCISES

Many factors, like pregnancy, childbirth, aging and obesity, can weaken the pelvic floor muscles. Kegel exercises are done to strengthen pelvic muscles to improve continence of urine and stools. Kegel exercises are easy to do and can be done anywhere and anytime of the day without any one knowing it. Identify your pelvic floor muscles while trying to stop urination and passage of stool. Once you have identified your pelvic floor muscles, empty your bladder and lie on your back. Tighten your pelvic floor or perineal muscles, hold the contraction for 5 seconds, and then relax for 5 seconds. Repeat it 4–5 times in a row. Increase the ability to contract and relax the muscles for 10 seconds at a time. Maintain your focus on pelvic floor muscles without contracting your muscles in the abdomen, thighs and buttocks. While doing the contractions, do not hold your breath, instead you should breathe in a relaxed manner. Try to do at least three sets of 20 repetitions of Kegel exercises daily. You can do Kegels or perineum-tightening exercises at virtually any time of the day—while sitting, standing, attending phone, watching TV, lying down or doing household chores. Apart from improving continence of urine and stools, Kegel exercises also improve the ability to achieve orgasm. It is important that you should not develop a habit of contracting pelvic muscles to stop the stream of urination. Doing Kegel exercises while emptying your bladder can actually weaken your pelvic muscles. It leads to incomplete evacuation of bladder with increased risk of urinary tract infection.

KERNICTERUS

When a neonate develops severe jaundice with serum bilirubin level exceeding 20 mg/dL, there is a risk of development of brain damage which is called as kernicterus. The features of kernicterus (acute bilirubin encephalopathy during newborn period) include lethargy, inability to take feed, shrill cry, downward rolling of eyeballs (setting-sun sign), convulsions and backward arching of neck and trunk. The manifestations are nonspecific in preterm babies who may die of apneic attacks.

During follow-up, these children have delayed milestones and develop rigidity of upper and lower limbs. There is sensory deafness as assessed by brainstem evoked auditory responses (BERA). Teeth are stained brownish-green in color. These children are managed by active and passive exercises (without any massage), early stimulation, occupational therapy and hearing aid. Kernicterus is prevented by early identification and prompt management of jaundice in the newborn by phototherapy and exchange blood transfusion.

KEROSENE POISONING

It is the commonest accidental poisoning in children. When kerosene is stored in a soft drink bottle, a thirsty child is likely to drink it by mistake. Due to unpleasant taste, child is likely to take a few sips but when taken in excess of one ounce (30 mL) it may prove fatal. Kerosene is readily aspirated into the lungs producing cough, breathing difficulty and fever due to chemical pneumonia. Drowsiness, lethargy, fits and coma may occur. The child will smell of kerosene.

No attempt should be made to induce vomiting because of increased risk of aspiration in the lungs. The child should be taken to the hospital without delay. Supportive management is provided by administration of intravenous fluids, electrolytes and oxygen. When X-ray chest is normal and there are no symptoms, the child can be sent home after 24 hours of observation.

KNOCK-KNEES

Most preschool children have knock-knees and it is not of any significance. When child stands erect with both knees touching each other, a gap of up to 5 cm between the feet is considered as normal. The knees may rub against each other and child may have difficulty in walking. Overweight children may have greater degree of knock-knees. Most knock-knees resolve by the age of 6 years. When knock-knees are severe (inter-feet distance >10 cm when child stands erect with knees just touching each other) or persistent, rickets (vitamins D deficiency), developmental bone defect, injury or infection of the knee joint should be excluded. When knock-knees persist beyond the age of 8–10 years and are affecting the gait or sports activities of the child, orthopedic surgeon should be consulted for surgical correction of the deformity.

K

LABOR PAINS

When a baby achieves full maturity, hormonal changes appear which initiate labor pains to deliver the baby. Most deliveries take place when baby achieves a maturity of 39–41 weeks. At times labor pains may start prematurely when conditions in the womb are unsatisfactory for further growth of the fetus or when there are some inherent problems in the fetus.

The first sign of true labor is usually "blood show" which is followed by crampy uterine contractions. The "show" is the protective plug of mucus which keeps the cervix closed. At the onset of labor, mucus plug is dislodged and is discharged through the vagina along with a small amount of blood. As the labor progresses, the "bag of water" (amniotic sac) ruptures with sudden gush of amniotic fluid or slow trickle of amniotic fluid through the vagina. When labor pains are true or genuine, uterine contractions become frequent and stronger with longer duration with each contraction. True uterine contractions are strong and persistent when mother changes her position and during walking. At times, the initial labor pains may be a false alarm. When uterine contractions are irregular and they are neither strong nor long lasting, they are indicative of false labor pains.

Labor is a physiological process and nature has so designed that when both baby and mother are normal, it does not impose any undue stress either to the mother or to her baby. However, when mother is anxious or unduly worried and unable to relax, the process of delivery is often slowed and prolonged. The fact that majority of women can go through the process of vaginal delivery without any problems should give you the confidence and assurance that you can also do it. You should learn and practice the art of relaxation and deep breathing during labor. During labor, you should relax and let go and your breathing efforts should coordinate with uterine contractions to push down. During child birth when vagina is markedly stretched, there is release of endorphins in the body which effectively cushions the pain and discomfort of delivery. The practice of allowing the husband to provide comfort and emotional support to the wife during delivery has gained wide popularity in the West and needs to be promoted in our country. Pain can be reduced by acupuncture, analgesics and subdural anesthetics. Above all humane and compassionate attitude of the health care providers in the labor room by showing genuine concern and providing encouragement and emotional support to her, boosts the morale during the most critical moments of her life.

LARYNGOMALACIA (Congenital stridor)

There is congenital softening of larynx (wind box) which gets sucked in or collapsed with each breath producing a crowing sound or stridor. Stridor occurs within a few days after birth and is low-pitched, loud and inspiratory, i.e. crowing sound occurs with each in-breath. There may be associated wet sounds in the trachea or wind pipe. Stridor may increase in intensity during feeding, crying or when baby is excited. The severity of stridor may depend upon the position of the baby—whether nursed supine (face up), prone (face down), turned to one side, neck flexed or extended, etc. Stridor usually disappears during sleep. The child may have feeding difficulty, increased risk of respiratory infections and aspiration of feeds into the lungs due to gastroesophageal reflux (GER).

Treatment The condition is benign and self-limiting and stridor usually disappears between 6 months and 1 year of age. Child should be nursed in a position of comfort which is associated with minimal intensity of stridor. The head should be kept raised during and after the feeding to prevent risk of aspiration. There is no role of mist therapy or steam inhalation. Administration of calcium syrup may facilitate recovery in some children. No investigations are needed except when obstruction is marked or associated with feeding difficulty.

L

LEARNING DIFFICULTIES

Most children are able to compete well with other children and have no problems in their schooling. About 10% of children face various types of learning disabilities with suboptimal academic performance. They are physically or apparently normal children without any obvious disability but an observant teacher or mother can identify the inherent limitation/s which may be interfering with the learning process. Child may have poor attention span, short memory, delay in development of language, and inability to appreciate temporal (time) and spatial (size and shape) sequence or relationships. There may be poor neuromotor ability, low intelligence (IQ), social and emotional quotients. At times the child may be under-age compared to other classmates which may lead to excessive pressure and stress to the immature child.

The child may have various grades of deafness or visual impairment which should be assessed and managed by an appropriate specialist. The child may be a slow learner due to compromised cognition or impaired fine motor skills and clumsiness. A detailed assessment should be done by a developmental psychologist for evaluation of global development and intelligence quotient (IQ) by formal tests. The child may not be able to express himself with clarity due to delayed or defective speech. A number of developmental disorders like dyslexia, dysgraphia, attention deficit hyperactivity disorder (ADHD) and autism spectrum disorders (ASD), may compromise learning process. These children should be evaluated by a child psychologist and a special educator. The specific learning disorders (SpLD) are discussed in detail at their respective alphabetic location in the book.

Instead of providing special attention and help by an educationist, these children are often labeled as 'lazy', 'stupid', 'careless', 'clumsy', etc.—further undermining their confidence and self-esteem. Children with learning disorders may develop frustration, loss of confidence and depression. It may lead to behaviour problems, like truancy (missing school without a legitimate reason) and delinquency (indulging in criminal acts). These children need a detailed assessment by a number of experts and special attention should be provided to them under the guidance and supervision of special educator. They should be taught in a mainstream inclusive school and not any special school, so that they can interact, compete and learn from other children. The Ministry of Human Resource Development, Government of India, provides certain benefits and exemptions to these children which should be availed to improve their confidence. They are exempted to learn a second language. The question paper is read out to them and they are provided one hour extra time because they are slow writers. They can even be provided with a "writer" from the junior class to write their answers. They may be allowed to use a calculator during the mathematics examination.

Some exceptional children may do poorly in an ordinary school because formal "bookish" process of learning may not interest or inspire them. Albert Einstein, the mathematical genius, never completed his schooling because his thinking and aspirations were much higher than what his teachers could teach him. The legendary microsoft wizard Bill Gates was a "slow" student and he dropped out from high school to become the most successful and richest man in the world. You should not, therefore, feel despondent when your child is not interested in his studies in the regular school—he may be an exceptional and unusual human being who will find his own destiny.

LEPROSY

It is a chronic disease due to infection with *Mycobacterium leprae* and is also called as Hansen's disease. The incubation period of the disease ranges from 3 months to several years and infection occurs by a close contact with the patient over several months or years. The common symptoms include white patches on the skin with loss of sensations. There are well-demarcated elevated pink skin lesions, sensory neuropathy with occurrence of deformities like claw hands and toes, loss of digits, and saddle nose deformity. The peripheral nerves may become thickened. Like tuberculosis, leprosy is also treated by multiple drugs which are given for 6–18 months duration. BCG vaccination (which is given for prevention against TB) is also partially protective against development of leprosy.

LEUKEMIAS

The cancer of white blood cells (leukocytes) is called as leukemia and it accounts for one-third of all childhood cancers. Acute lymphoblastic leukemia (ALL) is the commonest accounting for 75% of all leukemias. The etiology of leukemia is uncertain and may be related to exposure to ionizing radiation, therapeutic irradiation, certain chemicals and viral infections. Children with chromosomal (like Down syndrome) and certain genetic disorders are more prone to develop leukemia.

Clinical features The onset of disease is during preschool years with peak incidence between 3 and 5 years. The common symptoms include pallor, fatigue, fever, pains in the bones and small joints and bleeding manifestations. There is enlargement of lymph nodes, liver and spleen. Bone pains and tenderness over sternum are common. Enlargement of one or both testes may occur due to leukemic infiltrates.

Treatment Due to advances in chemotherapy and excellent supportive management, the survival rates of all childhood cancers have improved and over 80% children with ALL are now curable. Environmental sanitation and personal hygiene should be maintained to prevent risk of infection. Daily bath with soap and water, brushing of teeth twice a day, chlorhexidine mouth rinse after meals and use of mask are recommended to reduce the risk of infection. The child should be well hydrated and consume at least 2 liters of water daily. The specific treatment should be taken from the specialized center dealing with childhood cancers under the direct supervision of pediatric hemato-oncologist. Several chemotherapy protocols are available during phase of induction, maintenance of remission and treatment of relapse when it occurs. Bone marrow or stem cell transplantation from HLA-matched sibling is curative. Because of improved survival by effective chemotherapy, bone marrow transplant is reserved for patients who suffer from one or more relapses.

LOCK JAW (Trismus)

Inability to open the mouth is called lock jaw and it is the commonest manifestation of tetanus. Other causes include involvement of the joints of the jaw, tumor of the jaw, throat infection, involvement of the brain or brainstem and intake of certain drugs (phenothiazines and neuroleptics) and poisons (strychnine). Treatment depends upon the underlying cause. Feeding is given through a naso- or oro-gastric tube.

LOW BIRTH WEIGHT BABIES

Babies with a birth weight of less than 2500 g (<5½ lbs) are called low birth weight (LBW) babies. Baby may be LBW either because he is born early (premature) or fetus has suffered from intrauterine growth retardation (IUGR). About 10% of LBW babies are premature (<37 completed weeks) while a large majority in our country are term in gestation but have suffered from fetal malnutrition or IUGR. Premature babies are vulnerable to suffer from a large number of health problems due to immaturity of various organs of the baby. Depending upon the severity of prematurity, babies with a birth weight of less than 1800 g (<34 weeks) are looked after in the neonatal intensive care unit (NICU). The common clinical problems of babies with IUGR are discussed on **page 199.**

L

MACROCEPHALY

When head size is larger than normal-for-the-age, the condition is called as macrocephaly. Hydrocephalus due to dilatation of the ventricular system is the commonest cause of macrocephaly. Rarely, macrocephaly may occur due to certain metabolic disorders and space occupying lesions in the brain (subdural effusion, hematoma, abscess or brain tumor). At times, the head size appears large when skull bones are thick due to rickets, thalassemia major, achondroplasia, and osteopetrosis. In these conditions, there is no evidence of underlying brain damage or neuromotor dysfunction.

MALARIA

Malaria is the commonest mosquito-borne disease since times immemorial. It is caused by infection with parasites called as *Plasmodium vivax* and *Plasmodium falciparum* which involve the red blood cells of the patient. The infection is transmitted through the bite of infected female Anopheles mosquitoes. Some individuals are more prone to the bites of mosquitoes because of secretion of certain pheromones in their sweat. Transfusion of infected blood may also cause malaria. Malaria during pregnancy may affect the fetus by transmission of infection through placenta.

Common Symptoms

There is sudden onset of high grade fever with marked chills and rigors which is usually associated with headache, body aches and fatigue. There is marked sweating and weakness when fever drops down. In *P. vivax* infection, fever is typically intermittent occurring on every alternate day. Infection due to *P. falciparum* is a more serious causing continuous high grade fever which may involve the brain. The occurrence of convulsions with loss of consciousness and fall in blood glucose level (hypoglycemia) are suggestive of brain infection (cerebral malaria). Malaria in preschool children may be atypical producing continuous fever everyday and without any features of chills and shivering. *Malaria should be seriously considered whenever there is sudden onset of high grade fever without any associated features, like cough and cold, diarrhea and urinary symptoms.* The presence of chills alone is not suggestive of malaria because chills (feeling of cold) can occur in all blood-borne infections like viral fever, typhoid fever, urinary tract infection, septicemia, leptospirosis, etc.

Laboratory Investigations

Examination of thick and thin blood smears by an experienced and diligent technician is the gold standard to confirm the diagnosis. The blood smear should be taken during the height of fever and may be repeated after 12–24 hours when malaria is strongly suspected. Rapid diagnostic tests are available for detection of malarial antigens which do not require the services of a skilled technician and are not time consuming.

Treatment

The child should be encouraged to drink plenty of fluids (water, juices, soups) and given nutritious diet of his liking. During the bout of shivering, a blanket may be given to provide comfort. After shivering, the temperature is likely to shoot up followed by sweating and rapid drop in temperature. The child should be given a safe antipyretic (paracetamol, ibuprofen, mefenamic acid) for symptomatic relief of fever. Tepid water sponging (hydrotherapy) is advised, if fever remains above 102°F despite administration of optimal dose of paracetamol. Specific antimalarial drugs should be taken on the advice of your doctor when diagnosis is confirmed. Chloroquine phosphate is the drug of choice for treatment of malaria due to *P. vivax* but most strains of *P. falciparum* have become multi-drug resistant or unresponsive to conventional drugs. Administration of chloroquine in every case of fever is strongly condemned and is an important cause of emergence of drug resistant malaria. Patients with severe and cerebral malaria should be admitted to the hospital for management. After recovery, supplements of iron should be given to correct anemia.

Home Remedies

They are no longer popular because of availability of a large number of potent medicines to treat life-threatening malaria. They can be used as complementary supportive practices along with specific medicines under the supervision of a physician.

1. Drink plenty of water, orange juice or grape juice.
2. Boil one glass of water with honey, pepper and cinnamon powder, cool it and drink the concoction daily.
3. Take one glass of water with ginger and 3 teaspoons raisins, boil it for 5 minutes and drink the decoction after cooling it.
4. Roast alum on a hot plate or *tawa*. Give half to one teaspoon with a glass of water when patient feels feverish.
5. Take 2 freshly sprouted *dhatura* leaves, grind them with jaggery and make a pill. Take the pill with a glass of water.

Prevention

The preventive measures outlined under control of mosquito-borne diseases should be followed to prevent breeding of mosquitoes and ensure protection against their bites. As yet no vaccine is available for prevention of malaria although concerted efforts are being pursued since several decades. Chemoprophylaxis is recommended for travelers visiting endemic areas of the country. Intake of prophylactic medicines is started one week before the visit and continued for 4 weeks after leaving the endemic area. In chloroquine-sensitive areas, chloroquine is given in a dose of 5 mg base/kg once a week and in chloroquine-resistant regions, mefloquine is advised in a dose of 3.5 mg base/kg once a week.

MALOCCLUSION OF TEETH (Crooked teeth)

Normally, the upper jaw teeth are slightly in front of teeth of the lower jaw. In certain families, this difference may be more pronounced and upper jaw may look overhanging and prominent while chin may appear a bit receding. At times, chin may be prominent and jut forward while upper lip seems to recede. These are developmental or familial variations producing some cosmetic characteristics but without causing any difficulty in eating, chewing or biting. When teeth do not erupt in a symmetrical manner and they are too crowded and mal-aligned or they tend to protrude out, the help of a dental surgeon (orthodontist) should be sought. When management is delayed or ignored, it may cause a lot of embarrassment to the child later in life. Bracing and alignment procedures are delayed till the jaw is fully developed by the age of 14–16 years.

MANTOUX TEST

Mantoux or tuberculin test is done to assess delayed hypersensitivity response to tubercular antigens. Tuberculin (0.1 mL of 2 Tu of purified PPD) is injected on the upper part of anterior surface of left forearm. The test site is examined for the maximum diameter of induration or swelling (not redness or erythema) after 48 to 72 hours. The test is considered as positive when there is induration of more than 10 mm. Positive tuberculin test suggests that either the child had exposure to tubercular bacilli in the past or is currently suffering from tuberculosis. However, when tuberculin test is positive in a child less than 3 years of age, it is suggestive of recent tuberculous infection and should be treated.

MASSAGE

Body massage is popular in India and is credited to provide several health benefits. Massage improves circulation and muscle tone. It improves texture of the skin, reduces dryness and relieves fatigue. Some oil may get absorbed through the thin skin of the baby to provide some nutrition. Touch is believed to send stimulatory messages to the brain to enhance neuromotor development of the baby. Massage should preferably be done by the mother or grandmother with due concern and compassion to enhance bonding. The practice of asking a nurse aide or *dai* or *ayah* to massage the baby is not advised because they are likely to do it as a mechanical chore and often do it rather aggressively with a risk of causing potential harm to the baby.

Technique The baby should be at least 3 kg in weight and one month old before massage is given. Any mild non-irritating non-scented oil like olive oil, coconut oil or almond oil can be used. In some families, clarified butter (*desi ghee*) or milk with butter fat (*malai*) is used for massage. It is acceptable except its disadvantage of giving a long lasting odd smell to the baby. Mustard oil should preferably be avoided in infants because it is pungent to the eyes and irritating to the delicate skin of the babies. It is a common cultural practice to do body massage with olive or coconut oil in summer and mustard or sesame oil in winter.

Massage is usually done before giving a bath to the baby. The room should be warm and without any draughts especially during winter months. When weather is pleasant and not windy, baby can be massaged in the sun to provide additional benefit of vitamin D, which is produced in the skin under the influence of ultraviolet rays of sun. The oil should be rubbed between the palms to bring it to body temperature. Massage should be done by using gentle pressure and smooth rhythmical movements of fingers. Massage the baby first while he is lying on his back and then after placing him on his tummy. Start from the top of the baby and then move downwards to the toes. Massage the scalp by making, small circular movements with your fingers. The forehead is massaged with gentle movements of thumbs moving from center towards the periphery. Stroke and massage the baby's chest by gentle movements from the center toward the sides. Abdomen is massaged from above downwards and from center towards the sides. Roll the baby's arms between your hands and massage in both directions by "milking" action. Open the closed fists of the baby to massage the palms and fingers. Rub the lower limbs by using both upwards and downward movements of both hands. Move down toward the feet to massage soles and toes. Turn the baby on his tummy and stroke his back from side-to-side and then up and down. Make passive gentle movements at all the joints of baby during the procedure of massage. You must talk with your baby or make him listen to a melodious music during the massage session. Most children love to be massaged and often gigle and make various sounds during the massage. Take cues from your baby whether he is enjoying what you are doing or it is annoying or hurting him. Massage should be a fun both for the mother and her baby. Most babies enjoy taking a feed after the session of massage and bath, which is followed by a restful nap for several hours.

MASTURBATION

When a child learns to grasp objects around 5–6 months of age, he touches his own body organs including genitals. There is nothing wrong or bad about it and if it is ignored the child will stop it soon. He may touch the genitals as a signal to pass urine or it may be a symptom of local irritation because of nappy rash or anal itching because of pinworms. Many parents feel that it is dreadful for the child to touch his genitals and they may use aggressive tactics to stop it. Some children may rub their thighs together or make rhythmic rocking movements of the pelvis. During the episode, the child may appear to be lost in his own world, his face may be flushed and he may make certain moaning sounds of pleasure or self-gratification.

Treatment Parents should not create any fuss or scene when child manipulates his genitals. He should be distracted by interaction or offering a toy. If there is a local cause of irritation, it should be appropriately treated on the advice of a doctor. It must be remebered that touching the genitals is a phase of normal development (genital phase) when child explores his body organs and it should not be viewed as an evidence of sexual perversion. *It is important to remember that aggressive parental attitudes and actions are more harmful than the transitory phase of masturbation.* The unconcerned matter-of-fact attitude (intelligent neglect) on the part of parents is usually followed by discontinuation of the habit. The boredom of the child should be relieved by interaction, group activity (painting, music, dance) and play opportunities.

Masturbation with ejaculation in boys and orgasm in girls is extremely common among adolescents. The boys may have sexual fantasies and night emissions. Contrary to the common belief, it does not lead to any weakness, impotency, blindness, insanity or pimples. The physical act itself is not harmful but the associated guilt feelings and misconceptions may lead to depression and emotional disturbances. The child should be encouraged to channelize his energy for outdoor activities by cultivating friendships and participating in various group activities like body building, sports, swimming, dancing, music, painting, yoga and meditation.

MEASLES

Measles is an highly contagious viral infection. The incubation period (time taken from exposure to the onset of symptoms) varies between 8 and 12 days. The initial symptoms (prodromal phase) are characterized by fever, running of nose, sneezing, redness of eyes and dry cough. The skin rash appears after 3–4 days of onset of prodromal symptoms. Fever shoots up when rash appears and settles in next 2 days if no complications occur. Skin rash is characterized by diffuse redness with macules and pin-head sized papules which starts from forehead, behind the ears and spread downwards over the face, neck, trunk and extremities. Rash disappears in 4–5 days leaving behind brownish or coppery discoloration of skin with exfoliation or desquamation. Common complications include superadded bacterial infection, middle ear infection (acute otitis media), laryngitis (stridor) and bronchopneumonia. Rarely encephalitis may occur. Measles is known to suppress the immune system leading to flaring of tuberculosis infection. Due to prolonged convalescence, loss of appetite, respiratory and GI complications, it may lead to development of protein-energy malnutrition and vitamin A deficiency.

Treatment The child is provided with supportive and symptomatic treatment by maintaining good oral hygiene, ensuring adequate nutrition and giving supplements of vitamin A. Fever is controlled by administration of paracetamol and hydrotherapy (body sponging with tap water). Humidification and steam inhalation are useful for relief of upper airway inflammation and dry cough. Superadded bacterial infection is treated with an appropriate antibiotic.

Prevention Measles or MMR vaccine is given at 9 months followed by a booster dose of MMR (measles, mumps, rubella) vaccine at 15 months of age. The unvaccinated sibling who comes in contact with a case of measles can be given pooled human gamma-globulins (0.25 mL/kg) which may prevent or modify the severity of the disease.

MEDICATIONS

In ambulatory (outpatient) and consultancy practice, medicines are usually given orally or administered as aerosoles and for topical use. Oral medications are as effective as medicines administered through intramuscular injections. Some mothers (especially from rural areas) demand that injection should be given to the child for faster relief of his illness. It is a wrong belief that medicines administered through injections are more effective compared to oral medications. There is no need to give an injection unless the child is unable to take it orally or is having persistent vomiting and when the child is critically sick and admitted to the hospital. In day-to-day clinical practice, most medicines are equally effective when given by oral route and injections are given mostly for administration of vaccines. You should cross-check that the chemist has given the same brand of medicine which your doctor has prescribed. In case the pharmacist is offering an alternative brand, you must talk to your doctor before accepting it. Always make sure that you have bought the right medicine and in the formulation (like drops, suspension, kid tablet, mouth dissolving or dispersible tablets) and strength recommended by your doctor. Check the bottle label for name of the medicine, dose recommendations, side effects, expiry date and storage conditions.

How to administer medicines?

It is a daunting task to give medicines to a child. Most children hate to take medicines while some love to take them and may even demand them. It is convenient to administer medicines disbursed in "drops" formulation to infants (due to ease of administration because of small volume) and syrups and suspensions to pre-school children. The formulations which are available in syrup or suspension should be thoroughly shaken before administration. Those medicines which are available in a powder form and are reconstituted with potable water before use, have a short shelf life. They are meant for use for the treatment of a single disease episode and the left over medicine, if any, must be discarded. Some medicines are available as mouth dissolving or dispersible tablets which are convenient to use in pre-school children. They have a long shelf life and are cost-effective.

Most medicines are given in between the meals but few medicines are preferably given on empty stomach because they are non-irritating and absorption of medicine is enhanced when stomach is empty. The recommended amount of medicine should be administered with a dropper, graduated plastic dispenser, calibrated spoon or plastic syringe provided by the manufacturer. Teaspoons should not be used for measuring the quantity of syrup formulations because they are available in a variety of volumes. There is a potential risk of under and over medication by using teaspoons especially in case of antibiotics and life-saving drugs where administration of an accurate dose is mandatory. When dealing with small volumes like 0.5 mL or 1.0 mL, it is better to use a calibrated dropper or a plastic syringe for measuring the correct dose. It is not a good idea to mix medicine in a milk formula or baby food because the child may stop accepting those drinks and food. The medicine or crushed tablet can be mixed in honey or fruit juice.

The medicine should be offered without any fuss, pleading or bribing. Handle the child with firmness, confidence and sense of purpose. Shake the bottle before withdrawing the medicine in the dispenser for administration. Child's head should be slightly raised before administration of medicine. Infant can be held in the lap, mouth opened by pressing at the cheeks or depressing the jaw and medicine is offered with a dropper or a plastic syringe (without needle of course) or a small spoon. There is no need to pinch the nose to make him open his mouth. Most infants bring their tongue out when mouth is opened. Medicine should not be poured over the tongue, instead it should be delivered between the tongue and cheek. In a struggling child, due care should be taken to prevent choking and aspiration. If a medicine is vomited out immediately or within 5 minutes of administration, it is recommended to repeat the dose. Keep a wet towel or paper napkin in hand to wipe the face after giving the medicine. It is preferable to give a sip of water after administration of medicine to wash off odd or bitter taste and prevent any staining of teeth especially in case of medicines containing iron and colored preservatives. Most school going children should be encouraged to swallow a tablet but some children may refuse to swallow a tablet even during adolescence.

It is important that you should carefully follow the instructions of your doctor regarding the dose, frequency and duration of administration of medications. Keep a record of the time of administration of various medicines to reduce the risk of missing the dose or overdosing. When you do not follow the doctor's instructions strictly, the child's recovery from illness may be delayed or he may suffer from untoward side effects of medicine(s). If an adverse reaction has occurred following administration of a drug, you must keep a record so that the same medicine is not given to the child in future. In children, dosages of drugs are calculated on the basis of body weight, surface area or age of the child. The dosages of commonly used drugs, their frequency of administration and indications for use are listed in the **Box**.

Rectal Medications

Rectal medications are not popular or well accepted in Indian culture except insertion of glycerine suppositories for relief of constipation. Rectal route for administration of medicines is used in children with persistent vomiting and ambulatory or home treatment of convulsions. Certain medications are available in liquid form in prefilled syringe with a nozzle (diazepam) or a medicated suppository (paracetamol). The medicine is inserted through anus and delivered beyond the anal sphincter with the help of index finger. After insertion of medicine in the rectum, the mother is asked to hold the buttocks firmly for a few minutes so that medicine stays in the rectum.

Topical Medications

You must check the label of the bottle before oral or local instillation of any medicine. *Never commit the blunder of administering a topical medication through oral route and vice versa.*

Eye drops Let the child lie comfortably on the cot or mother's lap. Hold the head with one hand, gently pull down the lower eye lid and instil 2 drops in each eye in the space between the eyeball and lower eyelid. If a child is fighting, you may need the help of an assistant to hold and restrain the child. The same procedure is followed for administration of eye ointment. It is preferable to use ointment applicaps (which are meant for single use) to reduce the risk of cross infection. Even when one eye is infected, the drops should be instilled in both the eyes by putting the drops first in the normal eye and then into the infected one.

Ear drops Restrain the child on your lap or bed with head turned to one side. Pull the lobe of the ear firmly (backwards in an infant and upwards and backwards in an older child) and pour 2–3 drops into the ear canal. Let the child stay in the same position for 10–15 seconds and gently massage the ear canal before turning the child to the other side to instil the drops in the other ear. *Never instil urine or oil in the ear canal.*

Nose drops Hold the baby in your lap or on the bed on his back and tilt the head backwards. Gently but firmly hold the head with one hand and pour 2–3 drops of medicine in each nostril. It is preferable to use saline (0.6%) drops and avoid instillation of medicated nose drops which may cause chemical inflammation and rebound blockage of nose. *Never instil oil into the nostrils due to potential risk of development of aspiration lipoid pneumonia.*

Commonly used drugs in children

Drug	Dose (mg/kg/dose)*	Frequency	Indications
Antibiotics**			
Amoxycillin	7.0–12.5	6–8 hr	Respiratory and skin infections
Azithromycin	10 mg on day 1, 5 mg for next 4 days	24 hr	Respiratory, skin infections and typhoid fever
Cefixime	8.0	12–24 hr	Typhoid fever and urinary tract infection
Cephalexin	7.0–12.5	6–8 hr	Respiratory and skin infections
Norfloxacin	5.0–7.5	12 hr	Diarrhea/dysentery, urinary tract infection
Antihistamines			
Diphenhydramine hydrochloride	1.0	8 hr	Allergic conditions and insect bites
Hydroxyzine hydrochloride	0.5	6–8 hr	Allergic conditions
Cetirizine hydrochloride	<10 yr : 5.0 mg per dose > 10 yr : 10.0 mg per dose	12–24 hr	Avoid below 2 yr
Deworming			
Albendazole	200 mg/dose 1–2 yr 400 mg/dose > 2 yr 400 mg/dose/day	Single dose Single dose For 5 days	Covers all worms
Mebendazole	100 mg/dose	Single dose followed by repeat dose after 2 weeks	Giardiasis Pinworms
Pyrantel pamoate	100 mg/dose 11	Every 12 hr for 3 days Single dose	Covers all worms Covers all worms

(Contd.)

M

Commonly used drugs in children (contd.)

Drug	Dose (mg/kg/dose)*	Frequency	Indications
Niclosamide	< 6 yr:500 mg on empty stomach, repeat after 1 hr > 6 yr:1000 mg, repeat after 1 hr. Give a purgative 2 hr later	Two doses are given 1 hr apart	Tapeworms
Pain and fever			Pain and fever due to any cause
Paracetamol	15	4–6 hr	
Ibuprofen***	7.5 – 10.0	6–8 hr	
Mefenamic acid***	5.0 – 7.5	6–8 hr	
Sedation			Irritability and excessive crying
Chloral hydrate	5 – 10	6–8 hr	
Trichlophos sodium	10 – 12	6–8 hr	Avoid sedation in children with bronchitis, pneumonia and head injury
Promethazine hydrochloride	0.5	6–8 hr	
Vomiting			
Domperidone	0.2	6–8 hr	Give only a few doses
Ondansetron hydrochloride dihydrate	< 4 yr:2 mg/dose 4–11 yr:4 mg/dose > 12 yrs:8 mg/dose	4–6 hr	

*Unless specified otherwise in the box.
**Antibiotics are usually given for 5–7 days.
***Do not give ibuprofen and mefenamic acid in infants below 6 months.
For complete list of drugs, their dosages and trade names refer to Drug Dosages in Children by Dr Meharban Singh and Dr Ashok K Deorari, CBS Publishers & Distributors Pvt Ltd, New Delhi, 9th edition, 2015.

MENINGITIS

Inflammation of the membranes or meninges covering the brain and spinal cord is called as meningitis. It may be caused by bacterial (pyogenic and tubercular), viral and fungal infections. Meningitis is a serious disease, may manifest suddenly in a couple of hours (pyogenic and viral) or over a couple of days and weeks (tubercular). The classical symptoms are fever, headache, vomiting and convulsions. Neck stiffness and dislike for bright light (photophobia) are common. The child may become drowsy or unconscious. In infants, anterior fontanel (soft spot on the top of the head) may become tense and bulging with loss of pulsations. Skin rash due to small bleeding spots inside the skin (petechiae) and fall in blood pressure (shock) may occur in cases of meningococcal meningitis.

Treatment When child is suspected to have meningitis he must be admitted to the hospital without any delay. The diagnosis is confirmed by examination of cerebrospinal fluid (CSF). The spinal fluid is obtained by doing a lumbar puncture. It is a simple procedure wherein a needle is inserted in the lower part of child's back between L_4 and L_5 vertebrae and a small amount of CSF is obtained for biochemical and microscopic examination. The procedure is entirely safe and is mandatory to confirm the diagnosis of meningitis. Early and effective treatment of meningitis is associated with complete recovery. Children with pyogenic meningitis are treated with intravenous administration of antibiotics and excellent supportive care for a minimum period of 10 days. Tubercular meningitis (TBM) is treated with antitubercular drugs and steroids for a period of 9 months to one year. When treatment is delayed or is unsatisfactory, it may lead to permanent brain damage, deafness and neuromotor disability.

Prevention Several vaccines are available to provide protection against various bacteria which are known to cause meningitis. Hib vaccine provides protection against meningitis due to *H. influenzae type b* which is administered along with triple antigen. Meningococcal conjugate vaccine can be given as a single shot at the age of 2 years, while in case of meningococcal polysaccharide vaccine boosters are given every 2–3 years. Pneumococcal vaccine (PCV13) is given to infants in 3 primary doses at an interval of 4 weeks followed by a booster after one year. Bacille Calmette-Guérin (BCG) vaccine is given at birth and is creadited to prevent disseminated tuberculosis and tubercular meningitis. For details regarding these vaccines, refer to the section on immunizations.

MENSTRUAL PERIODS

Sexual maturity starts in girls between 10 and 12 years of age. There is enlargement of breasts, growth of pubic hair followed by appearance of hair in the armpits. Around the age of 12 years, most girls would have their first menstrual period (menarche). At this stage the body shape assumes a typical "feminine figure" with a full grown bust, narrow waste and broad hips. When menstruation is delayed beyond 15 years it is a cause for concern and consultation should be sought with an obstetrician.

Every month one ovum or egg is released (around the middle of menstrual cycle) and ovaries produce sex hormones (estrogens and progesterone) which cause thickening of the inner wall of uterus with increase in its blood supply. This is being done to prepare the womb (uterus) for nesting or implantation of the fertilized ovum. If fertilization of the ovum does not occur (ovum and sperm do not meet), the ovum dies and further production of hormones stops. The prepared thickened lining of uterus is shed off resulting in bleeding or menstrual blood flow through the vagina. The same cycle of changes are repeated every month till pregnancy occurs or menopause sets in after 45 years of age. The menstrual cycles are repeated on an average of every 28 days (range 21–36 days) and menstrual flow lasts for about 3–5 days. The initial menstrual cycles may be irregular and scanty, and may be associated with cramps but subsequently they become regular and do not cause any significant discomfort. The hormonal changes during menstrual cycle may be associated with mood changes. There is increased irritability, mental tension and headache just before the onset of menstrual flow.

Ovulation or release of ovum occurs sometime during the middle of menstrual cycle (10th–18th days after the onset of menstrual flow). After its release, the ovum remains alive for about 18–24 hours while sperms remain active for about 36 hours after coitus. The chances of sperm meeting the ovum and occurrence of conception are therefore best when sexual intercourse takes place in the middle of menstrual cycle, i.e. 12–16 days after the onset of last menstrual flow. It is difficult to predict the actual time of release of the ovum but maintaining an accurate record of body temperature during a couple of menstrual cycles may help. The resting or morning (soon after getting up) body temperature remains more or less steady after menstruation. The body temperature suddenly rises by 0.75°C (1.0°F) at or just around the time of ovulation. The body temperature continues to stay at a slightly higher level till the onset of next menstruation. When a menstrual period is missed in a married woman (sexually active girl) who has had regular monthly cycles, it is the most reliable sign of onset of pregnancy. The pregnancy can be confirmed by doing a urine test 5–7 days after the missed period. A sample of urine passed first thing in the morning is tested for the presence of human chorionic gonadotrophic hormone (hCG), which is produced by the placenta during pregnancy. If initial urine test is negative, it should be repeated one week later to exclude pregnancy. The menstrual period may become irregular, scanty or may even stop on account of a systemic illness, hormonal disorder, mental stress and air travel.

MENTAL RETARDATION

Children with mental retardation or mental subnormality have an impairment in their intelligence and they have limited ability to adapt and deal with day-to-day activities, social interactions and environmental situations. They have global delay in all the spheres of neuromotor development, namely motor (both gross and fine), adaptive, social and language. Mental retardation may occur due to a variety of causes. Brain damage may occur during fetal life (genetic, chromosomal, developmental defects, thyroid deficiency), during labor and delivery (birth asphyxia, birth injury), at birth or subsequently (meningitis, encephalitis and head injury). However, in over 50% cases of mental retardation, no cause is found. The severity of mental retardation can be assessed on the basis of intelligence quotient (IQ) which is calculated by the formula:

$$\frac{\text{Mental age}}{\text{Chronological age}} \times 100.$$

M

Clinical features Children with mental retardation are late in achieving all the milestones of development. They are late in acquiring motor skills and movements, recognition, speech, communication and learning skills. Some children with mental retardation may have additional problems like convulsions, spasticity of muscles (cerebral palsy), visual difficulties, deafness and behaviour problems. Head size may be small (microcephaly) or at times excessively large due to hydrocephalus. When mental subnormality is due to a chromosomal disorder (Down syndrome, fragile-X syndrome, Klinefelter syndrome), the specific features of the underlying disorders would be present. On the basis of severity, the child with mental retardation can be classified, from the most severe to the milder grade, as follows:

   (i) Not educable or trainable (IQ 21–35),

  (ii) Trainable but not educable (IQ 36–50),

 (iii) Educable with special efforts (IQ 51–70), and

 (iv) Educable in a regular school (IQ 71–90).

Treatment The child with mental subnormality should be identified early so that he is provided stimulation through his special senses namely music, lullabies, bright colored objects, lights, touch, caressing, smell, taste, etc. Detailed assessment and investigations are undertaken to identify the cause. Certain genetic defects and deficiency of thyroid hormone (cretinism) are managed by administration of specific medicines and dietary restrictions. Seizures should be controlled by administration of anticonvulsants. Visual and hearing aids should be provided if indicated.

The child should be handled with love, affection and compassion. They need active interaction, warmth, appreciation and guarded discipline. Instead of criticism, encouragement and motivation are more useful to improve learning and performance. Their specific capabilities, if any, should be identified and effectively harnessed. *It must be recognized that there are no specific drugs or tonics in any system of medicine to enhance intelligence and money and resources should not be wasted to buy them.*

MICROCEPHALY

When head size is small, the condition is called as microcephaly. The condition may occur due to poor growth of brain or because of early fusion of sutures or gaps between the skull bones (craniosynostosis) which does not allow the brain to grow. Microcephaly may occur due to developmental defect and intrauterine (TORCH) infection in fetal life or it may occur due to brain damage before birth, at the time of delivery because of birth asphyxia, brain injury, infection or subsequently due to a metabolic disorder (hypoglycemia or inborn error of metabolism). Depending upon the cause, microcephaly may be associated with neuromotor retardation, convulsions, cerebral palsy and mental retardation. Unfortunately no specific drugs or "brain tonics" are available to treat children with small or damaged brain. When microcephaly is due to craniosynostosis, it can be treated by an early surgical procedure to break the fusion between the skull bones so that brain can grow in size.

MICRONUTRIENTS

The nutrients which are required in small amounts for health and well-being are called micronutrients. They include minerals and trace elements, and vitamins which are required both for maintenance of health, prevention of diseases and convalescence following life-threatening diseases. Minerals and trace elements include sodium, potassium, chloride, iron, calcium, phosphorus, magnesium, manganese, iodine, fluoride, cobalt, copper, molybdenum, selenium, sulfur and zinc. Vitamins are subdivided into two groups, water soluble (vitamin B complex, vitamin C) and fat soluble (vitamins A, D, E, K). They are required for promotion of a wide range of metabolic processes and maintenance of integrity of immune cells to protect against infections and development of cancer.

MIGRAINE

Migraine typically causes episodes of one-sided headache which runs in certain families due to genetic predisposition. The disorder occurs in bright school going children who are prone to anxiety and stress. The attack may be precipitated by exposure to bright sunlight, loud noise, emotional stress, sleep deprivation or excessive sleep and menstrual period. Intake of nuts, chocolates, cheese, tea and coffee may trigger the attack. There may be initial symptom (aura) of seeing stars, flashes of light or zig-zag figures in the eyes. Headache is usually limited to one side and is often throbbing or pulsating in nature due to spasm and dilatation of blood vessels of the brain. Vomiting may occur when headache is severe. The child would prefer to lie down in a dark, cool and quiet room with eyes closed and head firmly strapped with a piece of cloth or elastic band. The episodes of headache may occur every week or after 1–3 months.

Treatment Administration of an analgesic like paracetamol or ibuprofen may reduce the severity or duration of pain. The child should lie in a dark quiet room with eyes closed. A tight bandage can be tied around the head. Specific antimigraine medicine can be taken on the advice of a pediatrician or neurologist. Common triggers like exposure to sunlight, stress, and sleep deprivation, should be avoided. When attacks of migraine occur frequently, preventive medicines can be taken on the advice of a doctor.

Home Remedies

- Tie a tight elastic band or cloth around the head to decrease blood flow to scalp to lessen the throbbing and pounding of migraine headache. The child should lie down in a dark, cool and quiet room with eyes closed.
- Wet a towel liberally and squeeze some water out. Fold it flat and keep in the freezer of frig for 5 minutes or till it becomes stiff. At the earliest evidence of migraine, apply the cold pack over the eye and temple on the affected side for 5–10 minutes, followed by hot fomentation on the back of neck.
- When attack is already advanced, pour 1–2 drops of ginger juice in the nostril on the affected side. In children it should be diluted with equal quantity of normal saline (or saline nose drops).
- Make a fine paste of cinnamon or sandalwood powder. Apply over the forehead and temples.
- Make a juice of carrots, spinach, beetroot and cucumber and drink it along with 8–10 almonds. Green leafy vegetables and nuts are a good source of niacin or nicotinic acid.
- Aromatherapy is useful for relief of migraine. Put any aromatic oil (peppermint, sandalwood, lavender, eucalyptus, primrose) in ice cold water. Dip a small towel in it and place it over the forehead and temples.
- A cup of chamomile tea taken at the onset of migraine may abort an attack.

MILESTONES OF DEVELOPMENT

Neuromotor development is assessed by various milestones which are achieved as the child grows. Every baby is unique and each develops at his or her own pace but within the broad range of normality. Developmental milestones are assessed in a wide range of fields like gross motor (locomotion), fine motor (skills), social and adaptive interactions, language or speech, vision and hearing. The process of development is continuous and child learns new skills as he grows. There is a wide range of ages for acquiring various milestones which are summarized below.

Social smile The baby tries to fix his gaze and look into your eyes by about 4–6 weeks of age when you talk to your baby or tickle his chin, he responds by smiling. He gives an interactive smile to everybody and does not differentiate between you and a stranger. After a few weeks, his smile becomes a broad grin and he expresses his pleasure by kicking his arms and legs, and by cooing, babbling or gurgling sounds. Social smile should not be confused with "spontaneous smile" (without any interaction) which many babies have soon after birth and they smile during sleep as if having a dream or while passing wind.

Head control When you pick up a young infant, you must support his head with your hand or elbow while holding or carrying the baby because he cannot hold his head. By about 4 months, when a child is made to sit in the lap, he can hold and support his head without any wobbling. At this stage, when a baby is lying on his abdomen, he can lift his head and shoulders off the cot and turn his head from side to side.

Rolling over When head control is achieved most babies can roll over to change their position. In India, since most babies are made to sleep on their back, they learn to roll over first from back to tummy and subsequently from tummy to back. The baby is gradually achieving mobility and you must be careful to protect him from any fall and injury. The cot should have side railings or pillows should be placed around the baby to protect him against the fall.

Sitting Most babies are able to sit with props of pillows or cushions by 5 months of age. Initially the baby is wobbly and takes the support of his arms to sit. By 6–8 months most children can sit independently without any support with their back straight and upright.

Crawling When a baby is able to sit stably, he tries to creep or crawl to explore his environment. Some babies crawl on their buttocks by giving themselves a push with their legs. Others crawl more gracefully on all the four limbs and try to reach virtually every corner of the house. The child is now ready to explore his environment by poking his fingers into every hole and "mouthing" every object that he can lay his hands on. At this stage, child needs constant supervision and vigilance round-the-clock so that he is protected against various hazards during the process of exploration and learning. During this phase, make sure that he has no access to small objects, beads, coins, removable parts of toys, electrical wires and sockets.

Standing Most children are able to stand with support around 9 months of age by holding on the furniture. He gradually learns to stand independently without any support in next one or two months. Most children are able to walk a few steps by holding your hand or furniture by 10–11 months of age.

Walking By first birthday, most babies are able to walk a few steps independently without any support. During 12–18 months, most children are able to walk fairly well but they are prone to frequent falls with minor bumps. Most parents buy a "walker" when baby is able to crawl so that he can move around on the wheels of the walker. But walkers are banned in many countries because they are fraught with dangers of accidents and injuries. Moreover, walkers eliminate the motivation and desire to walk independently because child can move around in the walker with a minimal effort. Around 18 months, the child can crawl up and down the stairs without any help. After 2 years, child can walk up the stairs by placing one foot on each stair, but comes down by placing both the feet on each stair.

Fine motor skills Newborn babies have a grasp reflex. When a finger is placed in their palm, they automatically and involuntarily grasp it firmly and do not release the hold as if to seek protection. By about 3–4 months, the baby tries to reach an object like a rattle and holds it crudely with his palm and fingers like a monkey. By 6 months, the baby can hold a spoon and tries to take it to his mouth. At this stage, his coordination is poor and he is unable to take food into his mouth and there is spillage and mess. His coordination improves gradually and he is able to eat with a spoon by 9 months of age. Around 10 months or so, most babies develop a fine grasp and can hold a small object like button or a bead in their thumb and index finger (pincer grasp). By first birthday, his grasp is mature, coordination is better and he can transfer objects from one hand to the other, and enjoys dropping and picking objects from the floor. He needs constant supervision and vigilance to reduce the risk of choking by putting small objects into his mouth.

Hearing Adequate hearing is essential for development of normal speech. You must carefully watch your child for his response to various sounds. In infants below 3 months, sudden loud sound may produce a startle response (Moro reflex). Around 4 months, the child would turn towards the sound of a rattle or temple bell. As the child grows, he will respond to the banging of door, sound of music, loud noises or roar of an aeroplane and car of the dad. After one year, he will respond to his name when called from behind or a different room. The best time to assess the hearing of the child is 3 months of age. A number of hearing tests namely brainstem evoked response audiometry (BERA), otoacoustic emission (OAE) and behavioural audiometry are available to precisely assess the hearing of the child.

Speech Crying is the only channel of communication during infancy. Babies are able to signal all their biological needs and physical discomforts through cries and gestures. The earlist speech of a baby is cooing and gurgling sounds which are produced around 3 months of age. By 6 months, the baby is constantly babbling and says simple words like ma-ma, ba-ba, pa-pa, da-da, na-na, etc. Between 9 months and one year, the jargon vocabulary increases and the child may use his own words for water, milk, mama and papa. By second birthday most children are able to talk meaningfully and use pronouns like "I", "me", "you", etc. Some children may continue to use "baby talk" much longer than others and it should be considered us normal. Most normal children develop meaningful speech by the age of 3 years.

Like other milestones of development, there is a wide age-range when normal children learn to speak. Girls speak earlier than boys and this capability stands them in good stead throughout life! High frequency deafness is an important cause of delayed speech. The child may respond to the whispers, tick-tack sound or clapping of hands but he is unable to understand normal speech. He may be

M

able to respond to a passing car, a banging door or a loud thud, so that parents can never believe that he is indeed deaf to certain high frequencies of sound. Whenever in doubt, hearing should be evaluated by formal hearing tests.

Delay in the development of speech is most commonly due to genetic or constitutional factors. In certain families children learn to speak rather late. Isolated delay in development of speech, when other motor and social milestones are normal, is most commonly due to deafness (deaf mutism). Delayed speech or at times regression of speech after having achieved reasonable speech, is an important feature of autism. These children lack social interactions and they live in a world of their own. Tongue-tie (*Tandua*), malocclusion of teeth, and cleft palate, etc. may affect the clarity of speech but they are never a cause for delay in development of speech.

Developmental Delay

In normal children, milestones of development are achieved within a wide range of ages. Children in certain families achieve neuromotor skills earlier and girls in general mature faster than boys especially in development of speech. At times, a child is advanced in development of a particular skill while he may be

Achievement of major milestones	
Milestone	Upper age limit*
Social smile	2 months
Stable head control	4 months
Ability to recognize mother	6 months
Ability to sit independently	8 months
Crawling	9 months
Standing without support	1 year
Walking without support	1½ year
Thumb-forefinger grasp (pincer grasp)	1 year
Disyllabic babbling (ma-ma, da-da)	1 year
Meaningful speech with sentences	4 years

*In prematurely born baby, you must use the corrected or conceptional age. For example, if a child, who was expected to be born on 15th August 2014, is born premature on 15th June 2014 (gestational age 32 weeks), his corrected age on 15th September 2014 shall be only 4 weeks. During first year of life his corrected age should be used for assessment of his physical growth and neuromotor development.

slow in achieving another. For example, it is a common observation that a child may start walking as early as 9–10 months but his speech may be delayed up to 3 to 4 years. The upper age limits for achievements of salient milestones are shown in the **Box**. When there is global retardation in all the milestones, it is suggestive of mental retardation. But isolated delay in walking may be due to malnutrition and poor muscle tone or due to dislocation of hips, and isolated delay in development of speech is most commonly due to deafness and autism spectrum disorder.

MINERALS AND TRACE ELEMENTS

In order to sustain rapid physical growth and mental development of children, they need higher amounts of micronutrients per unit body weight. They must be given balanced nutritious diet to ensure adequate intake of minerals and trace elements.

Calcium It is required for formation of bones and teeth, and integrity of neuromuscular units for maintenance of muscle tone. Milk and dairy products are excellent sources of calcium. Other dietary sources of calcium include millets, *bajra*, *ragi* and green vegetables like *cholai*, *methi* and drumsticks.

Iron It is required for formation of hemoglobin and its deficiency leads to anemia. Iron deficiency is extremely common among infants, adolescent children and pregnant women in our country. Iron deficiency may lead to poor growth, lethargy, fatigability, perverted taste (eating mud) and sluggish neuromotor development. The dietary sources of iron include meat, liver, egg yolk, green vegetables, lentils, fruits, jaggery (*gurh*), and cereals like wheat, *bajra* and *ragi*. Milk is a poor source of iron and children fed on milk alone for a prolonged period of time are likely to develop anemia.

Iodine It is an essential trace element which is required for production of thyroid hormones. People living in hilly areas develop swelling of thyroid gland (goiter) in the neck due to low content of iodine in the soil and water. The good dietary sources of iodine include fish (sea food), meat, green vegetables especially spinach, cereals, milk and dairy products. Common salt fortified with iodine is widely available and must be used.

Zinc Its deficiency can cause poor weight gain, frequent infections, poor sexual development and abnormalities of skin. Zinc intake is credited to promote recovery from diarrhea. The good sources of zinc include wheat, breast milk, eggs, cheese, grains, nuts and meat products.

Miscarriage (*see* Abortion)

MOLLUSCUM CONTAGIOSUM

There are discrete pearly, skin-colored, flat, smooth elevations on the skin with a central dimple or indentation. They may occur in clusters and may affect any part of the body. They are caused by a pox virus. There are no symptoms except mild itching. They are contagious and can affect other family members through close contact, sharing of towels, kerchiefs, and toiletry items. Children with poor immunity and atopic dermatitis may develop widespread lesions.

Treatment The lesions are benign and disappear spontaneously. The individual lesions may be burnt with chemical agents like salicylic acid, cantharidins or tretinoin. It is best to avoid use of any chemical cautery or curettage, which may leave behind pigmentation and scarring.

Mongol Baby (*see* Down syndrome)

MONGOLIAN BLUE SPOTS

In babies of African and Asiatic origin irregular slaty-blue patches of skin pigmentation are commonly present at birth over lower back and buttocks. Rarely, these patches may be seen over the extremities and any part of the body. The spots have no relation to mongolism (Down syndrome) and disappear spontaneously between 6 months and 2 years.

MOSQUITO-BORNE DISEASES

In tropical countries several parasitic and viral infections are transmitted to humans through bites of mosquitoes. In India, two parasitic infections, malaria (female Anopheles) and filaria (Culex species) are transmitted through bites of mosquitoes. Three viral diseases, dengue fever (*Aedes aegyptiae*, *Aedes albopictus*), chikungunya (*Aedes aegyptiae*) and Japanese encephalitis (Culex species) occur as epidemics of life-threatening and disabling diseases in various regions of the country.

Prevention

The mosquito-borne diseases can be prevented by effective control of mosquitoes by improving environmental sanitation, preventing collection of water in the puddles, flower pots, tyres, buckets, and garbage dumps. Avoid stagnation of water in the bathroom, kitchen, terrace, lawn, etc. All drains and sources of stored water should be kept covered. The water in the coolers should be frequently changed and treated with larvicidal chemicals (like kerosene). The dwellings should be provided with iron-mesh doors and windows. Window curtains can be treated with insecticides to prevent entry of mosquitoes. During night, use of mosquito nets treated with insecticides are most effective and safe option for prevention of mosquito bites. Alternatively, electrical vaporisers, mats, coils and sprays can be used at night. Insect repellent creams, lotions and sprays containing 30% DEET or herbal ingredients are available which can be applied over the exposed body parts (except face). Medicated bracelets and stickers are available which can be worn during day time. Children should be encouraged to wear full sleaved shirt and full pants during mosquito breeding season. During the transmission period of mosquitoes (during and after the rainy season), the public health authorities should launch special drives for spray or fogging of malathion at least twice at an interval of 7–10 days. In Vietnam, shell fish mesocyclops have been effectively used in the ponds and pools of water collection as they are credited to eat larvae of *Aedes aegyptiae*.

MOTION SICKNESS

In certain families children develop symptoms of motion sickness while traveling in a car, bus, ship or even an aeroplane. The symptoms occur due to discordance between visually perceived lack of movement inside the vehicle while the vestibular system of the inner ear perceives motion of the vehicle. The common symptoms include nausea, dizziness, vertigo, vomiting and fatigue while traveling in a car or bus especially through hilly terrain and culverts. These children are unable to see a map, read a book or play on an iPod or Tablet while traveling.

The child who is vulnerable to develop motion sickness should avoid intake of heavy fat-rich food before travel. He should preferably sit on the front seat and keep gazing towards the direction of travel or keep his eyes closed and dose off. Sucking dry ginger, sipping ginger tea, taking ginger biscuits or munching a chewing gum are useful for prevention of travel sickness. In severe cases, intake of certain drugs dimenhydrinate (dramamine) and a combination of cinnarizine and domperidone (domstal-CZ, vertigil) one hour before the start of journey are effective to prevent motion sickness. Promethazine (phenergan) and avomine are also useful but they produce drowsiness. When journey is prolonged, the medication should be taken every 4–6 hours during the course of travel.

MUMPS

It is a viral infection which has a predilection to attack salivary glands. After an incubation period (time taken from exposure to onset of symptoms) of 14–21 days, the illness starts with fever, headache, nausea and malaise. Within 24 hours of onset of fever, child develops pain and swelling over one of the parotid glands which is located below the lobe of the ear and infront and above the angle of jaw. Pain is aggravated by chewing and intake of sour food. The disease begins on one side but may involve the other parotid gland after 2–3 days. Common complications include aseptic meningitis, orchitis (swelling and pain in the testis which may lead to infertility) in adolescent boys and severe abdominal pain due to pancreatitis.

Treatment Paracetamol or ibuprofen is given for relief of fever and pain. Oral hygiene should be maintained by regular brushing and antiseptic mouth rinses. Intake of sour foods should be avoided. Orchitis is treated by bed rest and providing support to the testes.

Prevention Mumps can be prevented by administration of MMR (measles, mumps and rubella) vaccine at 9 months of age followed by a booster dose at 15 months. The child with mumps should be isolated until the parotid swelling has disappeared (about one week) to prevent spread of infection to friends and other school-mates.

NAIL BITING

Nail biting may start around 8–10 years of age and is more common in girls. The habit may continue in adult life or appear for the first time during adulthood. The common predisposing factors include insecurity, anxiety, jealousy and stress. Nail biting is socially unacceptable and is associated with increased risk of worm infestation or gastrointestinal infections. Inculcate the habit of keeping nails trimmed from early life. In children finger nails should be trimmed twice a week while toe nails once a week. In order to curb the habit, you should appeal to the sense of pride of the child because ridicule, teasing and scolding can do more harm. Anxiety, insecurity and stress should be relieved by active participation in sports, dancing, music, yoga and meditation.

NEBULIZATION

Nebulizer is an electrical device that converts the liquid drug into aerosol droplets of 1 to 5 microns in diameter. Nebulizers use either compressed air, ultrasonic power or oxygen (in hospital setting) to break up liquid drugs into small vaporized particles. Nebulization can be done either through a mask or mouthpiece. After the procedure, the face should be cleaned with a wet towel and child is asked to drink warm water to rinse the drug sticking over the oral mucosa and throat.

Nebulization is the treatment of choice for management of bronchial spasm or narrowing due to bronchial asthma, cystic fibrosis and other respiratory conditions with bronchospasm. In ambulatory cases, aerosol particles of drugs can be administered through a metered dose inhaler (MDI). A mask or mouthpiece is used for delivery of aerosol and child is asked to breathe through his mouth. A number of bronchodilators like salbutamol, terbutaline, ipratropium bromide and steroids are available which can be administered through inhalation. Aerosol or inhalation therapy is more effective because drug is directly delivered to the site of disease and side effects are lower because a relatively lower dose of medication is used. There is no evidence that inhalers or nebulizers are habit forming. Nebulization with non-medicated normal saline can be used for liquefaction of bronchial secretions and relief of nasal congestion.

NEPHROTIC SYNDROME

It is a chronic autoimmune disease of kidneys with leakage of large quantities of protein in the urine. The common age of onset is 1½ to 5 years. There is sudden development of marked swelling of whole body due to fall in serum albumin level. The swelling appears first on the face around the eyes followed by swelling of feet, legs and genital areas. Abdomen may be distended due to collection of fluid (ascites). Urine examination shows massive amounts of protein. There is marked fall in serum albumin and rise in cholesterol level.

It is a chronic disease with remissions (relief) and relapses (recurrence) and needs long term follow up and treatment. Child is given drugs to promote excretion of urine (diuretics) and corticosteroids. These children are prone to develop intercurrent infections which must be identified early and treated promptly. The child should be given high protein diet like milk and dairy products, *dals*, *chana* (chickpeas), lentils, soybeans, eggs, meat and fish. Supplements of calcium, vitamin D and zinc should be given. Urine should be examined regularly at home with the help of uristix or albustix strips for early identification of relapse. When child is receiving high doses of steroids, live vaccines (MMR, oral polio vaccine, chickenpox) should not be given. They can be given after 3 months of stopping prednisolone. The frequency of relapses decreases as the child grows and complete cure occurs in majority of children. Patients who are dependent or resistant to corticosteroids and those who are frequent relapsers should be under close follow-up by a pediatric nephrologist.

NIGHTMARES AND NIGHT TERRORS

N

Children start having bad dreams or nightmares between the ages of 3 and 5 years. The child may be scared of darkness or to sleep alone in a separate room. The exact cause is not known but they may occur due to stress and frustration during the daytime or after watching a scary program on the television or after unpleasant experience of sexual assault. Due to bad dream, the child wakes up crying and screaming. Mother should comfort and cuddle the child saying that everything is alright and he was just having a bad dream. After he is comforted and relaxed, you can ask him about the contents of the dream to identify the issue bothering him. You should given him the assurance and comfort that he should not worry because you are always close to him to protect him. You should stay with the child until he falls back to sleep. At times, young girls may scream at night when pinworms may wriggle into their vagina.

Night terrors are much less frequent and they tend to run in families. They are more common in boys and usually occur during the age of 5 and 7 years. During the night the child starts screaming loudly but his eyes are wide open with a blank stare. The child looks frightened, has a rapid breathing and marked sweating. The child does not respond to shouting or vigorous shaking by parents and it is difficult to wake him up unlike nightmares. *When the night terror goes off, the child has no scare or memory of the event because it is not dependent on a dream.* About one-third of children with night terrors also experience sleep walking. Mother should hold and cuddle the child during the episode of night terror till he goes back to sleep again. When a child is having frequent nightmares or night terrors, parents should consult a neurologist or child psychologist.

Nocturnal Enuresis (*see* Bed wetting)

NON-RETRACTABLE FORESKIN (Phimosis)

The foreskin (prepuce) is not retractable at birth in almost all newborns. Even by one year of age, foreskin is not retractable in up to 50% of boys. This does not cause any problem or difficulty in passing urine. Ballooning of prepuce while passing urine is normal in infants. There is no need to retract the foreskin during

1–2 years of age. After 2 years, efforts may be made to gently retract the foreskin while bathing the baby. Nappy rash should be prevented or promptly treated to prevent scarring of the foreskin. The boys should be explained to retract their foreskin and wash the penis with soap and water during bathing. When preputial opening is narrow and causing difficulty in passing urine, it can be treated by a minor procedure of dilatation of the orifice. When foreskin is scarred and there are frequent episodes of pus discharge from the urethral opening (balanitis) or recurrent episodes of urinary tract infection, circumcision is recommended. The procedure should be done by a pediatric surgeon under anesthetic cover.

NOSE BLEED (Epistaxis)

Nose bleeding is common in children especially during hot dry weather. It usually occurs spontaneously without any injury to the nose. Nose picking is an important cause of epistaxis. During an episode of cough and cold, bleeding may occur because of frequent cleaning or blowing of nose. Nose bleeding may rarely occur due to injury with a ball or insertion of a sharp object in the nose. Epistaxis may occur during acute viral illness (dengue fever), bleeding disorder or vascular malformation.

First-aid It is frightening to see a child bleeding from the nose. There is no need for any alarm or panic because bleeding stops spontaneously within a few minutes. Child should be asked to sit up with head slightly bent forwards. He should be asked to pinch both the nostrils firmly with a clean handkerchief or a paper napkin while breathing through the mouth. Apply a cold pack over the nose if the child is old enough to cooperate. When bleeding is massive or persistent lasting for more than 5–10 minutes and when it is occurring frequently, an ENT specialist should be consulted for management. In order to prevent recurrences, the nails should be kept trimmed and nostrils kept lubricated with a moisturizing cream or an antiseptic ointment.

NOSE BLOCK (Nasal congestion)

Nose block occurs most commonly due to swelling of the inner lining of mucosa of the nostrils either due to infection (viral, bacterial or fungal) or allergic rhinitis (nasal allergy or hay fever).

Persistent nasal blockage may occur due to enlarged adenoids, sinusitis, foreign body and deflected nasal septum.

Infants become miserable due to blockage of nose because it interferes with their sleep and feeding behaviour. Infants are facultative or compulsory nose breathers and they do not open their mouth even when the nose is blocked. Infant cannot effectively suck the breast or bottle and frequently stops sucking to take the breath from the mouth. The baby becomes irritable and cries during feeding. The swelling of nasal mucosa may block the Eustachian tube causing vacuum in the middle ear with retraction of drum/s or infection in the middle ear (acute otitis media) on one or both sides. When nasal discharge becomes thick and purulent, it is suggestive of superadded bacterial infection. The presence of blood in the nasal secretions is suggestive of local injury due to frequent aspiration or cleaning of nose, foreign body, nasal diphtheria and congenital syphilis.

Treatment

Nasal congestion makes babies miserable and it is difficult to treat because of small size of the nostrils. Avoid local instillation of medicated nose drops due to risk of develpment of chemical rhinitis and rebound nasal congestion, i.e. after initial temporary relief, the nasal congestion becomes worse. Cough mixtures containing antihistamines may also worsen the nose block by drying the nasal secretions.

Steam inhalation with a warm-mist humidifier or a steam vaporizer is useful to relieve nasal congestion. It should be given twice a day for about 10 minutes each time. After steam inhalation, the baby should be placed in a prone position (tummy position) to drain the nasal secretions. The nose should be kept clean with a cotton bud or nasal secretions sucked out with a soft bulb suction device because young children cannot blow out their nasal secretions. Squeeze the bulb of the aspirator and insert its tip into one of the nostrils. Slowly release the bulb to suck out the mucus from the nostril. Repeat the procedure on the other side. Saline nose drops (0.6% solution of sodium chloride in water) can be instilled for liquefaction of secretions before suction. Saline nose drops are better than medicated nose drops for keeping the nostrils wet and open. Placing the infant on abdomen (prone position)

Home Remedies

Steam inhalation can be done by adding eucalyptus, caraway or carom seeds (*ajwain*), holy basil leaves (*tulsi*), mint or sage leaves. The roasted *ajwain* seeds can be tied in a thin muslin cloth and kept near the pillow for the infant to inhale. The *ajwain* contained in a thin muslin cloth can be warmed on a *tawa* or hot water bottle and infant is allowed to inhale it.

may assist in draining the nasal secretions. Application of a rub liniment (over the chest and neck) containing eucalyptus and menthol is useful to relieve nasal congestion. To avoid irritation of the delicate skin of an infant, the liniment should be diluted with an equal quantity of cold cream, before application. Keeping the head raised and covered with a cap (especially in winter) is also useful to reduce nasal congestion.

OBESITY

Overnutrition and obesity are being increasingly recognized in children belonging to affluent families in our society. Over one-fourth of adolescent children attending private schools are obese. School going children are crazy to take calorie-dense unhealthy snacks and junk foods like soft drinks, canned juices, burgers, pizzas, French fries, noodles, *samosas*, chocolates, and desserts. There is changing lifestyle with poor participation in outdoor activities and sports. Children are seen munching snacks and taking cold drinks while sitting in front of TV and computer. According to WHO, body mass index or BMI [(weight in kg/ (height in meters)^2] of greater than 85th and 95th percentile of BMI-for-age and sex reference standard are used for the diagnosis of over weight and obesity respectively. Weight-for-height and abdominal girth-for-height are also used for the diagnosis of obesity.

Every mother is keen to see her baby plump and there is a constant urge to overfeed or force feed the child. Bottle or formula-fed babies are usually overweight compared to breastfed babies because animal milk is over dense in calories compared to human milk. Obesity runs in families and in these families the parents should be careful about the child's activity and his food intake. If both parents are obese, the chances of their child becoming obese are as high as 80%. Early onset of obesity leads to increase in the number of fat cells thus causing obesity in adult life. The constitutional predisposition to obesity occurs due to presence of an "ob" gene that regulates the production of a protein called leptin which controls metabolic rate and appetite.

O

Health Consequences

Obesity is most commonly due to constitutional factors and occurs because of imbalance between food intake and energy expended by physical activity. The yo yo, style of fasting or missing meals followed by periods of bingeing, is an important cause of obesity. When child becomes overweight, he becomes lazy and inactive thus establishing a vicious cycle of overeating-inactivity-obesity. These children may become unhappy and depressed when other children start nagging or making fun of them. Obese children are likely to be tall for their age and have a large body frame. In obese adolescent boys, small size of penis is of great concern to the parents. It is apparent and not real because two-thirds of the length of the penis is embedded in the pubic fat. Most of these boys have normal sexual development and many of them lose their excess weight at puberty. In some obese adolescent girls, obesity and hirsutism (appearance of facial hair) may be associated with polycystic ovarian disease (PCOD) which should be ruled out. Obese children are more prone to develop frequent respiratory infections. Obesity in adult life is a recognized risk factor for development of Type 2 diabetes mellitus, high blood pressure, heart disease, osteoarthritis and cancer. Obese children are more prone to develop snoring and obstructive sleep apnea (episodes of sudden cessation of breathing at night). Obesity due to hormonal causes is rare and occurs at a younger age. It is usually associated with short stature, poor sexual development, high blood pressure and mental retardation.

Treatment

- The whole family should be advised to change the lifestyle, i.e. increase the activity level and reduce the caloric intake. It is impossible to change the routine and habits of the child unless everybody in the family cooperates and participates.
- Healthy food habits should be practiced by taking plenty of green leafy vegetables, salads and seasonal fruits (except calorie-dense fruits like banana, grapes, mangoes and cheekoo). Food should be prepared in minimal oil or fat. Energy dense foods like soft drinks, *sherbats*, fruit juices, junk food, crisps and French fries, fried items (like *poories, samosas, kachoris, mathies, namkeen*, etc.) desserts, dry fruits, sweets, chocolates, etc. should be restricted or denied. Double-toned or fat-free milk should be

used for drinking or making curd, cheese and other milk products. It is desirable to adopt vegetarian diet and keep cooking oil to the barest minimum.

- Before eating the meals, salads like cabbage, lettuce, cucumber, carrots, tomatoes, etc. and water can be taken to fill the stomach. Food should be eaten slowly and not hurriedly so that satiety is achieved with lower intake of food.

- Missing of meals and "dieting" are strongly condemned. The common practice of fasting followed by excessive bingeing is detrimental to health and should be avoided. The use of drugs to reduce appetite and surgical treatment (bariatrics) of obesity are not recommended in children.

- TV viewing should be restricted to one hour and no food or snacks should be allowed while viewing TV. Healthy snacks like salads and fruits should be encouraged in-between the meals.

- The child should be encouraged to take part in outdoor activities and sports like running, jogging, skipping, cycling, and swimming. He should be encouraged to play badminton, tennis, football, basketball or cricket depending upon his interest. Aerobic exercises, yoga and dancing are extremely useful and health-friendly activities.

- If a child is depressed and unhappy, lacking drive or enthusiasm, the help of a psychologist should be sought to identify the underlying cause and treat it.

- The goal for weight reduction should be realistic, slow and sustainable. Motivation and will power are needed to stick to weight reduction program. It is reasonable to target a weight reduction of about 0.5–1.0 kg every 2–4 weeks.

- Treatment of endogenous or pathological obesity is symptomatic and depends upon the underlying cause. Hormonal replacement therapy (thyroxin, hGH and sex hormones) or surgical excision of an hormone-producing tumor are likely to be curative.

OMEGA-3 AND OMEGA-6 FATTY ACIDS

Omega-3 and omega-6 fatty acids are polyunsaturated fatty acids (PUFAs) which are essential fatty acids for promotion of health and well-being. Omega-3 fatty acids are heart-friendly as they reduce the risk of cardiac arrhythmia, keep the blood thin and reduce inflammation of blood vessels and risk of elevated blood pressure. The vegetarian dietary sources of omega-3 fatty acids include vegetable oils (flaxseed or linseed, canola or rapeseed, soya oil, olive oil, peanut oil), green leafy vegetables (fenugreek, broccoli), lentils (kidney beans, Bengal gram, *urad dal*, *bajra*) and dry fruits (walnuts, almonds, pistachios, peanuts, pumpkin seeds) and seaweed or algae. The nonvegetarian sources of omega-3 fatty acids and their metabolite DHA include human milk, egg yolk and sea food like oily fish (mackerel, sardine, *hilsa*, salmon, *seer*, *pasava*, *katla*) and fish oil. Omega-6 fatty acids are better than saturated fats (vanaspati, full cream milk, butter, cheese, coconut oil, palm oil) but not as good as omega-3 fatty acids. The dietary sources of omega-6 fatty acids include safflower oil, sunflower oil, corn oil, and sesame oil. They are cheaper than omega-3 fatty acids. It is recommended that omega-6 and omega-3 fatty acids should be consumed in a ratio of 5–10 : 1 to ensure optimal integrity of central nervous system and heart. Monounsaturated fats (MUFAs) or omega-9 fatty acids are also heart-friendly and they are obtained from olive oil, canola oil, peanut oil, mustard oil, clarified butter (*desi ghee*), and avocados.

ORAL REHYDRATION SOLUTION (ORS)

Oral rehydration solution is a life-saving treatment for replacement of fluids and electrolyte losses in children with vomiting and diarrhea. The child with fluid loss should be encouraged to take water, ORS or other home fluids like *dal ka pani*, coconut water, weak tea and butter milk. Fruit juices (fresh or canned) and cola drinks should not be given due to risk of aggravation of diarrhea and abdominal distension. WHO recommends ORS formulation containing glucose 13.5 g, sodium chloride 2.6 g, potassium chloride 1.5 g, and trisodium citrate 2.9 g per one liter. ORS can be prepared at home by taking 2 finger-and-thumb pinch (half a teaspoon) of table salt and 4-finger scoop of sugar (4 level teaspoons) and by adding few drops of lemon juice in one liter of RO or boiled safe drinking water. The properly prepared ORS should taste like tears.

The instructions printed on the ORS sachet for its reconstitution should be followed. To avoid risk of contamination, a small sachet (6 g) should be reconstituted in 200 mL or a glass of water. When one liter of ORS is prepared with a 30 g sachet, it should be properly covered and kept in a fridge or a cool room and used within

12 hours. The child should be given frequent sips of ORS with the help of a spoon. Large gulps of ORS with a cup or glass may lead to vomiting. Give extra fluids or ORS every time when child vomits or passes a loose motion. ORS must be continued during night to prevent dehydration. When a child refuses to drink ORS, he can be given plain water and home-available fluids. You should ensure that your child passes light-colored or water-like urine as frequently as he was passing before the onset of vomiting or diarrhea. Lack of passage of urine for more than 6 hours in an infant or 12 hours in an older child, is suggestive of severe dehydration and need for admission to the hospital for intravenous administration of fluids.

ORGANIC FOODS

Organic foods are non-genetically modified cereals, vegetables and fruits grown without the use of chemical fertilizers and pesticides. They are grown with the help of natural organic manure and protected with plant-based safe pesticides like neem and eucalyptus. The soil should be free of chemicals for at least 1–2 years before it is certified organic and produce can be labelled as organic. Organic foods are free from health hazards of chemicals and they taste better but their nutrient content is not superior to conventionally grown food products. Even milk, eggs, meat and poultry can be organically produced when animals and birds are reared in organic forms. Organic foods are sold in packages that are labelled as "organic". They are expensive and should be purchased if they are certified organic by a reliable licensing authority.

OSTEOMYELITIS

Infection of bone occurs most commonly due to pyogenic bacteria but may occur due to tubercular bacilli, fungi and viruses. It is characterized by fever and signs of inflammation over the affected bone/s. The signs of inflammation include swelling, redness, warmth, pain and tenderness. There may be preceding history of trauma or evidences of tuberculosis elsewhere in the body. The condition is treated by surgical drainage of pus and administration of appropriate antibiotic/s for several weeks due to poor penetration of antibiotics because of relatively poor blood supply of the bone.

Otitis Media (*see* Acute otitis media)

PACIFIER (Dummy nipple)

It is a common practice in the West to offer a pacifier or dummy nipple to the baby while mother is busy with her household chores. The use of a pacifier is associated with several health hazards and must be avoided in our setting. There is a risk of contamination of the pacifier by flies and when it falls on the ground, which may lead to frequent episodes of diarrhea. The sucking of empty dummy nipple leads to swallowing of air with intestinal colic. When a pacifier is used with a sweetening agent (sugar or honey), it may cause damage to the teeth. Above all, mother ignores the signals of hunger and discomfort by quieting or comforting the child with a pacifier. The child may become malnourished because his hunger cries are satisfied with a pacifier rather than by giving him milk. In Indian setting, a pacifier should never be given to the baby due to several health hazards.

PAIN ABDOMEN

Pain abdomen is an extremely common symptom in children. When pain is acute, severe and of sudden onset and associated with fever, vomiting, abdominal distension and disturbances in passage of urine or stools (constipation or diarrhea), the child must be immediately taken to a doctor for proper evaluation.

School going children often complain of frequent, vague, momentary episodes of pain. Pain lasts for a brief period, child is generally well, takes his food normally, goes to school and participates in play activities. Child does not cry due to pain and points the site of pain vaguely over the navel region. Pain mostly occurs at home and not in school or during play time. The pain may be due to a prank by the child to miss the school or avoid drinking milk. There are no associated symptoms pertaining to bowels or urinary system. Some children may also complain of aches and pains over the head, chest and limbs. These episodes of pain are usually an attention seeking behaviour or blackmailing tactics to seek attention or avoid intake of food or milk. These children do not need any investigations and episodes of pain disappear by "intelligent neglect" (not showing excessive concern and anxiety), distraction, denial of any "gain" like missing the school or sleeping with parents and administration of home remedies like *pudin hara* or *ajwain*. Some children may have genuine abdominal pain and flatulence after drinking milk because of deficiency of lactase enzyme (lactose intolerance). The episodes of pain disappear on stopping milk. These children, however, can tolerate intake of milk products like yoghurt, custard, *kheer* and cheese.

The common physical or genuine causes of recurrent abdominal pain in children include worm infestation, giardiasis, urinary tract infection, gastroesophageal reflux, acidity or dyspepsia. The pain may occur due to excessive food indulgence, food allergy or intolerance. These children have associated symptoms like nausea, vomiting, retrosternal burning sensation, constipation or loose motions, frequency of micturition and failure to thrive. The child may wake up at night and pain is usually severe enough to make the child uncomfortable or cry. The pain is usually located at a site other than mid-abdomen and generally pointed by the child with his finger tip rather than the whole hand. These children should be investigated to identify the underlying cause of pain abdomen and managed appropriately. It is true that worm infestation is common in our country but many a times it does not cause abdominal pain. Nevertheless, it is advisable to deworm the child every 6 months or whenever stool examination shows ova or cysts of worms.

PEPTIC ULCER

Peptic ulcer is uncommon in children but may occur in school going children or adolescents. Ulcer develops in the second part of duodenum due to imbalance between pepsin, acid and enzymes of stomach. It is caused by an infection with bacteria called *Helicobacter pylori*. Pain is usually aggravated by intake of spicy and fried food, pickles, chocolates, cola drinks, tea and coffee. Stress, anxiety and worry are recognized aggravating factors.

P

The common symptoms are dyspepsia, bloating, burning pain in the upper abdomen and behind the chest bone or sternum. The symptoms occur more commonly when stomach is empty (before meals) and during sleep due to gastroesophageal reflux. Discomfort and burning sensation are relieved by intake of cold water, milk, yoghurt, and bland food. Symptomatic relief is obtained by intake of antacids, sucraflate and ranitidine or omeprazole. In resistant cases, *Helicobacter pylori* should be treated by administration of specific medications like amoxicillin, metronidazole and omeprazole.

PICA (Mud eating)

During 1–2 years when children are passing through the "oral" or "mouthing" phase of development, they try to put their fingers and every object into their mouth. It may be a sign of lack of attention or boredom, birth of a younger sibling or irritation of gums due to teething. The child may pluck his hair and swallow them or eat inedible objects like mud, scrapings of wall, chalk, crayons, paint of toys, etc. virtually anything that he can lay his hands on. When perverted habit persists, it poses a risk for development of diarrhea, worm infestation and lead poisoning (paint of toys and furniture). It was originally believed that pica may be a sign of calcium deficiency but there is no scientific basis for this. There is some evidence that perverted apptite or behaviour may be a symptom of iron deficiency.

The condition is best managed by distraction, providing more opportunities for play and by reducing his chances to play with clay and mud. The child should not be left alone in the garden where he would have ample opportunities to eat mud. Scolding and frightening the child does not serve any purpose. Administration of iron supplement is associated with faster recovery. The child should be encouraged to take iron-rich foods like green vegetables, fruits (banana, apple, pomegranate), egg yolk, chicken, liver and jaggery. In due course of time most children abandon the habit as their "mouthing" tendency gradually decreases.

PERIANAL ITCHING AND SORENESS

The commonest cause of anal itching, which mostly occurs at night, is pinworm infestation. Other causes of anal itching include constipation, anal fissure, rectal prolapse and insertion of foreign body in the anus. Perianal redness and soreness is common in bottle fed babies due to passage of acidic stools and it becomes worse following a bout of diarrhea.

Local application of a bland oil (coconut or olive oil), moisturizing cream or calamine based anesthetic cream provides symptomatic relief. The underlying cause of anal itching should be identified and appropriately treated under the guidance of your doctor. The baby with perianal soreness or redness should be cleaned gently and lightly with wet cotton after passage of urine and stools. Keeping the baby in a prone or tummy position and exposing the buttocks to the air (preferably sunlight) is followed by prompt recovery. You can apply zinc and titanium containing baby cream which hastens recovery. Never apply mustard oil which can produce irritation and smarting.

PHIMOSIS

When foreskin (prepuce) of the penis cannot be retracted it is called phimosis. During first 2 years of life, foreskin is normally not retractable and it should not be labelled as phimosis. Some children cry before passing urine (due to unpleasant sensation of full bladder), become quiet while passing urine and start crying again after having passed urine due to wet napkin. It is normal and should not be considered as difficulty in passing urine. Phimosis occurs due to inflammation and scarring of foreskin because of constant use of diaper and infrequent cleaning of bottom. It leads to difficulty and straining while passing urine. The urine may dribble in drops rather than a forceful stream. When child has definite phimosis after the age of 2 years, it is managed by circumcision (excision of foreskin). The procedure should be done by a pediatric surgeon under anesthetic cover.

PHYSIOTHERAPY

Therapy by physical means like active and passive exercises, body massage, heat therapy, wax bath, hydrotherapy, diathermy, infrared rays, nerve stimulation, and occupational therapy, etc. is commonly harnessed for management of developmental disorders and neuromotor disabilities which are common in children. Facilities for developmental screening, assessment of cognition and special senses (hearing and vision), physiotherapy and early

stimulation or intervention program should form an integral part
of all neonatal intensive care units.

POISONING

Children are at an increased risk of accidentally drinking or
swallowing toxic drugs and chemicals. The commonly ingested
agents include kerosene, insecticides or agricultural pesticides, rat
poison, acids or alkalies, naphthalene balls and drugs. Children
in the villages are at risk to eat poisonous seeds (*dhatura* and castor
seeds), fruits and leaves. Most of the household cosmetics (except
nail polish, after shave lotion, depilators and skin color lighteners)
are safe and non-toxic. Poisoning as a suicidal attempt may occur
in adolescent children.

When poisoning is suspected, try to induce vomiting by tickling
the throat, giving him a glass of milk or a mixture of milk with
egg white which helps to dilute and delay absorption of most
poisons. Vomiting should not be induced if child has consumed a
hydrocarbon agent like kerosene, petrol, cleansing agent or thinner
and when child is drowsy or unconscious. Every episode of
suspected poisoning should be taken seriously and child must be
taken to the hospital. The empty bottle of medicine must be taken
along with to show to the doctor. Parents must take necessary
steps and exercise vigilance at home to prevent occurrence of
poisoning.

Predicted Adult Height (*see* Ultimate adult height)

PROBIOTICS AND PREBIOTICS

Probiotics in Greek language means "for life" and they refer to
health-friendly bacteria in the gut which promote health and well-
being. They are present in plenty in human milk (*L. acidophilus*
and *Bifidobacterium bifidum*) and yoghurt. Human gut contains
a large quantity of probiotics which are made up of at least
500 species of health-friendly bacteria. Probiotics are credited to
prevent the entry of harmful or pathogenic (disease-producing)
bacteria and food allergens, promote digestion and absorption of
food, stimulate immunity of the gut and promote endogenous
production of vitamin K. Excessive intake of antibiotics and poor
dietary choices may lead to imbalance between health-friendly

and disease-producing bacteria which is called dysbiosis. A number of food products (like milk, yoghurt and milk supplements) are available in the market which are fortified with probiotics. They are safe and useful and can be consumed by healthy children.

Prebiotics are fructo-oligosaccharides which are obtained from carbohydrate fibers (fruits, vegetables, legumes, and whole grains) and they promote the growth of probiotics. Synbiotics are commercial preparations that contain both prebiotics and probiotics.

Therapeutic benefits The indications for use of probiotics in clinical practice are controversial. They have been found to be useful for prevention of antibiotic-associated diarrhea, hospital or community acquired diarrhea and necrotizing enterocolitis (NEC) in newborn babies. They have a controversial role in the treatment of a large number of clinical conditions like acute infectious diarrhea, lactose intolerance, irritable bowel syndrome, inflammatory bowel disease, evening colic and allergic rhinitis. A number of prebiotic and probiotic formulations are available in the market. Their beneficial effects are related to the dose and type of probiotics. A combination of *Lactobacillus GG*, *Saccharomyces boulardi*, *L. acidophilus* and *Bifidobacterium bifidum* have been found to be most useful. They are generally safe but should be avoided in sick immunocompromised children.

Q FEVER

Q fever (query fever) is caused by *C. burnetii* belonging to the genus of Legionellales. The infection is transmitted from domestic livestock or contact with products of conception of sheep, dogs, cats and rabbits. The infection is common in people working in the farms and slaughterhouses. It may occur as acute fever with influenza like symptoms or chronic Q fever with involvement of several body organs including valves of the heart. Most cases are self-limiting and resolve spontaneously. Doxycycline is useful to shorten the course of disease.

QUICKENINGS

The movements of the baby in the womb are called quickenings. They appear around 14–16 weeks (after 3 months) of pregnancy. You are excited to feel the kicks of your growing baby. They can also be felt by your partner or elder sibling by placing their hand or cheek against your tummy.

Fetal kick count after 28 weeks of pregnancy is useful to assess the well-being of the fetus. The fetus must produce at least one movement per hour or 10 kicks during the day. Excessive movements or sluggish movements are equally bad. If there are less than 10 movements for two consecutive days, you must report to your doctor. Excessive fetal movements are indicative of fetal hypoxia. When fetus does not get enough oxygen in the womb, it behaves like a strangulated individual and makes desperate physical efforts and movements. The exaggerated fetal movements are gradually followed by slow and reduced fetal movements which finally stop when fetus dies in the uterus.

QUINSY

It is a rare complications of acute tonsillitis due to *Group A beta-hemolytic streptococci*. The infection spreads beyond the tonsils to cause peritonsillar abscess or quinsy. There is high grade fever, marked toxemia, difficulty in swallowing, drooling of saliva, hoarseness of voice and lock jaw. There is asymmetrical enlargement of tonsils with bulging of tonsils on one side. The child should be admitted to the hospital and managed under the guidance of an ENT specialist. Amoxicillin-clavulanic acid is given intravenously and abscess is drained by needle aspiration or open surgical drainage is done along with removal of tonsils (tonsillectomy) during acute stage.

RABIES

Rabies is caused by a viral infection which is transmitted by the bite of a rabid dog, cat, monkey, bat, mongoose and jackal. The incubation period is long and varies between 20 and 40 days (rarely up to one year). The disease may occur early when bites are on the face or upper limb. The initial symptoms include fever, muscle pains, headache, easy fatigability and changes in the mood. This is followed by changes in behaviour, agitation, restlessness, excessive tears and salivation. *The associated symptoms of tingling sensations or fasciculations at the site of bite are highly suggestive of impending rabies.* Hydrophobia (fear of water) is the most characteristic feature of rabies. When shown a glass of water, patient develops violent spasms of muscles of swallowing. A draught of air over the face may cause similar symptoms (aerophobia). There is no specific treatment and rabies is an invariably fatal disease. It is, therefore, crucial to prevent occurrence of rabies by effective antirabies vaccination and administration of antirabies immunoglobulin (RIG) following the bite of a potentially rabid animal (refer to dog bite).

Rabies in animals Rabies in dogs take two forms, namely furious and dumb rabies. In the commoner furious rabies, dog becomes restless and develops tendency to bite any object or person without any provocation. There may be drooling of saliva and inability to bark. Over the next few days, the stage of restlessness subsides and the animal seeks a secluded place and dies of rapidly progressive paralysis. The dog with dumb rabies becomes depressed and withdraws itself and lapses into coma. Following development of clinical signs of rabies, the dog generally dies within a week. The manifestations of rabies in cats, resemble furious rabies of dogs. The cat hides in an isolated corner and attacks unprovoked anyone coming near it. The cat may strike forepaws in air as if it were catching imaginary mice.

RECTAL PROLAPSE

There is abnormal descent or prolapse of rectal mucosa through the anus after passing the poop. It appears like a bright pink glistening swelling with leakage of few drops of blood. The condition is mostly seen in infants and preschool children. The predisposing conditions include malnutrition, constipation, recurrent or persistent diarrhea, worm infestation, inflammatory bowel disease (IBD), and celiac disease.

The prolapsed rectum should be manually pushed back after defecation. The nutritional status should be improved by giving balanced diet and nutritional supplements. Sitz baths are useful to strengthen perineal muscles. The child is made to sit in a plastic basin containig warm water and he is asked to contract (as if trying to stop urination or defecation) and relax perineal muscles for 5–10 minutes three times in a day. In severe cases the buttocks can be strapped with leukoplast after reduction of the prolapse. Injection of sclerosing agents into the submucosa of rectum and surgical repair (rectopexy) are rarely needed in children.

REGURGITATION OF FEEDS

Most healthy babies regurgitate some curdled milk after a feed but they continue to gain weight satisfactorily. During feedings, baby swallows some air which causes distention and discomfort till baby is able to eructate. Regurgitation is more common in bottle fed babies compared to breastfed infants. After each feed (sometimes even when only one-half of the feed is given) mother should make the baby sit in her lap or hold the baby against her shoulder to help him eructate the swallowed air. After burping, the baby should be placed in the cot in the right lateral position with head end slightly raised. When regurgitation is persistent and frequent, and weight gain is unsatisfactory, gastroesophageal reflux due to lax gastroesophageal sphincter should be ruled out.

RETINOPATHY OF PREMATURITY

Retinopathy of prematurity (ROP) is characterized by proliferation of small blood vessels of retina in premature babies. The condition is by and large limited to preterm babies with a birth weight of less than 1500 g or gestational age of less than 32 weeks. The leading cause of ROP is exposure to high concentrations of oxygen leading to marked elevation of oxygen tension in the arterial blood. Other risk factors include exposure to bright light, episodes of "no breathing" or apneic attacks, anemia, acidosis, blood transfusion, patent ductus arteriosus and assisted ventilation. Hyperoxia (excessive concentration and tension of oxygen in the arterial blood) leads to vasoconstriction of retinal vessels which is followed by formation of new blood vessels and retinal damage due to scarring and retinal detachment. ROP is one of the leading causes of preventable blindness in children.

Oxygen is life-saving but it is potentially toxic drug and should be given in the lowest concentration and for as short a period as required. All infants with a birth weight of <1500 g or gestational age of <32 weeks should be screened by a pediatric ophthalmologist in the NICU for early diagnosis of ROP. Timely laser photocoagulation is associated with reduced risk of retinal damage and blindness.

Reproductive Health Education (*see* Family Life Education)

RETRACTED NIPPLES

There are wide variations in the shape and size of breasts and nipples. When nipples are flat, retracted or inverted, it causes serious feeding difficulties leading to engorgement of breasts. The condition should be identified during pregnancy and mother can be asked to roll the nipple/s between thumb and index finger and pull it out. If manual eversion fails to correct the abnormality, syringe method is usually effective to treat the condition. Take a 10 ml plastic syringe and remove its piston. Cut the barrel of syringe half a centimeter from the nozzle and insert the piston from the cut end of the barrel. Place the smooth or non-cut side of the barrel of the syringe around the nipple and withdraw the piston gently. The nipple will slowly protrude into the barrel. After 30–60 seconds, push the piston gently to release the hold of the syringe on the nipple. The procedure should be repeated 5–8 times before each breastfeeding. As soon as the nipple becomes prominent or everted, hold the nipple and areola in your thumb and index finger to form a teat and put the baby to the breast. You should wear a breast shell under the bra to avoid compression of nipples.

Avoid the use of a nipple shield, which is usually ineffective and may be harmful.

RHESUS ISOIMMUNIZATION

When an Rh-negative mother is carrying an Rh-positive fetus, the leakage of fetal red blood cells into the maternal circulation may invoke an antibody response in the mother. Enough anti-D (rhesus antigen is called D antigen) antibodies are not produced during the first pregnancy but each subsequent pregnancy with Rh-positive fetus leads to increasing titers of anti-D antibodies. The anti-D antibodies being IgG in type, they readily cross over to the fetus through placenta and destroy Rh-positive or D-positive fetal red blood cells. the Rh-isoimmunization can be suspected during antenatal period by identifying the blood group of the mother (Rh-negative mother) and estimating the titer of maternal anti-D antibodies by indirect Coombs' test.

Rhesus isoimmunization leads to development of rhesus hemolytic disease (Rh-HDN) of the newborn. There is increasing severity of disease with each subsequent pregnancy. Jaundice occurs within 24 hours of age and rapidly increase in intensity and is managed by phototherapy or exchange blood transfusion. In a severely affected baby, there is severe anemia, marked increase in the size of liver and spleen, generalized swelling (hydrops fetalis) and at times the baby may die in the uterus.

Rhesus isoimmunization can be effectively prevented by pro-phylactic administration of anti-D immunoglobulins (500 μg IM) to an unsensitized (indirect Coombs' test negative) Rh-negative mother within 72 hours of delivery or after a procedure in following situations: (i) Delivery of Rh-positive baby, (ii) abortion or stillborn Rh-positive fetus and (iii) after conducting certain procedures like amniocentesis, chorionic villus sampling and external podalic version in an Rh-negative woman. The anti-D immunoglobulins should only be given to the mother whose indirect Coombs' test is negative. It should be given as early as possible after the delivery, abortion or procedure, but preferably within 72 hours. In order to improve its efficacy it is recommended to administer 500 μg anti-D immunoglobulins to all unsensitized Rh-negative women during 28–32 weeks of gestation. When delivery occurs more than 4 weeks later and the infant is Rh-positive, the mother should receive additional 500 μg anti-D immunoglobulins IM within 72 hours of delivery.

RHEUMATIC FEVER

Rheumatic fever occurs when Group A beta hemolytic streptococcal infection of throat (strep throat) or skin (pyoderma) is inadequately treated or not treated at all. The common age of occurrence is between 5 and 14 years. After about 2 weeks of sore throat or skin boils, the child develops high grade fever with pain and swelling in several joints. The commonly affected joints include wrists, elbows, knees and ankles. The joint pains migrates or shifts from one joint to the other, wherein previously affected joint becomes normal. The child may develop skin rash and subcutaneous nodules over bony prominences. Jerky, purposeless, "dancing-like" incoordinated movements due to chorea may occur in adolescent girls. Chorea is usually not associated with joints pains. The main danger of rheumatic fever is damage to the heart because of myocarditis, involvement of cardiac valves and heart failure.

The child should be under careful observation of a pediatrician and pediatric cardiologist. Streptococcal throat infection must be treated with pencillin or amoxycillin for at least 10 days. Bed rest and salicylates are used for relief of joint pains. Corticosteroids are used for treatment of carditis. Recurrence of rheumatic fever can be prevented by administration of long acting penicillin (600,000 units < 6 yr and 12,00,000 units > 6 yr) every 3 weeks deep IM for at least 5 years or up to the age of 18 years. In patients with carditis or rheumatic heart disease, penicillin prophylaxis is continued lifelong or at least up to the age of 40 years. When valves of the heart are permanently damaged, the child would need a surgical repair or replacement of affected valve/s later in life.

RICKETS

Rickets is the disease of growing bones and occurs in children with vitamin D deficiency. Breast milk is relatively deficient in vitamin D and infants who are exclusively breastfed should receive supplements of vitamin D. Other causes of vitamin D deficiency include dark skin, poor exposure of skin to sunlight, chronic diarrhea and poor dietary intake of vitamin D. Rickets usually occur in actively growing or chubby children between 6 months and 2 years of age. It causes various deformities of bones and delayed eruption of teeth. The head looks large and square and soft spot on the crown or top of the head is large and its closure is delayed. The chest may be narrow and project forward like a pigeon. The bones become soft and curved (bowed legs or knock knees) and ends of long bones become enlarged and wide at wrists and ankles. Spinal deformities may occur. Muscle tone is reduced and child develops pot belly. These children are likely to have iron deficiency anemia and frequent respiratory infections. The diagnosis is confirmed by estimation of vitamin D level, serum calcium, phosphorus and alkaline phosphatase and skiagrams of wrists or knees. The condition is treated by weekly administration of oral vitamin D_3 60,000 i.u. for 10 weeks. The child should be encouraged to play outdoor for adequate exposure to sunlight and given a diet rich in calcium and vitamin D.

RINGWORM

R

Fungal infection of skin in hot and humid climate causes ringworm. The typical skin lesion is ring shaped coin-sized red colored plaque with elevated margins. There is marked itching. The central area shows clearing with formation of thin scales. The common sites of occurrence of ringworms include scalp, trunk, groins, upper and inner sides of thighs, feet and nails. Ensure strict personal hygiene and avoid sharing of towels, caps and scarves. Topical application of antifungal cream twice a day for 2–4 weeks is curative. Fungal infection of scalp, feet and nails is treated by oral antifungal agents (griseofulvin, fluconazole, ketoconazole, terbinafine) which are given for at least 8–12 weeks.

ROAD-TO-HEALTH CARD

During first five years of life, weight and length/height should be recorded on a Road-to-Health card. These measurements should be recorded every month (during visits for vaccinations) during first year, every 2 months during second year and every 3 months subsequently. The periodic and regular weight record provides valuable information regarding physical growth and well-being of the child. The trend or slope of the weight and height curves is more important than its location on the chart. The growth curve of the healthy child should be directed upwards or it should run parallel to the 50th percentile line. The card also gives simple messages regarding immunization, feeding and developmental milestones. You should understand the significance and importance of growth charting, and keep the Road-to-Health card in your safe custody.

Rubella (*see* German measles)

SCABIES

Scabies occur due to infection by a tiny flea *Sarcoptes scabiei var hominis*. Infection occurs because of poor standard of personal hygiene. The child may get scabies from his classmate or during out of town school trip. When one member of the family gets scabies, it is common for others to get cross infection. The child develops small pin-sized pimples especially over creases of skin (neck, armpits, groins), genitals, wrists and webs between fingers and toes. The classical lesion is a burrow, a grey thread-like serpentine tunnel with a minute papule at the end. The face is usually spared except in infants. There is marked itching which is worse at night.

Ensure good standard of personal hygiene to prevent scabies. Child should be given a bath everyday and his underclothes changed daily. The bed sheets should be washed frequently and sun-dried. The bed may have to be placed in the scorching sun to get rid of fleas. The whole family should be treated at the same time to prevent cross infection. A number of lotions and creams containing 25% benzyl benzoate, gamma benzene hexachloride or crotamiton and permethrin 5% are available for local application. A single application (whole body except face) after a bath with hot water at night followed by a repeat application after one week is usually enough. Itching can be relieved by oral administration of promethazine hydrochloride (phenergan) or hydroxyzine hydrochloride (atarax). The nails should be kept trimmed and clean to prevent superadded bacterial infection. It is recommended that all members of the family and close contacts should be treated with anti-scabies cream or lotion even if they do not have any skin lesions.

Seborrhea (*see* Dandruff)

Seizures (*see* Convulsions)

SEX DETERMINATION

The sex of the baby depends upon the sex chromosome pattern of the fetus. The sex chromosome in man (sperm) carries XY-chromosome while in a woman (egg or ovum) it is XX-chromosome. During conception, sperm can contribute either X or Y-chromosome while ovum or egg has no choice but to contribute only X-chromosome. When an X-carrying sperm fertilizes the egg, the baby will be XX or a girl. And when a Y-carrying sperm fertilizers the egg, the baby will be XY or a boy. In every conception there is a 50 : 50 chance of either having a daughter or a son.

Reliable techniques are available to correctly identify the sex of the baby during early pregnancy. It is possible to identify the sex of the baby around 8 to 10 weeks of gestation on sonography. Sex of the child can be accurately determined by examination of amniotic fluid after amniocentesis. *However, it is illegal and unethical to determine the sex of the baby in utero for selective abortion of a female fetus.* It is against the basic tenets of nature and maternal instinct and no couple should be a party to this calculated criminal act. However, fetal sex determination is legally permitted in families having the burden of life-threatening sex or X-linked disorders (hemophilia, Duchenne muscular disorder) wherein male fetuses are selectively aborted on medical grounds. We are now having more accurate and sophisticated techniques like chorionic villus sampling (CVS) for definitive antenatal diagnosis of a genetic or metabolic disorder for undertaking selective termination of a pregnancy.

Sex Education (*see* Family Life Education)

SEXUAL ABUSE

Children are innocent and vulnerable to sexual abuse. Sexual exploitation is not limited to girls alone, it is equally common in boys. Sexual abuse may occur in children of all ages including infants. A variety of sexual molestations like kissing, touching or fingering the sensitive parts, rape and unnatural sex (oral or anal sex) are reported. The sexual abuse is most common at home but may occur in a friend's or relatives or neighbour's place, school, coaching class and dance academy. The sexual abuser is most commonly a "trusted" relative, friend, neighbour, teacher, tutor or a servant. The victim may be too young to complain or may feel embarrassed to confide with parents. At times the victim may suffer the ignonimity of the sexual abuse in silence for several months or years.

How to reduce the risk of sexual abuse?

The parents must have high index of suspicion that their child is at a risk of sexual abuse. The child should never be left alone with a stranger or someone whom you do not trust completely. Many a times a "trustworthy" person is the perpetrator of the abuse. The children should be educated that they should not allow anybody to get over-familiar with them and touch their sensitive or private parts such as chest (breasts), bums on the back (potty side) and front side of bottom (urine side). And if anyone tries to do it, they should resist, shout, leave the place and inform their parents. The abuser must be confronted and appropriate legal action taken against him. In an unfortunate event of rape in a grown-up girl, contraceptive pills should be administered without delay and child followed-up for development of pregnancy and STDs (sexually transmitted diseases) including AIDS. The screening for STDs is also required in boys who are victims of anal sex or sodomy.

SEXUALLY TRANSMITTED DISEASES (STDs)

Adolescents or teenagers are highly vulnerable to develop STDs due to unhygienic and unnatural sexual practices, lack of awareness, sexual promiscuity, sexual abuse and lack of sex and family life education in school or at home. The sexual exploitation is further aggravated by smoking, consumption of alcohol and substance abuse. Women are more prone to develop venereal diseases than men. The common STDs include infections by *Candida albicans*, Chlamydia, Mycoplasma, *Trichomonas vaginalis*, genital herpes, genital warts, gonorrhea, syphilis, AIDS (HIV infection) and infection by human papillomavirus (precursor for carcinoma cervix and genital warts).

STDs are important cause of serious morbidity like fever, genital ulcers, discharge from vagina and/or urethra, pelvic inflammatory disease, pain during sexual intercourse (dyspareunia), infertility and death. Whenever STD is suspected, both the partners should be examined, investigated and treated. There is a greater need for family life and sex education in India because of early marriages and high incidence of teenage pregnancies. Effective use of condom by the male partner is mandatory to prevent the occurrence of sexually transmitted diseases. *It is important to remember that use of oral contraceptives can prevent unwanted pregnancy but not STDs.*

SINUSITIS

The sinuses are air-filled spaces which are situated around the nose in the cheek bones (maxillary sinuses) and above the eyes in bones of forehead (frontal sinuses). Frontal sinuses are not present in preschool children and develop after 5–6 years of age. These air-spaces provide resonance to the voice. In children with persistent cough and cold, the sinuses may get infected because they are connected to the nose and throat. The cold symptoms become persistent with continuation of fever, cough, headache with tenderness over the forehead or cheek bones and yellowish-green pus discharge from the nostrils. There may be soggyness with black discoloration under the eyes, blocked nose and non-resonant voice with nasal twang.

Treatment Steam inhalation and instillation of saline water drops in the nose are useful to relieve nasal congestion and help in drainage of pus from the sinuses. Paracetamol or ibuprofen can be given for relief of headache. Appropriate antibiotic and decongestant should be taken on the advice of your doctor.

SKIN RASH

Occurrence of skin pimples or diffuse pink spots over the trunk and extremities are common in children. It may occur due to bacterial (boils, impetigo), viral (measles, German measles, chickenpox) and fungal (ringworm, nappy rash) infections. Skin rash with bleeding manifestations (purpura) may occur due to life-threatening viral (dengue fever) and bacterial (meningo-coccemia) infections. Skin rash may occur as an adverse reaction to a variety of drugs. Rash may occur as an allergic manifestation to certain foods. Allergic reaction to insect bites may produce generalized skin rash (papular urticaria). Itching is common if skin rash is due to allergy. Waxing and waning type of skin rash may occur in certain autoimmune or rheumatic diseases.

When a child develops skin rash, all medications should be stopped. Viral rashes disappear spontaneously while allergic skin rash responds to oral administration of antihistamines. Measles, rubella and chickenpox can be prevented by timely administration of specific vaccines.

SKIN-TO-SKIN CONTACT

Direct skin-to-skin contact of the baby with mother (or any other family member) is a useful and cost effective strategy for providing care to stable babies with a birth weight between 1500 g and 1800 g or gestation of 32–34 weeks. It is based on the marsupial care concept of keeping the off-springs warm in a maternal pouch (kangaroo-mother-care or KMC). It enhances infant–mother bonding, provides biologically controlled warmth and promotes breastfeeding. There is reduced risk of infections, better stability of vital signs, faster weight gain and earlier discharge from NICU. Above all, mother can transmit electromagnetic vibrations of healing, love and compassion to her baby.

KMC is started when baby is stable and receiving oral feeds. The baby is dressed with a front-open sleeveless shirt, cap, socks, mittens and a diaper. The baby is placed between mother's breasts by keeping the head in upright position. The head is turned to one side and kept straight to keep the airway open. The hips and arms of the baby are kept flexed and abducted to maintain frog-like position. The bottom of the baby is supported with a sling or binder. The back of the baby is covered with a woolen shawl. KMC is continued till baby achieves a body weight of 2500 g or gestational maturity of 37 weeks. The baby is weaned from KMC when baby shows discomfort by crying or wriggling movements or there is sweating.

SLEEP PROBLEMS

Sleep is essential for well-being of everyone but much more so for children. Physical growth occurs much faster during sleep because human growth hormone (hGH) production is at least 3 times more during sleep than during waking hours. Children have greater need for sleep because they have intense physical activity when they are awake and they need to sleep more to augment their physical growth. Children differ widely regarding their physiological need for sleep. The duration of sleep depends upon the age, personality, intelligence and constitution (genetic factors) of the child. The newborn baby sleeps most of the time. At 3 months most babies are likely to have 2–3 sleeping sessions. Most children drop their afternoon nap by about 3 years (entry to play school). The active, energetic and brighter children tend to sleep less while placid, slow and relatively inactive children are likely to sleep more.

The bedroom The newborn baby often sleeps with mother in her bed or in a baby cot placed next to her bed. The baby needs constant care, breastfeeding and change of nappies. After 6–9 months his cot is often moved to a corner in the same room. In our country due to shortage of space and cultural practice, children continue to sleep in the same bed with their parents or in a separate cot in the same room till the age of 7–8 years or even longer.

Disturbed night sleep The depth and duration of sleep decreases as child grows. Newborn babies sleep soundly but are awakened by hunger as they need to be fed at night during first 8–10 weeks. Sleep may be disturbed by wet nappy, insects and mosquito bites. Hot weather, over clothing and exposure to cold are common causes of sleep disturbances. Sleep may be disturbed by anal itching due to pinworms. Children are known to awaken up at night with a sudden scream due to nightmare or at times by entry of pinworms in the vagina. Night crying may occur due to excessive wind or colic. During teething the child may be cranky at night. Sleep may be disturbed due to a blocked nose because of cough and cold or use of a heater or hot air blower. Diaper rash is a common cause of night crying. The child may wake up at night, arch his back and cry because of gastroesophageal reflux disease (GERD) due to a lax sphincter at the junction of esophagus with stomach. A common causes of sleep disturbance is the presence of parents in the same room. The child is likely to be disturbed by their talking, late night TV watching, bright light, coughing, snoring or other noises. Whenever feasible, it is desirable that when a child is older than 3 years he should preferably sleep in a separate room.

Sleep-time rituals Most babies are fussy and fretful while falling asleep because they are more keen to play rather than sleep. The fussiness becomes worse if the child is unwell, tired or hungry. Some children are more active, wiry and alert, and they take a long time for "winding down" at the end of the day. The child may be desperately sleepy but he wants to remain active and enjoy the overtures of doling parents and grandparents. Some children put their fingers into their mouth, bang or roll their head while falling asleep. Many children want to be carried, rocked or patted on the back or taken for ride in the car before they sleep. After one year, the child may like to hug a favourite teddy bear or a doll while falling sleep. The list of sleep-time rituals and demands may go on increasing during this phase, e.g. child may ask for a drink, like to have light music, may want dim light or TV on, etc. Most children discard these rituals after the age of 3 years (entry to play school).

How to handle sleep problems?

It is important both for the child and parents to have a good night's sleep to wake up fresh, charged and energetic to enjoy another day. A child who has had an enjoyable daytime activities without undue frustrations and had a "healthy fatigue" (not too tired or over stimulated), he is likely to have less difficulty in falling asleep. He should not be hungry and preferably given a cereal feed last thing at night to prolong satiety and reduce the need for a night feed. Many children fall asleep while listening to a story or a lullaby. You should identify the best time when your child falls asleep with least fuss. The best time, place and "harmless sleep-time rituals" should be exploited to facilitate the process of sleeping. You must stick to his established sleeping routine, otherwise the child will become cranky and irritable. Avoid playing exciting games before bed time. The child should have a comfortable and loose night dress. The bedroom should be cool, comfortable, dimly lit and well ventilated. The child should be adequately covered and nicely tucked by avoiding both over clothing and exposure. Ensure that there are no mosquitoes and insects in the bedroom. It is unwise to leave a crying child alone in his bedroom to teach him a lesson or break the habit. Many a times, father comes home late at night when the child has gone to sleep or getting ready for it. The father may want to spend some time with child whereas the mother is anxious that the child should go to bed. At times, the tired mother becomes helpless and she is at her wits end and needs all the understanding and sympathy of her husband to cope with the challenging process of putting the child to sleep. The parents should handle the "night time blues" together with common sense, patience, good humor and matter of fact manner. *Sedatives should never be used to break a bad habit or for putting a healthy child to sleep.* When a toddler is waking up several times at night for a milk feed, the habit can be broken by offering him water and denying the milk feeds. When a child is suspected to have a painful condition which is interfering with his sleep like intestinal colic, teething, pinworms, nappy rash, gastroesophageal reflux disease (GERD), etc., he should be managed appropriately under the guidance of a pediatrician.

SLEEP WALKING (Somnambulism)

Sleep walking runs in certain families and is usually a self-limited condition. During sleep, the child stands up with vacant stary eyes and starts walking. He may walk through the stairs, wander out-of-the house or walk over a dangerous place like a parapet without any risk of falling. He may have mumbling speech and semi-purposeful activity like passing urine or opening a cupboard. After the ritual, the child goes back to his bed on his own and sleeps for the rest of the night. He will have no memory of the event next day. Most sleep walkers give up the habit after a couple of months. When sleep walking is frequent, child can be given diazepam at bed time under the supervision of a child psychologist.

SLEEPY BABY (Lazy baby)

Most newborn babies sleep for 16–18 hours in a day and they wake up only for feeds or after passing urine and stools. But most of the time they are in a light or REM (rapid eye movement) sleep where in they have occasional blinking of eyes, spontaneous smiling and random movements of arms and legs. During the first few days of life, many infants keep their eyes closed most of the time and they readily go to sleep after taking only a few sucks at the breast. This excessive sleepiness may be aggravated by heavy sedation of the mother during labor. Barbiturates and opium derivatives when taken by the nursing mother may cause sleepiness in her suckling infant. Infants with Down syndrome and hypothyroidism (cretinism) are often lazy and lack spontaneous activity due to low tone of muscles. *The sudden appearance of lethargy, inactivity or lack of interest in feeding, in a baby who had been active and feeding adequately before, is ominous and may be the sole indicator of a serious illness and he must be taken to a pediatrician to exclude an underlying sepsis or metabolic disorder.*

SMOKING (Passive or Secondhand)

It is well known that smoking is injurious to health of the smoker (active smoking) through a variety of health hazards. What is generally not known is the fact that passive or secondhand smoking is equally harmful and associated with adverse health consequences. When a child (or adult) is exposed to cigarette smoke either in a public place or at home, he or she is more prone to develop (i) cough or aggravation of bronchitis or wheezing, (ii) coronary artery disease, (iii) lung cancer, (iv) cognitive impairment, (v) dementia and (vi) early death. It is important that parents must realize that smoking is not only bad for their own health but also for the health of their children and spouses. Incidentally, the habit of smoking generally starts at adolescence or teenage by social influences like watching their friends or parent(s) smoking or exposure to movies in which their favorite actors smoke. The studies have shown that almost 35% of the established smoking habit can be attributed to exposure to smoking in the movies. It is important to remember that other modes of smoking (pipe, cigar, *hookah*, etc.) and tobacco chewing are equally harmful. Life years lost to cigar and pipe smoking have been estimated to be 4.7 years, compared with 6.8 years for cigarette smoking. It is interesting to know that toe nails can be analyzed for nicotine level to assess the severity of active and passive smoking and the likely risk of health hazards.

SNAKE BITE

There are about 200 species of poisonous snakes in the world, of which around 50 are in India. Even when bitten by a poisonous snake, 20–50% victims may have little or no poisoning. There is severe pain, marked swelling and fang mark at the site of bite. In Cobra and Krait bites, there are neurological manifestations like ptosis (drooping eyelids), paralysis of muscles of eyes and difficulty in swallowing. The bite by a viper or pit viper causes widespread bleeding manifestations, hemolysis and circulatory collapse.

The situation should be handled calmly and without any panic because majority of bites are by non-poisonous snakes. The child should be given moral support because most victims suffer due to fear and mental shock. The bitten limb should be splinted to prevent movements which facilitates absorption of poison. There is no need to apply a tourniquet above the site of bite. The child should be lifted and not allowed to walk. There is no role of local application of ice pack or oral suction of venom.

The child should be promptly rushed to a nearest hospital without wasting any time in rituals and folklore remedies. If the snake has been killed, it should be taken along with to identify whether it is poisonous or non-poisonous. The victim needs excellent supportive and nursing care. Booster shot of tetanus toxoid is given. Polyvalent antivenom serum is administered intravenously after conducting hypersensitivity skin test. The dose of antivenom in children is the same or dose is higher in children compared to adults. The outcome of snake bite is poor in children because the same amount of venom is injected into the small body size of the child.

SPINA BIFIDA

There is a gap in spinal cord through which coverings of the spinal cord (meningocele) or part of the nervous tissue of the cord (myelomeningocele) may protrude out. There is a soft round swelling in the midline over the lower back which may be covered with skin or it may be open with oozing of cerebrospinal fluid (CSF). The baby may not have any spontaneous movements of legs and may not withdraw the legs on pin prick. At times there may be constant dribbling of urine or incontinence of feces. Hydrocephalus may be present at birth or appear later in life after repair of the spinal defect.

The baby should be nursed on tummy position. When swelling is covered with skin, it can be operated electively after a few days. The open or uncovered swelling should be protected against development of infection by local application of betadine or mercurochrome. The bottom should be kept scrupulously clean and effectively covered with a plastic sheet to minimize chances of superadded infection. Surgical repair should be done as early as possible before it gets infected. It is futile to do a surgical repair if defect is associated with severe paralysis of lower limbs, incontinence, marked deformity of the spine and severe hydrocephalus. The occurrence of a similar defect (neural tube defect) in the next pregnancy can be prevented by administration of folic acid during periconceptional period, i.e. before missing the period and during first 8 weeks of pregnancy.

STAMMERING (Stuttering)

Some children, who have developed normal speech, may start stammering during 3–4 years of age or any time subsequently. The child loses the rhythm and flow of words, gets stuck, stumble and repeat certain words in an explosive and disjointed manner. About 5% of preschool children stutter at some point of time and most children grow out of it without any special help. The disorder may run in families and is more common in boys than girls. Most children have normal speech for sometime and then suddenly develop stuttering without any obvious cause or due to stress and emotional upset. The stuttering becomes worse when child is anxious, worried or excited and the situation becomes worse when either mother or father is tense. The child is frustrated when he feels that you are not paying any attention to what he is saying. Stutterers often speak normally when alone and when singing, talking to animals or reciting nursery rhymes.

Treatment Stuttering is usually a temporary speech defect and can be resolved by proper handling.

- Parents must pay full attention and listen patiently to what the child has to say. The child must feel that you are interested in what he is saying, not in how he is saying.

- He should not be hurried but encouraged to speak slowly and loudly. He can be asked to sing a song or recite nursery rhymes infront of a mirror or when he is alone.

- You should try to build his self-esteem and confidence by praising him for all the activities he is doing correctly without drawing any attention to his speech difficulties.

- The child should never be chided or shamed by making fun of him or imitating him. You should set aside some relaxed time each day to play and talk with him slowly and clearly in a simple language.

- Always speak to the child in a clear, loud voice and in a slow manner while maintaining eye contact.
- Identify the factors that make the stammering worse and those that make it better.
- Exercise the muscles of the cheeks, tongue, palate and mouth by games like blowing out candles at increasing distances, blowing soap bubbles, puffing the cheeks out, rotating tongue in various directions, making sounds of various birds and animals like roar of a lion, or the purr of a cat by vibrating the tongue.
- Yogic postures are useful for relaxation of the body and mind. Lion pose (jutting out the tongue maximally with force) provides strength to throat and tongue muscles.
- You should seek the help of a speech therapist if stammering persists for 2–3 months. It is desirable that the child should have normal speech by the time he starts regular school because he may feel embarrassed or humiliated by other children.

S

Home Remedies

Soak in water 7–10 almonds overnight and peel off their skin. Crush them with 5 black peppercorns and make a paste with honey or jaggery. Give daily on empty stomach for 1–2 months.

Stridor (*see* Croup)

STUNTING (Short stature)

Every parent want their child to be tall and smart. In our society there is an over concern and craving to have a tall child. The height of a child is dependent upon the genetic potential (height of parents, grandparents, uncles, aunts, etc.), freedom from any developmental defect (chromosomal or genetic disorder), systemic disease or endocrinal disorder, adequacy of nutrition and availability of a health-friendly environment like love, emotional support, play and fun activities, and lack of pollution. Early growth pattern of the child and height of parents can be used to predict the ultimate adult height. Length (below 2 years of age) and height of the child should be taken on a periodic basis and charted on the Road-to-Health card. The growth curve of a healthy child is directed upwards or it should run parallel to the 50th percentile line. The height achieved at 3 years is a good predictor of ultimate adult height

Boys = 0.545 H_3 + 0.544 P + 14.84 inches

Girls = 0.545 H_3 + 0.544 P + 10.09 inches

(Wherein H_3 is height at 3 years and P is mean parental height in inches)

The likely or target height of the child, when he grows to become an adult, can be calculated from the mid-parental height (± 6 cm) as follows:

Boys = Mean height of parents + 6.5 cm

Girls = Mean height of parents – 6.5 cm

In a school going child, when height velocity is less than 4 cm per year, it indicates slow linear growth and a cause for concern. Stunting or short stature is diagnosed when height is less than 2 standard deviations or below 3rd percentile of the mean height-for-age as per reference standard. The short stature of adults in developing countries is largely due to poor growth during the first 3 years of life due to suboptimal nutrition.

Causes

Nutritional disorders and systemic diseases are likely to have greater adverse effect on body weight than the linear growth. Stunting or dwarfism occurs more commonly due to endocrinal disorders (growth hormone deficiency, hypothyroidism), skeletal dysplasias (achondroplasia, chondrodystrophies, rickets), gonadal disorders (delayed puberty, Turner syndrome, precocious puberty), chromosomal and genetic disorders (Down syndrome, Turner syndrome). *In any girl with short stature and/or delayed puberty, Turner syndrome should be ruled out.* When one or both parents have short stature, the child is likely due to be stunted because of familial or genetic short stature.

Treatment

The child with short stature should be investigated and managed by a pediatric endocrinologist because of complex nature of diagnostic techniques and therapeutic regimes. Bone age must be assessed in all children with short stature. When bone age is retarded, the child is likely to have good prognosis for ultimate adult height. Dietary advice should be given to ensure intake of balanced nutritious diet. Supplements of proteins, vitamins and minerals should be provided. There are no miracle medicines, products or exercises which are credited to increase linear growth. Administration of anabolic steroids is condemned due to risk of premature fusion of epiphyses with early arrest of linear growth. Availability of recombinant human growth hormone (rhGH) has revolutionized the management of children with short stature but it is often misused or over used. The definite indications for use of rhGH include growth hormone deficiency, Prader-Willi syndrome, small-for-gestational age babies, chronic renal failure, Turner syndrome, and idiopathic short stature. Growth hormone therapy must be taken under the guidance and supervision of a pediatric endocrinologist. The cost of rhGH is prohibitive. The estimated cost for gain in 1.0 inch or 2.54 cm height in children with idiopathic short stature is estimated to be around US $ 35,000.

S

STYE

A stye is an inflammation of the eyelid caused by infection of the follicle of the eye lashes. This may occur due to rubbing of eye with dirty hands, putting *kajal* in the eyes or as a result of rundown condition of the child who may get frequent styes. There is a localized swelling, pain or redness at the margin of the eyelid. Warm fomentation or compresses with cotton soaked in warm water containing a pinch of boric acid or coriander (*dhania*) seeds provides relief to pain and swelling. Stye may rupture with release of pus followed by prompt recovery. Antibiotic containing eye drops during the day and an ointment at night, as recommended by your doctor, would control the infection. Frequent hand-washing with soap and water and splashing of eyes with tap water on coming home from school or playground helps to keep the eyes clean and free from infection.

SWADDLNG

In temperate or cold countries, it is a common practice to swaddle the baby. The baby is tightly packed with warm sheets and blankets and tied like an "object or a baggage". During early life swaddling is soothing to most babies beause it safeguards against startling due to loud sound and it produces a cramped up but comfortable nest for the baby which is similar to his position in the womb. Swaddling should be limited to initial couple of weeks or months because it interferes with natural cycling and swimming movements and freedom of the baby. It is not recommended in hot and humid conditions because it is uncomfortable to the baby.

SWINE FLU

It is also known as influenza A (H1N1) or H1N1 influenza 09 which occurred as a pandemic in 2009. Infection occurs through air-borne droplets or direct contact with infected humans or by handling of infected pigs. The infection is not spread through food products or eating cooked pork. The symptoms are similar to seasonal flu and include high-grade fever, chills, headache, watering from nose and cough. History of travel to an epidemic area, contact with a known case of swine flu and bimodal course, i.e. period of brief recovery followed by return of worse symptoms of fever, toxemia and cough with blood-tinged sputum, are highly suggestive. The diagnosis can be confirmed by examination of nasopharyngeal secretions by real-time transcriptase polymerase chain reaction (rRT-PCR) and elevation of H1N1-specific neutralizing antibodies.

Most patients recover spontaneously and are treated with supportive measures like administration of paracetamol, fluids, nutritious soups and antibiotics for control of super added bacterial infection. The role of antiviral agents is controversial but they do reduce the period of infectivity and risk of cross-infection. Oseltamivir (Tamiflu) and Zanamivir (Relenza) may be given but they are available only through specified government health care facilities. A combined swine flu (H1N1) and seasonal flu (H_3N_2) vaccines (Vaxigrip, fluarix) are available. Two doses are given IM at 4-week interval, 0.25 ml during 6 months to 3 years and 0.5 ml above 3 years. In children above 9 years, a single primary dose is given. Boosters with a newly formulated vaccine are given once a year after the rainy season. Their protective efficacy against swine flu is doubtful.

SYNCOPE

Syncope or fainting occurs due to temporary reduction of blood flow to the brain. There is transient partial or complete loss of awareness followed by spontaneous recovery. It is uncommon in children and is usually seen among adolescent girls. The common triggers include pain and anxiety (vaccine shot or taking blood sample), sudden change in posture (rising from sitting or lying down position), fasting or dehydration. Syncope may occur during an attack of migraine and may be invoked by Valsalva maneuver due to bout of coughing, straining (urination, defecation) and swallowing. The attack may occur because of sudden fall in blood pressure or change in cardiac rhythm. There is transitory loss of consciousness or light headedness or a "blackout", pallor, dizziness and cold extremities. Episode is brief and recovery occurs spontaneously and can be facilitated by making the child lie flat with head low and by raising his legs. Headache may occur during recovery.

S

TEETH GRINDING (Bruxism)

It is generally believed that teeth grinding (whether during the day or during sleep) is a sign of worm infestation though there is no scientific basis for it. Even children in developed countries, where there is hardly any incidence of worm infestation, grind their teeth during sleep. The exact cause of teeth grinding is unknown but it may be a symptom of tension due to unexpressed anger or resentment during the day. Teeth grinding may occur due to irritation in the teeth. In some children, teeth grinding may be accompanied by talking during sleep. Excessive teeth grinding may cause, malocclusion, reduction in the size of teeth and pain in the jaw. The child should be encouraged to participate in group activities (like sports, dancing, music, yoga, etc.) and he should learn to express his anger and resentment without any restraint. Bed time should be made enjoyable by narrating a story or by talking with the child regarding various pleasant and unpleasant events of the day so that he is able to unwind himself. It is important to remember that praise and encouragement boost the confidence of the child and reduce mental tension.

TEETHING

Teething is a physiological process and is not expected to cause any significant problems in the child. Some babies may be born with a tooth or tooth may appear soon after birth, which is considered as a bad omen without any basis. This is a primary tooth which has erupted early and not an extra tooth. If a natal tooth is loose or causing difficulty in breastfeeding, it should be removed because of risk of aspiration.

Teething troubles

According to Indian folklore , teething has been blamed to cause a large number of ailments including fever, cold, diarrhea, convulsions and even death! The truth is that teething is a harmless physiological process and is not associated with any serious health consequences. Teething (6 months – 2 years) may be associated with irritability, disturbed feeding, drooling of saliva and mouthing, i.e. child putting his fingers or every object in his mouth. These symptoms occur due to irritation of gums when tooth is erupting. Discomfort is worst when child is cutting his first tooth or molars (around one year). At times, the toddler may touch or pull his ear when pain of tooth eruption is referred to the ear. *Teething is never a cause of watery diarrhea or fever*. However, in some children stool frequency may increase when tooth is erupting (say from 1–2 stools/day, the child may pass 3–4 stools/day) and stools may become green in color. The child may wake up more often at night due to discomfort. The eruption of primary teeth continues during the age of 6 months to 2½ years. During this period, the inquisitive and restless toddler is likely to put many dirty objects in his mouth (including his fingers and toys) which may lead to development of watery diarrhea. During the prolonged period of teething, the child is also likely to suffer from common day-to-day infections (like common cold, measles, pneumonia) and teething is wrongly blamed for it. A large majority of children do not manifest any "teething troubles" and teeth erupt as a mother of routine. Therefore, whenever a child is genuinely sick, it should never be attributed to teething and the child should be taken to a doctor for the diagnosis and treatment of underlying disorder.

Care during teething

There is really no medicine which is known to promote or facilitate teething though practically every mother gives homeopathic medicine calcarea phosphonica! All sorts of teething powders and syrups are advertised but they have no proven utility. Due to irritation of gums, the baby likes to chew on a rubber ring or plastic toy. Avoid giving toys having small loose parts which can dislodge and cause aspiration. Alternatively, a big piece of hard biscuit, rusk, toast or a peeled carrot can be given to the child to chew. If a child is cranky and irritable, he can be given a safe analgesic like paracetamol and/or a sedative like phenergan. A gel containing a mild anesthetic can be rubbed over the swollen gums to relieve itching. Just rubbing or massaging the gums with your index finger (after washing the hands with soap and water) usually provides comfort and relief. You can put one drop of clove (*laung*) oil in one teaspoon honey, almond or olive oil and massage over the gums. During teething, the child should be given soft nutritious home-made weaning foods containing calcium (milk and milk products), vitamin D (fats, oils, exposure to sunlight), and vitamin A (green leafy vegetables and yellow colored fruits).

Eruption of teeth (dentition)

The human dentition, like most of the mammals, consists of two generations of teeth. The first generation of teeth is known as the deciduous or temporary dentition (milk teeth) and the second as the permanent dentition. The logic for two sets of dentition is based on the fact that the jaw of an infant is small and it can accommodate only a limited number of teeth (20 milk teeth). Primary teeth are delicate and required for eating soft semi-solid food. A second set of permanent teeth erupt, which are stronger, larger in size and greater in number (28–32) to fill the bigger jaw of an adolescent child and adult.

Milk teeth (primary, temporary, deciduous teeth)

The time of eruption of milk teeth is in accordance with genetic clock. In some families children erupt their teeth by 6 months of age while in others it may be delayed till the first birthday. Delayed or early dentition are not related to the nutritional status or neuromotor development of the child. It is not unusual to see a healthy and chubby infant without any tooth by 9 months or 1 year of age because his parents cut their teeth late. However, when eruption of teeth is delayed beyond one year, the child should be investigated to rule out rickets (vitamin D deficiency) and hypothyroidism (sluggish thyroid gland).

In general, eruption of teeth in the lower jaw (mandible) usually precede the dentition in the upper jaw (maxilla). Usually teeth in both the jaws appear in pairs, one on either side. The lower central incisors are usually the first teeth to erupt around 6 months of age. Subsequently, the child on an average is likely to gain one tooth every month (for example, one year old child is likely to have 6 teeth, if first tooth erupted at 6 months of age) till the complete set of 20 milk teeth (four incisors, two canines and four molars in each jaw) have erupted by the age of 2–2½ years **(Box)**. Milk teeth are white in color and have a smooth edge. They can be kept clean with wet piece of gauze or damp cloth after feedings. If milk teeth are well looked after, then it is more likely that the permanent teeth will grow in their correct position. Avoid giving a bottle feed or fruit juice during sleep as it may facilitate the process of tooth decay. Occasionally milk teeth may erupt in a crooked manner but fortunately it has no implications for eruption of permanent teeth.

Timing for eruption of teeth				
Teeth	Milk teeth		Permanent teeth*	
	Lower jaw	Upper jaw	Lower jaw	Upper jaw
Central incisors	5–7 mo	6–8 mo	6–7 yrs	7–8 yrs
Lateral incisors	7–10 mo	8–11 mo	7–8 yrs	8–9 yrs
Canines	16–20 mo	16–20 mo	9–11 yrs	11–12 yrs
First premolars	—	—	10–12 yrs	10–11 yrs
Second premolars	—	—	11–13 yrs	10–12 yrs
First molars	10–16 mo	10–16 mo	6–7 yrs	6–7 yrs
Second molars	20–30 mo	20–30 mo	12–13 yrs	12–13 yrs
Third molars	—	—	17–22 yrs	17–22 yrs

*Milk teeth are shed first before any permanent teeth erupt except in case of first permanent molars which erupt before any milk teeth are shed.

Permanent teeth

In school going children, milk teeth are shed followed by eruption of permanent teeth. The first molars of permanent teeth appear at the age of 6 years without loss of any deciduous teeth ("6-years molars"). There is no pain or discomfort when a milk tooth is shed. In order to console the child, as a ritual the shed tooth is often hidden under the pillow and replaced by a tiny toy as a gift by the fairy. Around 6 years of age, lower central incisors are shed followed by eruption of permanent teeth. During 10–11 years, due to eruption of permanent canines, the teeth in the center of upper jaw become crowded giving an appearance of "ugly duckling". You should not be worried about this temporary physiological appearance because in due course of time, the teeth become well aligned. By the age of 12–13 years, a set of 28 permanent teeth are usually well in place **(Box)**. Third molars or wisdom teeth do not erupt in all individuals but only in some by the age of 17–22 years. Eruption of wisdom tooth may be associated with discomfort and pain due to constraint of space in the jaw. The complete set of 32 permanent teeth comprises 4 incisors, 2 canines, 4 premolars, 6 molars (teeth in both the jaws appear in pairs). In contrast to milk teeth, permanent teeth are ivory-white or off-white in color and have a finely serrated edge.

Care of teeth

Children need healthy, well aligned, sparkling white teeth for chewing, clarity of speech, pleasant breath and a charming smile. Teeth care should begin as soon as the milk teeth start erupting **(Box)**. You can clean the teeth of your baby with a gauze piece or muslin cloth rolled around the index finger.

Tips to keep the teeth healthy and sparkling

- Establish the habit of regular brushing of teeth twice a day after the age of 2 years.
- Avoid bottle feeding while toddler is asleep.
- Avoid giving any tinned juices and fizzy drinks.
- Do not give chocolates and candies as rewards. Color-free and sugar-free (containing xylitol or sorbitol) chewing gum is teeth-friendly and can be given after 4–5 years.
- Encourage eating a crunchy fruit (apple, guava, pear) after meals and after "sweet encounters".
- When a colored medicine (like iron) is given, it should be followed by a bite of crunchy fruit or vegetable (carrot, cucumber) or by a few sips of water.
- Caries of primary teeth should not be ignored and must be treated to ensure eruption of healthy well-aligned permanent teeth.
- The age old Indian custom of rinsing the mouth after meals or snacks should be encouraged.
- Consult a dentist every 6 months!

After 2 years, when a complete set of milk teeth has appeared, brushing of teeth with extra soft bristles is advised. A bright colored baby brush with favorite cartoon characters is more readily accepted by the child. It is desirable to establish the habit of brushing the teeth twice a day, morning and before going to bed, right from the preschool years. In case of infants, it is convenient for the mother to place the baby's head on her lap so that she can see the teeth better. You should use correct circular movements of brush so that healthy habit of brushing the teeth is established **(Box)**. Use a tiny bit of flouride-free toothpaste so that there is no harm even if it is swallowed by the baby. There is no need to use a flouride-rich toothpaste because in several parts in India, the flouride content of water is high. Due to tropical climate we also tend to drink a lot of water. Moreover, tea and certain Indian spices like *jeera*, turmeric (*haldi*) and black pepper are rich in flouride. Baking soda or common salt has no virtue to keep the teeth white and shining. The correct technique of brushing teeth is more important than the brand of toothpaste but it should have a pleasant acceptable taste and flavor. The child should not have any foul breath. Avoid use of battery-operated brushes. The child should not do any pranks or run around with a toothbrush dangling in his mouth, as it may cause serious injury to the oral cavity. Eating fruits with a hard pulp (like apple, guava, pear) after a meal or snack are useful to "floss out" food debris stuck in

Correct method of brushing the teeth*

- Hold the toothbrush just under the gum line at an angle of 45°. Gently jiggle the brush (short jerky up and down and to and fro motions) or use tiny circular movements over the teeth and gums. Brushing for 2 minutes is adequate.
- Use tip of the toothbrush to clean the insides of each tooth both in the upper and lower jaws with the same jiggling movements.
- The chewing edges of upper and lower teeth should be cleaned by using back and forth light movements of the brush.
- Tongue should be cleaned gently with the brush or a tongue cleaner. Avoid use of a sharp metallic tongue cleaner.
- Massage the gums with your fingers after brushing.
- School going children should be taught flossing of teeth, i.e. cleaning the spaces in-between the teeth with a thread.

*Avoid use of hard brush which can damage the enamel of teeth. It is not so much the brand of toothpaste but the correct technique of brushing which is more important to have trouble-free healthy teeth.

between the teeth. The age-old cultural practice of rinsing the mouth after every meal is a most "teeth-friendly habit" and must be promoted. It effectively removes food particles, starches and sugars which are known to cause proliferation of germs. When a child is given any chocolate, candy or a colored medicine like iron tonic, it should be followed by a sip of water as a safeguard against discoloration of teeth.

TELEVISION VIEWING

It is an unfortunate fact that TV remote, computer mouse, play stations, iPhones, iPads are gradually replacing the toys and outdoor play activities of children. Some parents use TV as a "baby sitter" for their toddlers. Watching violence, aggression, dangerous stunts, cartoons and even commercials can have adverse effects on the mind and psyche of children. Soap operas, prime time TV and many other popular programs may expose children to sexuality, smoking, drugs and alcohol at a time when they are too young to understand.

Hazards of TV

Apart from waste of time, excessive TV watching is associated with a large number of health hazards **(see Box)**. Children sitting in front of "idiot box" often drink cola drinks and munch on potato chips and crisps which are recognized risk factors for obesity. Watching TV is a passive habit and it does not help the child to acquire the most important skills such as communication,

---

Hazards of excessive TV viewing

- Violent, excessive or bullying behavior (*Dadagiri*).
- Sleep deficit, poor attention span, decreased intellectual ability and failing grades in school.
- Reduced physical activity, greater munching of snacks and taking fizzy drinks or canned juices may lead to obesity.
- Eye strain and headaches.
- Early exposure to sex, violent, antisocial behavior and substance abuse.
- Increased incidence of nightmares, night terror and bed wetting.
- Risk of injury by imitating "stunts" shown on TV.
- Reduced communication, socialization, lack of cooperation and inability to build friendship.

cooperation and leadership. It has been shown that kids who grow up watching TV rather than playing outdoors are more likely to commit crimes later in life. The way a child handles a car in video games will be reflected in the way he is going to drive the real car later in life.

Guidelines for viewing TV

Television viewing is habit forming and may isolate the child from his classmates, teachers and even parents. You should encourage your child to join enjoyable and constructive activities like sports, swimming, dancing, music, group activities like picnics and trekking. Parents should restrict their own TV viewing and child should be encouraged to watch appropriate child-friendly programs for a maximum of one hour in a day. Like other daily activities, child should have a time slot for watching TV so that you know in advance what options he has to watch. Whenever feasible parents should watch television with their child to guide him to become a critical and discerning viewer. Parents should make him understand that the violence shown on television is "make believe" or just "made-up" and not real. They should criticize the characters that are dishonest, drink alcohol, smoke, use drugs and indulge in fights and wreckless car driving. The child should be made to realize that most commercials are misleading and are merely advertisement stunts to promote their

Guidelines for TV viewing

- Parents must serve as role models to their children for censored and sensible viewing of TV.
- Never keep a TV set in the children's room.
- TV viewing should be a family activity.
- Turn-off TV during meal times.
- Set time limits and monitor the programs being watched by your child.
- Explain that watching television is not the best way to spend leisure time and emphasize the need for various sports and social activities.
- The child should be made to understand that advertisements and associated stunts are commercial gimmicks and they do not reflect the true virtues of the product.
- Explain and make the child understand that TV programs are "created" and they do not depict real life situations.

sales and child must appreciate the difference between "healthy" and "unhealthy" or undesirable foods **(Box)**. Parents must spend a quality time with their children involving active interaction, play and fun activity. Reading a book to a child, telling a story of valour, courage or compassion is far more useful to stimulate mental faculties and develop humanistic qualities in children.

TEMPERATURE RECORDING

A clinical glass thermometer containing mercury (35–42°C or 95–108°F) or a digital thermometer is used to record body temperature. The clinical thermometer is provided with a constriction at the bottom end of the mercury column. Due to constriction, the mercury column does not fall after recording the body temperature. Thermometer must be vigorously shaken to let the mercury column drop below 37°C or 98°F before recording the next temperature. Hold the thermometer firmly by its upper end (the end opposite the bulb) between thumb and index finger. Shake the thermometer vigorously with a sharp, snappy or jerky motion to drive the mercury down. In infants and preschool children, skin temperature is recorded and is fairly reliable. Axilla (armpit) or groin should be dried with a cloth and bulb of thermometer is placed and kept snugly in contact with the skin by tightly holding the arm against chest or flexing thigh over the abdomen. Thermometer should be left in place for at least 2 minutes before reading the temperature. It needs some practice to read a conventional glass thermometer. Roll the thermometer gently in your fingers till you see the mercury column. Skin temperature of forehead can be recorded with the help of thermo-crystal strips. They are convenient to use but are unreliable. Temporal artery thermometers record the skin temperature with the help of a transducer that rolls across the forehead and are accurate and reliable. By practice and experience you can reliably assess the temperature of your child by touching his forehead, chest or abdomen. Most normal children have relatively warm forehead because of high flow of blood to the brain. Some children have warm hands while others may be endowed with less warm or cold hands.

In school going children oral temperature is recorded by placing the thermometer under the tongue and asking the child to breathe through the nose: Rarely, some children may bite and break the thermometer with a risk of exposure to mercury. Digital thermometer is safer, easy to read and gives an audible signal when temperature has been recorded. Be careful not to wet the digital display, on-off button or battery cover of digital thermometer. Oral temperature should not be taken immediately after intake of a hot or cold drink.

There is no need to record rectal or core body temperature at home which should be undertaken by a nurse in a hospital setting. Rectal thermometer has a short and bulbous mercury end. The child is restrained in lateral or side position and upper leg is flexed against the abdomen. A lubricated thermometer is gently inserted through the anus by directing it posteriorily, i.e. towards the back. *To safeguard against rectal perforation, thermometer should be directed posteriorly (towards back) and should not be inserted beyond 2 cm.* The child is kept restrained by holding him firmly for 2 minutes. Ear drum temperature can be recorded with a thermoscan ear sensor which works on the principle of infrared technology. It is a useful device in a busy clinic of the doctor because read-out is obtained within one second. Tympanic thermometer is difficult to use in infants, need accuracy of technique and necessary skill and gives unreliable reading if there is wax in the ear. Oral temperature is considered as the standard or reference body temperature, it is higher than the skin temperature and lower than core temperature. The skin temperature is about 0.5°C (0.75°F) lower than oral temperature while rectal or ear drum temperature is 0.5°C (0.75°F) higher than the oral temperature.

TEMPER TANTRUMS

The sudden outbursts of anger in young children are called temper tantrums. The usual expression of anger is that the child drops on the floor and starts yelling and pounding with his hands and feet or banging his head. At times temper tantrum may be followed by a breath holding spell. Children are stubborn and likely to have frequent and violent tantrums. The only child or over indulged and pampered child is more likely to have tantrums. It helps the child to "let off his steam", frustration and helplessness. The tantrum may be sparked off when some demand of the child is unfulfilled, he is being forced to eat or his clothes are being changed or he is being given a bath, or merely for seeking attention. Temper tantrums are the expression of ego and individuality of the child who is trying to send a message that "he cannot be taken for granted".

Treatment

When a child throws a tantrum, the best way to handle it is to show "intelligent neglect". Mother should get away from the scene without showing any concern and reaction, and the child should be left alone. The child often cools off quickly and meekly if mother goes about her own business in a matter-of-fact manner. It is unwise to counteract his tantrum by showing your own temper or frustration. Never scold the child or argue with him but handle the situation with common sense and patience. You should not shout but be firm and considerate. Every wish of the child should not be fulfilled because "there is no end to wishes" and child must learn to handle frustration from time-to-time. You should not feel helpless or at his mercy, otherwise he will "blackmail" you and make it a habit to get what he wants. When the drama is over, the mother should try to explain to the child the reality of the situation and futility of the prank. It is important to remember that young children understand a lot more language than they can express. Hunger, fatigue and boredom are common causes of outbursts of temper tantrums. Try to ensure that the child is getting enough

T

Strategies to cope with tantrums

- Give a toddler lots of praise and encouragement for his good behavior.
- Ignore some of his bad behavior as a means to "let off steam".
- Give him choices whenever you can so that he can feel as if he has some control over the situation.
- Do not take a firm stand or make it a prestige issue on unimportant concerns like what he wants to wear or eat.
- Do not accede to each and every demand—there is no end to it.
- Use positive phrases to get him do certain things instead of continually saying "No" to everything.
- Stay calm keeping in mind "child is a child" and you are an adult.
- Remain calm and concerned but be firm—if you "give in" to each and every demand, your toddler learns that tantrum works.
- Handle your child with love, tact and common sense—you cannot win a fight with a child!

sleep, having his meals on time and is occupied playing with his toys. After the age of 4–5 years, temper tantrums are replaced by other ways and means to express their anger and frustration. Some children may start abusing or hitting the parents which should never be allowed and handled firmly. Instead of hitting back the child, he should be firmly reprimanded and ignored for sometime and denied his favorite demand or need.

TETANUS

It is caused by spore bearning bacilli C. *tetani* which reside in the soil contaminated by the excreta of animals. Tetanus can occur in a newborn baby when umbilical cord is cut with a dirty knife or blade and mother is not immunized and lacks protective antibodies against tetanus. In older children, infection occurs by roadside injury, sports accidents, cuts by sharp object, nail piercing through the sole and chronic suppurative otitis media with pus discharge from the ear.

The common symptoms of tetanus include lockjaw (inability to open the mouth), inability to feed, spasm of muscles when child is touched or handled, stiffness of whole body and difficulty in breathing. Patient is not contagious to others. Tetanus is a life-threatening emergency and is managed in an intensive care unit. Patient is nursed in a quiet and dark room, and provided with excellent nursing and supportive care. Crystalline penicillin is given IV for 10 days to eliminate C. *tetani*. Human tetanus immunoglobulins 250 iu are administered IM and intrathecally through lumbar puncture. Diazepam and chlorpromazine are given through intravenous route in high doses to control muscle spasms. Mechanical ventilation and tracheostomy may be required in some cases.

Tetanus in a newborn baby is prevented by vaccination of mother by giving two doses of tetanus toxoid (TT) or tetanus-diphtheria toxoid (Td) 4 weeks apart. The second dose of tetanus should be taken at least 4 weeks before the expected date of delivery. The cord should be cut with a sterile knife or blade (even a new blade should be boiled for at least 5 minutes before use) by following strict aseptic precautions. The cord should be left open without any dressing or application of any home antiseptics. Triple antigen (DTaP or DTwP) should be given to children as per recommended schedule. After completing DTP schedule, TT or Td is given every 10 years to maintain adequate protection against tetanus.

TETANY

Hypocalcemia, i.e. fall in serum calcium below 8 mg/dL or ionized calcium below 4 mg/dL is associated with neuromuscular irritability and spasm of skeletal muscles. There may be seizures, twitchings, muscle cramps and rarely spasm of larynx leading to breathing difficulty and stridor. The child remains fully conscious. The common causes of hypocalcemia include prematurity, sick baby, feeding with cow's milk (high phosphate content), vitamin D deficiency and disorders of kidneys and parathyroids. Tetany is treated by intravenous administration of calcium gluconate followed by oral supplements of calcium and vitamin D.

THALASSEMIA

It is a form of hereditary anemia where patient cannot form enough amount of normal adult type of hemoglobin. Instead there is excessive production of fetal hemoglobin. Both the parents may carry the defective gene and they usually hail from Pakistan. The disease is common in countries wherever Alexander the Great and his forces went and conquered.

Clinical features The carriers of defective gene (for example, parents of patients with thalassemia major) are designated to have thalassemia trait or thalassemia minor. They have mild anemia without any symptoms and their HBA_2 is elevated. When both parents have thalassemia trait, there is 1:4 chance that their child may have thalassemia major. The child appears normal at birth and develops gradually increasing severity of anemia between 3 months to 2 years of age. Anemia does not respond to any drug and as the disease progresses there is progressive enlargement of liver and spleen. When hemoglobin drops below 5 g/dL, there is increasing breathlessness due to congestive heart failure. Because of repeated blood transfusions, accumulation of iron can cause damage to several body organs.

Treatment The patient with thalassemia major needs repeated blood transfusions to maintain hemoglobin between 10 and 12 gm/dL. Iron chelators (to remove excessive load of iron) are given orally or through a mini-infusion pump to prevent accumulation of iron in various body organs. *The patient should never be given any iron supplements*. The disease can be cured by bone marrow transplant or stem cell transfusion which is available in a few advanced centers in the country. Children with thalassemia trait do not need any treatment. They should not be given any supplements of iron but administration of folic acid off and on may help. Parents can join Federation of Indian Thalassemics to interact and share information and knowledge with parents of thalassemic children (www.thalassemiaindia.org and thalind@ndf. vsnl.net.in).

Prevention During premarital counseling, the would-be-couples can be screened for thalassemia trait, if they belong to high endemic region for thalassemia. If only one of the potential parents is carrying thalassemia trait, there is no risk of transmission of thalassemia major to the offsprings. When both the parents are known to have thalassemia trait (as diagnosed on the basis of premarital blood test or because the couple has earlier given birth to a child with thalassemia major), it is advised to conduct specialized test on their unborn baby during 10–18 weeks of pregnancy by doing a chorionic villus biopsy. If baby in the womb is found to be suffering from thalassemia major, the mother is offered the option of undergoing an abortion on medical grounds.

THRUSH

There are discrete white patches with red margins over the tongue, gums and inside of cheeks (buccal mucosa). It is caused by a yeast or fungus (*Candida albicans*) which is commonly transmitted through feeding bottles but at times from mother's vaginal tract or nipples of her breasts. Prolonged administration of antibiotics is a common predisposing factor. Recurrent episodes of thrust may occur in children with poor immunity due to malnutrition, AIDS, chemotherapy for malignancy, etc. Oral thrush may cause difficulty in feeding and swallowing especially when infection has spread to the food pipe (esophagus). Local application of anti-fungal lotion after each feed, gives prompt relief in 5–7 days. The mother should also receive appropriate treatment if there is any evidence of fungal infection of vagina or breast.

THUMB SUCKING

Putting fingers in the mouth or opening the mouth is usually a signal for hunger in some newborn babies. Around 3 months of age most infants put their fingers or thumb in the mouth because of "oral phase" of development. When child has learnt grasping the objects at 5–6 months, he tries to put every object into the mouth (oral or mouthing phase). The habit becomes more persistent because of irritation of gums due to teething. Thumb sucking is often a symptom of hunger, boredom, shyness, teething, fatigue and sleep. The habit reaches its peak around 18–24 months and gradually disappears by the age of 3 years.

Finger and thumb sucking is a normal developmental phase but may become a habit in some children. In some children thumb sucking becomes a "sleep ritual" and they cannot sleep without sucking their fingers or thumb. Persistent and compulsive sucking of thumb in an older child is a sign of insecurity, dependence, boredom or unmet need for sucking. Bottle fed (or spoon fed) babies are more likely to suck their thumb because they are able to finish their feed quickly from the bottle and they resort to thumb sucking to fully satisfy their sucking urge. Thumb sucking has been blamed for a variety of ailment by grannies without any basis. It may produce soreness or callus formation over the thumb and occasionally it may cause malocclusion of teeth if habit persists beyond 5 years.

Treatment

The habit should be handled with care and compassion rather than aggresion or disdain. The application of bitter substances over the thumb and use of restraining devices is condemned. They may cause psychological disturbances and do more harm. Nothing needs to be done in young infants who put their fingers or thumb in their mouth while sleeping. Most children will grow out of the habit in due course of time. When thumb sucking is excessive and occurs both during the day and night in a child over 2 years of age, one should look for the cause. The common causes are insecurity, boredom and sibling jealousy. The child should be distracted and provided with greater opportunities for interaction and play activity. Children have a lot of energy and mother should give them paper, pencil, blunt scissors, clay or mud for modelling, toys, and building blocks, to keep them occupied. Constant nagging, reprimands and forceful removal of thumb from the mouth cause unhappiness, resentfulness and more insecurity. The child should not be rediculed, teased, shamed or given threats. When parents make a lot of fuss about his thumb sucking, he may continue to suck the thumb as an attention-seeking behavior. In an older child, a direct appeal can be made to him that he is no longer a "baby" and he is now a big boy or a grown-up girl. The dangers of thumb sucking lie not in the act of thumb sucking but the way you perceive or handle the habit. Thumb sucking does not cause any harm to the permanent teeth because most children leave the habit by the age of 5 years when they join the regular school.

TICS (Habit spasms)

Tics are sudden stereotyped, awkward, purposeless and repetitive movements of a particular part of the body. Tics are more common in boys and usually start between 8 and 10 years of age. They may start as an imitation of an awkward mannerism of another family member, friend or a teacher. At times they may start as a symptom of a physical ailment and then continue thereafter. The common examples of tics are shrugging of shoulders, blinking of eyes, twitchings of face, twisting of neck, producing dry hesitant cough or throat clearing noises. Sometimes one tic disappears, only to be replaced by another. They are likely to occur in a child who is tense and whose parents are very strict and demand high standard of performance and discipline. When a child gets attention due to tics, their frequency increases. At times tic-like movements may occur as an early sign of a serious psychological or mental disorder. Gilles de la Tourette syndrome (TS) is a life long condition which has onset between 2 and 20 years of age. There are multiple major tics involving face, eyelids, neck and shoulders with vocal tics like throat clearing, sniffing, barking, repetition of words or use of obscene gestures and words (coprolalia). It is a progressive disorder and commonly associated with obsessive-compulsive disorder (OCD) and attention deficit hyperactivity disorder (ADHD).

Treatment

Most tics are benign and usually disappear spontaneously within a few days or weeks. The child should not be given undue attention or scolded because tics are beyond his control. Teasing and nagging should be avoided because they will aggravate the tics. Efforts should be made to identify any factors that may be causing anxiety and stress. The child should be made to relax at home and school, and kept engaged in physical activities such as outdoor games and competitive sports. Participation in various group activities like music, dance, yoga and meditation are useful. When tics are marked and persistent or associated with additional physical symptoms, a psychologist must be consulted. In Tourette syndrome administration of haloperidol may provide some relief but must be taken under the guidance of a pediatrician.

TOE WALKING

The child walks on toes without putting any pressure on the heel or any other part of the foot. Toe-walking is common in toddlers when they start walking. They usually adopt normal walking pattern as they grow older. If a child continues to walk on the toes beyond the age of 3 years, he should be evaluated by a doctor. The common causes of toe walking include spastic child (cerebral palsy), Duchenne muscular dystrophy, foot drop (peripheral neuropathy) and autism.

Treatment The majority of cases of toe walking are habitual and they usually resolve without any treatment. When Achilles tendon (tendon behind the ankle) is stretched or shortened, stretching exercises are advised by forcibly dorsiflexing the foot (trying to touch the upper surface of the foot to the shin). When toe walking is marked and unrelieved by stretching exercises, a brace or splint can be worn to keep the Achilles tendon stretched. In severe cases when physical measures fail to relieve the condition, surgical procedure can be done by an orthopedic surgeon to lengthen the Achilles tendon.

TOILET TRAINING

Toilet training should neither be aggressive nor left to the whims or fancies of the child but a common sense approach should be followed. There are no rigid rules and mother should follow a flexible approach depending upon the development of the child.

Bladder Control

Newborns pass urine almost after every feed with a frequency of 8–10 times in a day. As the child grows, the capacity of bladder increases, the child is able to hold urine for a longer period of time. Mother should be observant and identify the time when child is most likely to void. Most babies are likely to pass urine an waking up or soon after a feed. The child may indicate urge to pass urine by subtle gestures like touching or holding the genitals, becoming restless, uncomfortable or still. The observant mother holds the baby over the wash basin to encourage the infant to void. If a child is unwilling to void, he should not be forced and mother should handle the situation in a relaxed manner. Avoid using unnecessary force and coercion which may lead to rebellious and defiant attitude. After the age of 2 years, the child can be taken to the washroom to void. When proper toilet training is given, most children become dry by the age of 2–3 years. At this stage, most boys learn the art of voiding while standing by observing their elder sibling and friends. Even after achieving bladder control, occasional accidents may occur when child is engrossed in play, is unhappy, tired or unwell and when he is in an unfamiliar environment.

Bowel Control

During early life, passage of urine and poops are involuntary activities without any control to initiate the process, delay it or stop it at will. When rectum is full of feces, further increase in pressure following a feed, leads to opening up of the anal canal and evacuation of stools. The child may become still, stop playing, or look intently into mother's eyes. There may be some straining efforts or facial grimaces before or while passing stools. The mother must be observant to identify the subtle "signals" and "best time" for placing the child on the potty. During potty session the child should be kept busy with a toy or picture book. When attempts at potty training are rewarded, the child should be appreciated to strengthen the process of conditioning.

Aggressive potty training is counter productive and is likely to make the child rebellious. When adequately trained, most children become independent and can look after their toilet needs by 3 years (entry to play school) of age. At this stage the child can wash his bottom with a toilet spray or when water is poured by the mother or school maid. Girls should be taught about the importance of washing bottom from "front-backwards" to avoid potential risk of soiling vulva with feces as a safeguard against ascending urinary tract infection. After washing the bottom, the child should be trained to wash his hands with soap and water and explained about the importance of personal hygiene.

TONGUE-TIE (Tandua)

There is a fold or frenulum on the under surface of tongue which fixes it to the base of the oral cavity or mouth. When the frenulum is too thick or tight it is called tongue-tie. The condition is over diagnosed and wrongly suspected by the grandmother when the child has difficulty in feeding or delay in the development of speech. Genuine tongue-tie is uncommon and should be suspected when child is unable to protrude the tongue beyond the lips or he is unable to lick his upper lip or touch the roof of oral cavity (palate) with tip of the tongue. The presence of a midline notch at the tip of tongue due to traction by the tight frenulum is diagnostic. Tongue-tie is neither a cause for feeding difficulty nor it is responsible for the delay in the development of speech. However, the child with tongue-tie may lack clarity in speech due to inability to clearly pronounce certain syllables like na, la, ta, da, tha, etc. which need free mobility of tongue. A genuine tongue-tie may be snipped between 6 months to one year of age by a qualified pediatric surgeon under anesthetic cover.

TONSILS AND TONSILLITIS

Tonsils are two pads of lymphoid tissue, one on either side, deep in the of throat. They can be seen as small rounded glands in the throat on asking the child to widely open the mouth and say "*Aah*". They serve as protective sentinels in the throat to prevent the entry of the germs into the body. Tonsils are relatively large in size in children between 3 and 8 years of age to provide extra protection during the vulnerable period of life. The large size of the tonsils does not indicate that they are diseased and should not be a cause for concern. They shrink in size and assume adult proportions by the age of 8–10 years.

Tonsillitis

The infection of tonsils may occur by a number of bacteria and viruses and is called acute tonsillitis. Tonsillitis usually occurs after the age of 2 years and is commonly caused by *Streptococcus hemolyticus* which is also called "strep-throat". The child develops high grade fever, pain in the throat, and headache. The tonsils become large, walnut sized, angry-red in color with whitish patches or pus points in their follicles. The soft palate is also inflammed and there may be pin point bleeding spots. The lymph glands in the neck may become enlarged and tender. Unlike common cold, there is no watering in the nose or eyes and cough is either minimal or absent. When "strep-throat" is inadequately treated, there is a potential risk of development of serious complications like rheumatic fever (and rheumatic heart disease) or acute glomerulonephritis (AGN) during recovery.

Treatment "Strep-throat" should be promptly treated by administration of an appropriate antibiotic on the advice of a doctor. The antibiotic must be given for at least 7–10 days to prevent development of complications. The symptomatic treatment induces administration of paracetamol or ibuprofen for relief of fever, sore throat and headache. Gargles with saline warm water are useful for relief of irritation and pain in the throat. Hot vegetable or chicken soup (without chillies) provides nutrition and local fomentation to the throat. The child should be asked to avoid intake of cold water, cold drinks, ice cream, condiments and ketchup.

After the advent of antibiotics, there are limited indications or justifications for removal of tonsils. Tonsils should not be removed because they look large because they do perform an important function of preventing the entry of pathogens in the body. There is a wrong belief that removal of tonsils would improve the growth of the child. Tonsillitis can be easily treated these days with administration of penicillin or an alternative antibiotic and tonsillectomy is unnecessary. A child with frequent episodes of tonsillitis can also be managed by long term administration of penicillin therapy orally or through injections on the advice of a doctor. In current medical practice there are limited indications or justifications for removal of tonsils.

TOOTHACHE (Caries and Cavities)

The common causes of toothache include caries or cavities in teeth, infection, injury and eruption of wisdom teeth. Toothache is generally boring in character, extremely severe in intensity and may be referred to the forehead, eye or ear of the same side. The pain may be aggravated by intake of a hot or cold drink. When teeth and gums are not properly cleaned, bacteria and food particles combine with saliva to form a sticky material called dental plaque that sticks to the surfaces of teeth. Bacterial growth (*Streptococcus mutans*) is facilitated when oral cavity is loaded with starchy food and sugars (chocolates, sweets, soft drinks, fruit juices, etc.). In order to reduce the risk of caries, sucrose has been replaced by xylitol and sorbital in chewing gums, liquid and solid formulations of medicines. Bottle feeding, especially when milk feed or fruit juice is given during sleep, is an important risk factor for caries. When plaque is not removed and there is continued growth of bacteria and production of acid, it dissolves the mineral content of teeth (enamel and dentin) leading to development of caries and formation of cavities. There may be toothache with swelling and bleeding of gums. Caries teeth is an important cause of foul breath and bad taste in the mouth. It may lead to formation of tooth abscess, headache and even sepsis. Their is recent evidence

T

Home Remedies

A number of home remedies are useful for temporary relief of toothache but consultation must be sought with a dentist for definitive treatment of caries teeth.

- Soak a piece of cotton wool with a few drops of clove (*laung*) oil. Keep it pressed over the affected site.
- Crush 2–3 cloves and fry them in a spoonful of coconut oil. Make a paste and apply over the affected tooth.
- Apply a mixture of powdered black pepper (*kali mirch*) and clove oil over the affected site.
- Pound asafoetida (*Hing*) in a mortar and pestle and add some lime juice, warm it and soak a swab of cotton wool and hold it against the affected tooth.
- Make a tooth powder by burning mango leaves and apply it over the site of toothache. A decoction of fresh mango flowers or henna leaves can be made by boiling them in water and used as a mouth rinse to relieve inflammation and pain.
- Take a table spoon of mustard oil and add a teaspoon of common salt and use it for massage of gums. Alternatively, make powder of alum (*phatkari*) burnt in a non-stick pan and massage it over the gums. Rinse or gargle with warm plain water after 5 minutes.

to suggest that decay of teeth and diseases of gums are associated with increased risk of heart disease later in life due to chronic inflammation.

Treatment Pain and infection are treated by administration of paracetamol or ibuprofen and an appropriate antibiotic on the advice of a dentist. The help of a dentist must be sought for proper management of the affected teeth (root canal) and prevention of further spread of caries to other teeth. In children dental appointment should preferably be sought in the morning when child is fresh after a good night's sleep because he is likely to be tired and irritable in the evening. It is often argued as to what is the need to treat carious milk teeth because they are eventually going to fall off and get replaced by permanent teeth. But it is recommended that they must be treated for two reasons. Firstly they are used for biting and chewing food for 5–6 years and secondly early loss of milk teeth may deform the jaw with a risk of malocclusion of permanent teeth.

TORCH infections (see Intrauterine infections)

TORTICOLLIS

Torticollis (wry neck) is an asymmetric deformity of the neck and head which is characterized by flexion of head toward the affected side and rotation of chin toward the opposite shoulder. In normal infants the head can be rotated so that chin can touch the opposite shoulder and the ear can be made to touch the shoulder on the same side. Torticollis may occur in a newborn due to swelling or shortening of neck muscles on one side (sternomastoid tumor). It is treated by gentle movements of the neck by tilting the head and rotating the chin to the other side to correct the abnormality. Sudden exposure to cold may lead to development of wry neck which recovers spontaneously in a few days. Torticollis may occur due to abnormalities and infection in the cervical spine or spasm of neck muscles. Children with double vision (due to squint) may tilt their head to avoid double vision. Torticollis is treated with an analgesic (paracetamol, ibuprofen), muscle relaxant, hot fomentation with a wet towel and gentle movements or physiotherapy of the neck.

TOXIC ERYTHEMA

About one-third of healthy term newborns may develop a pink rash with a pale central papule on the second or third day of life. The rash usually starts from the face and spreads to the trunk and extremities in about 24 hours. The rash disappears spontaneously after two to three days without any specific treatment. The exact cause of rash is not known but it is believed to be an earliest marker of atopy or allergic tendency.

TRADITIONAL BELIEFS IN CHILD CARE

Every community has its own way of rearing children, which are ingrained in the society through traditions established over centuries. The customs and cultural practices pertaining to mothercraft and child care are passed from one generation to the other, from grandmother to mother and to their daughters and grandchildren. The ancestral or conventional child care practices are by and large based on core knowledge, experience and wisdom although some of them may have emerged purely from intuition and superstition. The traditional practices are influenced by the education level, socio-economic status and value system of the family and society. There is evidence to suggest that traditional child care practices and home remedies are based on the practice and principles of Ayurveda. It is

T

Useful traditional health care practices

1. Delivery at mother's place.
2. Isolation of mother–baby dyad for 40 days.
3. Oil body massage of the mother and baby.
4. Universal and prolonged breastfeeding and wet nursing.
5. Instillation of colostrum in the eyes of the baby to prevent conjunctivitis.
6. Use of a cup and spoon or *paladay* for top feeding.
7. Baby sleeping on mother's bed and latter avoiding to turn her back towards the baby.
8. Use of honey, holy basil (*tulsi*) and ginger tea for treatment of common cold.
9. Washing hands before taking meals.
10. Rinsing mouth after taking a meal.

neither possible nor feasible to provide modern medical care to all people of a developing country, which is bogged by numbers, illiteracy and economic poverty. It is, therefore, desirable that a combination of modern and traditional health care practices should be harnessed to serve the health needs of people.

Traditional health care practices can be categorized into four groups, i.e. useful, harmful, inoccuous and of uncertain utility. A number of traditional health care practices are useful and based on sound scientific basis and logic **(see Box)**. There is a need to systematically study the utility, futility and possible dangers of traditional health care practices. The blind faith in the traditional health care practices of doubtful utility may lead to delay in seeking health care from professionals dealing with modern system of medicine. Nevertheless, there is a need to preserve the good and useful traditional practices for the care of children and weed out the harmful cultural beliefs and practices by health education.

Travel Sickness (*see* Motion sickness)

TRIPLE TEST

In high risk mothers (age above 35 years and previous baby with a developmental defect) a blood sample is taken at 16–18 weeks of pregnancy for estimation of alpha-fetaprotein (AFP), human chorionic gonadotropin (hCG) and unconjugated estriol (μE_3) to screen for neural tube defect and Down syndrome. Inorder to improve the sensitivity of triple test, quadruple test (Quad screen) is done by estimating the level of dimeric inhibin A (DIA). When AFP and estriol levels are low, while hCG and inhibin A levels are raised, it is suggestive of increased risk of Down syndrome. When triple or quad screen shows high risk (1:200 or more) of Down syndrome, sonography of the fetus, amniocentesis or chorionic villus sampling are done to confirm the diagnosis of Down syndrome.

TUBERCULOSIS

It is caused by *Mycobacterium tuberculosis* and remains a public health problem despite the availablity of BCG vaccine. Infection may occur at any age through droplets disseminated by breathing and coughing by an adult patient who discharges bacilli in the sputum. Most cases of tuberculosis in children occur below 5 years of age or during adolescence. Young children are more likely to have disseminated tuberculosis like miliary tuberculosis and tubercular meningitis. Tuberculosis can virtually affect any organ of the body. Infection is more likely to occur when body defences are weakened by undernutrition and viral infection like measles. The diagnosis of tuberculosis should be seriously considered when child has prolonged fever (> 2 weeks), failure to thrive, irritability, loss of appetite, poor weight gain or weight loss with or without cough. History of contact with an adult patient of tuberculosis is usually present.

The diagnosis is supported by markedly elevated erythrocyte sedimentation rate (ESR), positive tuberculin or Mantoux test and radiological evidences of tuberculosis on X-ray chest, ultrasound abdomen, CT scan of chest and brain. The diagnostic utility of MTB-serology is doubtful. BACTEC MGIT (mycobacteria growth indicator tube) 960 is useful for rapid isolation and detection of mycobacteria. Line probe assay (LiPA) can be used for rapid screening of smear-positive specimens for identification of MDR-TB patients. The diagnosis is confirmed by findings of histo-pathological features (FNAC of lymph node and liver biopsy) and isolation of tubercular bacilli from the sputum, CSF, gastric or bronchoalveolar lavage.

The child is managed by adequate rest, exposure to sunshine, and intake of nutritious balanced diet. The source of infection should be identified and family members screened to identify any infected subject/s. The patient is treated by a combination of 3 to 5 antitubercular drugs for a period of 6 months to one year depending upon the extent and severity of the disease process. In order to ensure compliance and reduce the duration of antitubercular therapy to 6 months, Government of India has launched DOTS (directly observed therapy schedule) wherein health worker administers medicines to the patient 3 times in a week under her direct supervision. Bacillus Calmette-Guérin (BCG) a live vaccine is given intradermally (inside the skin) with a special 26 G needle and a syringe on the top of left shoulder. A single dose of vaccine is given soon after birth (within 4 weeks of age) and there is no need for any boosters.

The vaccine site develops a papule or nodule after 4–6 weeks which may ulcerate and take several weeks to heal. BCG is not very effective vaccine but it prevents occurrence of severe and disseminated disease.

Tuberculin Test (*see* Mantoux test)

TYPHOID FEVER (Enteric fever)

Typhoid fever is caused by infection due to *Salmonella typhi*. It can occur at any age but is relatively uncommon below 2 years. It is a water-borne bacterial disease and infection occurs through oro-fecal route by taking contaminated food or water. The bacteria enter the blood stream through the Peyer's patches of small intestine.

Common features

It is characterized by prolonged fever, chills, headache, constipation or loose motions and toxemia. The fever starts as low grade or moderate in intensity and gradually increase in severity (step-ladder pattern). There are no symptoms of cough and cold, difficulty in passing urine or body aches. Mild distension of abdomen and enlargement of spleen are commonly associated. *When fever persists for more than 5 days and there are no specific symptoms, typhoid fever should be seriously considered.* The common complications include abdominal distension, bleeding from intestines, circulatory collapse (shock) and encephalopathy. At times two water-borne diseases like typhoid fever and hepatitis A may occur simultaneously causing difficulty in the diagnosis and management.

Laboratory investigations

During early phase of the disease, laboratory investigations are not helpful and they should be delayed for 4–5 days when most viral fevers would have settled. Complete blood count shows low leukocyte count (including absence of eosinophils), typhi dot IgM and widal test may be positive. The definitive diagnosis is based on positive blood culture for *S. typhi* which also provides information regarding the utility of various antibiotics.

Treatment

Most cases of typhoid fever can be managed at home under the supervision of a pediatrician. The child should be kept in a cool room and given plenty of fluids and nutritious diet. Fever should be kept under control by administration of a safe antipyretic like paracetamol and ibuprofen. If despite antipyretic therapy, fever remains above 102°F, tepid water sponging of the trunk and extremities can be done to bring down the fever. *The child with fever should never be starved.* He should be given nutritious diet of his liking including vegetable or chicken soup and broth. Eggs, chicken, rice, lentils (without covering), *lauki*, *tori*, potatoes, peas, etc. can be given. Avoid intake of high fiber and gas producing vegetables (okra, bitter gourd, spinach, corn, cruciferous vegetables like cauliflower, cabbage, turnips, radish and salads) and fried food items. Intake of chillies, condiments, sauce and vinegar should be restricted. Fruit juices should be avoided but fresh seasonal fruits like banana, apple and chikoo can be given. Specific antibiotics (like cefixime, ofloxacin, azithromycin, ceftriaxone) can be taken on the advice of a physician. Even after start of a specific antibiotic, it may take 3–4 days for the fever to settle. The antibiotic should be continued till the patient remains afebrile for at least 4–5 days. Vitamin supplements should be given during antibiotic therapy and convalescence.

Prevention

Drinking safe potable water (boiled, filtered, RO water, bottled) and maintenance of strict standard of personal hygiene are important to reduce the risk of infection. Avoid intake of food and juices from roadside hawkers, street vandors and *dhabas*. Food should be kept covered and taken steaming hot. Children should be encouraged to develop a habit of washing their hands with soap and water whenever they return home from school, market or playground, after attending their toilet needs and before taking their food. The vegetables and fruits should be thoroughly washed under running water and preferably taken after peeling. Typhoid vaccine is given as a single primary dose after the age of 2 years. Booster doses are given after every 3 years to maintain protection. A newer conjugated typhoid vaccine (Typbar TCV) is available which is given during 9–12 months followed by a single booster dose at 2 years of age for life long protection. The protective efficacy of available vaccines is around 60–70%. Typhoid fever may occur despite intake of typhoid vaccine but the disease will be mild and without any complications.

ULTIMATE ADULT HEIGHT

Every parent is keen and concerned to know about the likely height of their child when he grows to become an adult. Every mother wants that her child should be as tall and as smart as Amitabh Bachchan. The ultimate or adult height depends upon the health and velocity of linear growth of a preschool child, freedom from any developmental defects and systemic diseases and genetic potential of the child (height of parents and relatives). In a healthy child, who has no constraints (like congenital defects, systemic disease, dietary deficiency, and emotional deprivation), his adult height can be predicted as follows:

1. Adult height = Height at 2 years × 2
2. Adult height = Height at 3 years × 1.37
3. Adult height in inches:
   Boys = 0.545 H_3 + 0.544 P + 14.84
   Girls = 0.545 H_3 + 0.544 P + 10.09
   H_3 is height of the child at 3 years and P refers to mean height of parents in inches
4. Adult or target height of the child can be calculated on the basis of mid-parental height:
   Boys = Mean height of parents in cm + 6.5 cm
   Girls = Mean height of parents in cm − 6.5 cm
   The predicted or likely adult height of the child has an accuracy of ± 2 inches (5 cm).

UMBILICAL GRANULOMA

It manifests as a flesh colored or pale nodule at the base of umbilical stump with persistent discharge. It is usually benign and disappears after local application of betadine lotion or surgical spirit. When it persists, it can be managed by cautery with silver nitrate or application of common salt for 3 to 4 days.

UMBILICAL HERNIA

In some babies, when umbilical cord falls off after 7–10 days, the gut may protrude through the navel. Umbilical hernia is more common in infants with poor tone of abdominal muscles due to cretinism, rickets and Down syndrome. It is more likely to occur or become large in size when there is increase in intra-abdominal pressure because of excessive crying, constipation and persistent cough. Most umbilical hernias disappear spontaneously by 6 months to one year of age. Application of coin and bandage over the hernia is not recommended, as it may further weaken the abdominal wall and may cause damage to the gut. The underlying predisposing and aggravating conditions should be identified and managed appropriately. Rarely when hernia is large or it persists beyond 3 years, surgical closure is advised.

UNDESCENDED TESTIS (Cryptorchidism)

In premature babies, testes may be undescended at birth but gradually descend to the scrotum within a few weeks. The testes are retractable and get easily pulled up when scrotum is touched with cold hands. About 1% of boys may have undescended testis by first birthday. The condition is usually unilateral. The scrotal sac may be small and under developed on the side of undescended testis. The testis may be located in the groin or inside the abdomen. The condition may be associated with inguinal hernia. The undescended testis poses serious psychological embarrassment to the child and may lead to infertility and development of cancer. There is no role of hormonal treatment. Surgery is recommended to bring down the testis in the scrotum (orchiopexy) at the age of one year. When testes are undescended on both sides, it is likely to be associated with ambiguous genitalia because of serious developmental or a chromosomal disorder.

Upper Respiratory Infection (*see* Common cold)

URINARY TRACT INFECTION

It is usually caused by fecal *E. coli* and is more common in girls than boys. Ascending infection occurs in girls due to close proximity of anus and vulva. In infants, the incidence of urinary tract infection (UTI) is identical in children of both sexes because it occurs as a consequence of blood-borne infection. Urinary infection is more likely to occur in children with persistent constipation due to stasis of urine because of compression of bladder. Boys with nappy rash, inflammation of foreskin and tight prepuce are at an increased risk of UTI. Associated developmental defects in the genitourinary system should be looked for in children with recurrent UTI. In a boy when urinary stream is narrow or child strains while passing urine and there is dribbling of urine in the end, it is suggestive of bladder neck obstruction.

There is sudden onset of fever with feeling of chills and shivering. There may be difficulty or smarting (dysuria) and frequency of urination when infection is limited to bladder (cystitis). When infection ascends and involve kidneys (pyelonephritis) it is associated with high grade fever, toxemia, discomfort and tenderness over the back just below the rib cage at the renal angles. In infants, urinary symptoms are either absent or difficult to identify. Therefore, whenever a young child has fever without any obvious cause, UTI or viral infection should be seriously considered. Diagnosis is confirmed by finding pus cells in the urine and growth of pathogenic bacteria in a properly collected sample of urine. The sample of urine for routine examination and culture must be collected before starting antibiotic therapy.

Children with cystitis (fever, dysuria and frequency of urination) are treated with oral amoxicillin, cefixime or norfloxacin for 7–10 days. Infants with pyelonephritis are treated with parenteral (IM or IV) ceftriaxone and an aminoglycoside (gentamicin or amikacin). The antibiotics may be changed on the basis of culture report. In children with recurrent UTI, underlying cause should be identified and appropriately treated. The child is encouraged to drink plenty of fluids and if there is associated constipation, it should be relieved. Long-term prophylaxis with cotrimoxazole or cephalexin is advised in children with reflux of urine from bladder into the ureter (vesicoureteric reflux). Girls must be taught to wash the bottom (after each urination and defection) from front-backward to prevent the risk of contamination of vulva with stools.

Urine Collection

The sample for urine examination and culture must be collected before starting antibiotic therapy. Genital area should be washed with soap and water (without using any antiseptic) before collection of urine sample. A "clean catch" midstream sample of urine should be collected straight into a sterile container at the collection center. The urine sample collected with a collection bag in girls or condom in boys, is not suitable for culture studies. A reliable urine sample for culture can be obtained by percutaneous suprapubic aspiration or by passing a urethral catheter into the bladder. In order to ensure best yield on urine culture, the urine sample should preferably be collected in the laboratory and plated for culture studies without any delay. The colony count of 10^5 (100,000 colonies/mL) is considered as diagnostic of UTI. When colony count is low or there is isolation of multiple bacteria, it is considered as contaminants.

URTICARIA (*Chhapaki*)

It is a type of skin allergy to intake of certain foods, drugs, insect bites, animal dander, infections or worm infestations. In many cases no cause is found. There may be a family history of skin allergy. The child may have other associated allergic disorders like allergic colds (hay fever), eczema, and bronchial asthma. There is sudden development of blotchy red patches (wheals) on the skin with raised irregular margins. The central areas are relatively pale. There is intense itching which makes the child extremely uncomfortable. Rarely, it may be associated with swelling of the voice box (edema of larynx) with stridor (noisy breathing) and breathing difficulty. When swelling occurs around the face, lips, eyes and voice box, it is called angioedema. The skin lesions may disappear on its own and comeback on and off. Emotional stress, exposure to cold or sunlight and excessive perspiration may trigger the attack.

Treatment If child is taking any drug, it should be stopped immediately. The itching and skin lesions respond to administration of antihistaminic drugs. During daytime hydroxyzine hydrochloride, diphenhydramine hydrochloride or citirizine dihydrochloride are given while a long activing antihistaminic like loratadine or fexofenadine hydrochloride is given as a single dose at night. In severe cases, coticosteroids may be given on the advice of a doctor. Local application of soothing skin cream or lotion provides temporary relief. Avoid intake of chillies, condiments and hot foods. Avoid hot baths and showers, and tight fitting clothes. The associated infection and worm infestation should be treated. The antihistaminic drugs should be stopped gradually over a couple of days or weeks to prevent relapse.

Vaccination Schedule (*see* Immunizations Schedule)

VAGINAL BLEEDING

Monthly or menstrual period during adolescent phase is the commonest cause of vaginal bleeding which continues till pregnancy occurs or menopause sets in. About 20–25% of female babies may develop menstruation-like vaginal bleeding after 4–5 days of birth. The baby was exposed to high levels of female sex hormones during pregnancy which suddenly fall after birth leading to withdrawal vaginal bleeding. The bleeding is usually mild and lasts for 2 to 4 days. It does not need any specific therapy apart from local aseptic cleaning of genitals.

VEGETARIAN VERSUS NON-VEGETARIAN DIET

There is a popular saying that "you become what you eat". There is a profound influence of food on our memory, comprehension, thinking, judgement, intellect and emotions. Human beings by virtue of their evolution and nature of teeth are vegetarian. In view of greater health benefits of vegetarian diet, there is increasing trend to adopt a vegetarian food style in many countries of the world. Albert Eeinstein was a staunch vegetarian and he said "*Nothing will benefit human health and increase the chances of survival of life on earth as much as evolution to a vegetarian diet*". There is a wide variety of plants, cereals, vegetables and fruits to choose our daily diet. Fresh vegetables and fruits are loaded with anti-oxidants, phytochemicals, flavonoids, polyphenols, micronutrients and fiber. There is enough scientific evidence to suggest that vegetarian diet is more health-friendly with reduced risk of various age-related diseases like high blood pressure, coronary artery disease, cerebrovascular strokes, cancer and gout. They can be as muscular and athletic as non-vegetarians, infact they are endowed with greater stamina compared to non-vegetarians. Vegetarians are more likely to have greater poise, peace of mind, serenity and spirituality in life. They are likely to have better control on their emotions with reduced risk of vices like lust, anger, greed, possessiveness and arrogance. Vegetarian diet provides all the essential nutrients except vitamin B_{12}. Most vegetarians, however, do take milk and milk products (and sometimes eggs) which are rich sources of vitamins B_{12}. Children should be encouraged to adopt vegetarian diet style by informing about its virtues but they should never be forced or cajoled to become pure vegetarian against their wishes.

Virtues of Veggies

Both vegetables and fruits are health-friendly and loaded with micronutrients, phytonutrients, fiber and antioxidants. Fruits are rich in carbohydrates (glucose and fructose), vitamin A (carotenes), vitamin C, fiber and antioxidants. Vegetables are more health-friendly and less fattening (if taken raw, steamed or boiled) because of their low glycemic index (blood glucose level rises slowly and not sharply) due to presence of complex carbohydrates. Veggies are a good source of vitamins A, C, B complex, E and K apart from minerals, antioxidants, phytochemicals and fiber. Onions, garlic, ginger, green chillies and cruciferous vegetables (cabbage, cauliflower, turnips, knol khol) are loaded with anticancer and anti-inflammatory compounds. No doubt fruits are delicious but they are no match to the nurtritional power of veggies. Your child needs a mix of both, at least 5 helpings of fruits and vegetables in a day to keep diseases at bay.

VISION

Newborn babies respond to bright light by blinking and turning their head towards diffuse source of light. The neonate can see clearly up to a distance of one foot and can appreciate different colors but red and black are perceived best. Around 4–6 weeks, the child is able to fix his gaze and look into your eyes and give an interactive or social smile when talked to. He can fix his gaze and follow a dangling red ring. By 3 months of age he can see objects up to a distance of 10 feet. The acuity of vision gradually improves as child grows and reaches the adult level by the age of 6 years.

When a baby is unable to see, he will not blink in response to bright light, may have purposeless roving eye movements and persistence of squint (crossed eyes) beyond the age of 6 months. The child may not give any blink response when you suddenly bring your finger towards his eyes. A blind infant is extrasensitive to noise and gets easily startled by a loud sound. Whenever there is a doubt about the vision of the child, a consultation must be sought with an ophthalmologist for evaluation of vision by a variety of modern tests like indirect ophthalmoscopy, opticokinetic nystagmus and visual evoked response (VER).

Visually Handicapped Child (*see* Blindness)

VITAMINS
Vitamins are essential for maintenance of good health and their deficiency can lead to several health problems. They are broadly divided into two classes, fat soluble and water soluble.

Fat Soluble Vitamins
They are present in fatty food and their absorption is facilitated by fats. They are stored in the body and excessive intake (especially vitamin A and vitamin D) may lead to adverse effects due to toxicity.

Vitamin A Vitamin A is needed for healthy eyes and it is credited with anti-infective and anti-oxidant role to prevent occurrence of acute respiratory and gastrointestinal infections. Night blindness (inability to see in the dark) is the earliest manifestation of vitamin A deficiency. The rich dietary sources of vitamin A include butter, *ghee*, cod liver oil, vegetable oil, green leafy vegetables, yellow vegetables (carrots) and fruits (papaya, mango, apricot), egg yolk and dairy products.

Vitamin D It is essential for growth of healthy teeth and bones. Its deficiency leads to development of rickets with various deformities of the bones. Recent evidence suggests that vitamin D is credited with a large number of non-skeletal health benefits like modulation of immunity with reduced risk of autoimmune disorders, type 2 diabetes mellitus, coronary artery disease and various cancers. Vitamin D is formed in the body by the action of ultraviolet rays of sun on the skin. Children should be encouraged to play in the open for adequate exposure to sunlight. The dietary sources of vitamin D include butter, *ghee*, margarine, fish, liver, egg yolk and vitamin D fortified dairy products. Infants who are exclusively breastfed during first six months of life must be given supplements of vitamin D (400 iu/day) because breast milk is relatively deficient in vitamin D.

Vitamin E It is a potent antioxidant, improves fertility, memory and muscular activity. The dietary sources of vitamin E include wheat, vegetable oils, green leafy vegetables, eggs, liver, nuts and dairy products.

Vitamin K It is required for production of prothrombin in the liver which is needed for normal clotting of blood to stop bleeding. Vitamin K is produced in the intestines by friendly bacteria (probiotics) in the gut. The dietary sources of vitamin K include milk and milk products, green leafy vegetables (spinach, kale or *karam ka sag*, cabbage, cauliflower), beans, peas, potatoes, carrots and liver. Breast milk is relatively deficient in vitamin K. All newborn babies are given one dose of vitamin K (0.5–1.0 mg IM) soon after birth to prevent hemorrhagic disease of the newborn.

Water Soluble Vitamins

They are relatively unstable and may be destroyed by heat and exposure to light. Unlike fat soluble vitamins, they are endogenously produced in the gut by probiotics. They are not stored in the body and when consumed excessively, they are excreted in the urine (passage of yellow-colored urine) without any risk of toxicity.

Vitamin B complex There are at least eight vitamins grouped together under vitamin B complex. They include thiamine (B_1), riboflavin (B_2), niacin (B_3), pantothenic acid (B_5), pyridoxine (B_6), cyanocobalamin (B_{12}), biotin and folic acid. They are necessary for normal functioning and protection of central nervous system, lining of oral cavity and gut. The dietary sources of vitamin B complex include milk and dairy products, wheat, parboiled or unpolished rice, green leafy vegetables, meat, fish, nuts and seeds. Strict vegetarians get their quota of vitamin B_{12} from dairy products. Sprouted *dals* and legumes are extremely rich in vitamin B complex.

Vitamin C Vitamin C is essential for development of bones, teeth, integrity of blood vessels and healing of wounds. It helps in the absorption of iron from gut. Its deficiency leads to development of scurvy which is characterized by bleeding from gums, irritability due to bone pains, inability to move a limb and anemia. Dietary sources of vitamin C include citrus fruits (orange, sweet lemon, *kinoo*, grape fruit), Indian gooseberries (*amla*), guava, tomatoes, potatoes and green vegetables. Breast milk provides sufficient quantities of vitamin C but bottle fed babies are likely to have poor intake of vitamin C because it gets destroyed by heating the milk.

VOMITING

Vomiting is a common symptom in children and occurs due to a variety of causes. It is very frightening for the parents though most of the time it is either due to benign or non-serious causes, or is a self-limiting disorder. Some children are prone to vomit on a minor pretext like a bout of coughing, during temper tantrum or after a feed.

Benign causes Regurgitation of curdled milk may occur due to improper technique of feeding (bottle feeding with a tiny or wide hole in the rubber teat, lack of burping), forced feeding or over feeding. These children continue to have a satisfactory weight gain. Some infants may vomit following a bout of cough due to asthmatic bronchitis or wheezing. Administration of oral medications may be associated or followed by vomiting.

Serious causes Vomiting is commonly the first or a sole symptom of acute gastroenteritis or food poisoning. Vomiting is a common symptom of systemic infection or sepsis and may occur due to infection and inflammation of any organ of the abdomen like kidney, liver, pancreas and appendix. The triad of fever, headache and vomiting is suggestive of meningitis (brain infection) but may occur because of non-specific acute viral infection. Vomiting is an important symptom of raised intracranial pressure. Persistent and forceful green-colored vomitings in association with abdominal distension and constipation is suggestive of intestinal obstruction. Persistent regurgitation of milk feeds from early infancy may occur due to gastroesophageal reflux. In normal children, regurgitation of stomach contents is prevented due to presence of a sphincter at the junction of esophagus (food pipe) and stomach. In some children gastroesophageal junction is lax or lacks a sphincter leading to regurgitation of feeds and poor weight gain. At times the regurgitated feeds may be aspirated into the lungs with frequent episodes of aspiration pneumonia or wheezing during infancy. The child with vomiting should be encouraged to take sips of water or milk (not gulps with a glass) immediately after a bout of cough or vomiting. When vomiting occurs due to bitter taste of the medicine, changing the formulation may help. Children with gastroesophageal reflux disease (GERD) respond to administration of thickened feeds and restraining them in a propped-up position in a special chair after every feed. Antiemetics (domperiodone 0.2 mg/kg/dose and ondansetron hydrochloride 2–4 mg/dose) are useful for symptomatic relief of vomiting. Additional water and ORS should be given to replace loss of fluids in the vomitus. When vomiting is persistent or there are associated symptoms or development of dehydration (lack of urination for more than 6 hours), the child should be taken to a hospital.

WARTS (Massa)

Warts are caused by infection of skin with human papillomavirus (HPV). They affect about 10–20% children and are more common in girls. There are rough, raised or flat, skin or flesh colored irregular skin lesions resembling a "cauliflower". They can occur on any part of the body but are more common over the hands, feet, knees and elbows. Warts over the soles may be painful and cause difficulty in walking. Warts are contagious and can spread to other family members through contact or sharing towels, kerchiefs or toiletries.

Treatment Warts are self-limiting and disappear spontaneously. They can be destroyed by freezing with liquid nitrogen, cryosurgery or laser therapy. Palmar and plantar warts are treated by application of 40% salicylic acid lotion. Cimetidine has been used for treatment of multiple warts in children.

Home Remedies

- Crush a garlic clove and rub it over the wart/s at night and cover with a band aid.
- Apply organic apple cider vinegar on the wart/s with a cotton swab or toothpick twice a day and cover with a band aid. To improve its efficacy you can apply a paste of baking soda in water over the wart/s before application of the vinegar.
- Rub lemon juice over the wart/s twice a day.

Wasp Sting (*see* Bee and Wasp Sting)

WATERING OF EYES (Epiphora)

Tears are constantly produced by the lacrimal or tear glands to keep the eyes moist. The excess tears are normally drained off through a duct or a tube which connects the inner corner of the eyes with the nose (nasolacrimal duct). When ducts are blocked by debris, the newborn baby may develop persistent watering of one or both eyes. The duct can be cleared by regular massage. Trim your nails and apply moisturizing cream over the thumb and index finger of your dominant hand. Place them over the inner angles of baby's eyes and press gently but firmly the lacrimal sacs and slide them downward along the outer surface of the nose by maintaining a constant pressure to massage the nasolacrimal duct. You can repeat this procedure several times in a day when you are playing or fondling with your baby. Antibacterial eye drops should be instilled after massaging the nasolacrimal duct. If watering of eyes persists beyond the age of 3 months, you should consult an ophthalmologist who may clear the duct by probing and syringing.

WEANING FOODS

Milk is a complete food and exclusive breastfeeding is able to maintain normal growth of children during first 6 months of life. After 6 months, infant must be gradually weaned off (changed over) to take semi-liquid or semi-solid complementary food otherwise his weight gain will slow down and he is likely to develop nutritional deficiencies. Timely weaning is crucial to maintain adequate nutrition of the infant and it demands considerable time, effort and ingenuity on the part of the mother. It is recommended to give home-made nutritious weaning foods with utmost care by maintenance of personal hygiene to prevent the risk of bacterial contamination. Hands should be washed with soap and water before preparing or serving food to the child. During weaning, as milk intake gradually dcreases, child is given sips of water after intake of semisolid food. The water must be safe and free from contamination. Depending upon the source of water supply, the family may have to filter the water, use RO system or boil the water. It is preferable to use a cup or a glass rather than a sipper to give water to reduce the risk of infection.

6 Months

Breastfeeding is continued for at least one year or even longer but after 6 months, the child is offered gradually increasing amount of semi-liquid or finely mashed or pureed weaning food. Offer one food item at a time (by replacing a milk feed) and watch for tolerance or any allergic reaction for a week or so before introducing another food. It is useful to have a hand blender or mixer to thoroughly mash and blend the semi-solid food. There is no need to introduce milk feeds at this stage but child can be given milk products like custard, curd, *kheer*, *dalia* and cheese. You can start weaning with a precooked rice-based cereal which is prepared in water and given with a small spoon by holding the baby in the lap. The child is gradually introduced home-based weaning food like thin porridge, and *kheer* made from *suji* or rice flour. It is recommended to use less salt and sugar so that child develops a healthy habit of taking less salt and sugar when he grows to become an adult. Offer the weaning food when baby is awake, hungry and in good mood. The breastfeeding can be replaced by a weaning food or child can be offered a breastfeed after feeding with a semi-liquid gruel. Give small amount of weaning food and gradually increase the quantity. There is no virtue in giving thin watery soup like *dal ka pani*, instead *dal* should be mashed in the soup and given to the child as thin gravy. Freshly prepared fruit juice (sweet lemon, orange, kinoo) can be given at this stage but they are time consuming to prepare and are associated with potential risk of bacterial contamination. It is useful to give fresh fruit juice if child is constipated. It is much better to give mashed (soft fruits like banana, *cheekoo*, papaya), stewed or pureed whole fruit to the child rather than fruit juices. Tinned fruit juices and fresh fruit juice procured from the road-side vendors should be avoided.

7–8 Months

The child is gradually introduced to a variety of cereals, vegetables and fruits. In certain communities weaning is delayed till "*Anna Prashasan*" ceremony is held. It is a wrong belief that child must have teeth before he can accept or digest semi-solid food. A variety of foods can be offered at this stage like rice and *dal* gruel (*khichdi*), rice and *dal* with mashed vegetables. You can add a pinch of salt, butter or clarified butter (*ghee*) to improve the taste and caloric density. If you are non-vegetarian, egg can be introduced in the diet at this stage. Raw egg should not be given due to the risk of Salmonella infection. Start by giving egg yolk of a full boiled egg because it is less likely to cause allergic reaction. After a few weeks, egg white can be given and child watched for any allergic reaction like vomitng, skin rash, abdominal discomfort or sudden pallor. If child is allergic to egg protein or any other food, he should be taken off the offending food. Depending upon the cultural and regional food habits, children can be offered foods of their region like *dosa, idli, sambar, upma, dhokla, suji, ragi, and besan ka halwa.* In north India, *choori* is prepared by mashing a fried *chapati* (*parantha*) with clarified butter (*desi ghee*) and powdered jaggery or *chhakkar.*

9–11 Months

At this stage child can accept a variety of foods and fruits 3–4 times in a day. He is able to chew and swallow the food. He can accept bits of *chapati, prantha* or bread soaked in milk, *dal* or vegetable gravy. Hand-eye coordination has improved by this age and because of irritation of gums due to teething, the child enjoys to have finger foods like butter toast, soup stick, cake rusk, French toast, cake piece, biscuits, apple slice or a piece of carrot. Non-vegetarian foods like chicken soup, minced chicken or fish can be introduced after the age of 9 months.

12 Months–1 Year

By first birthday, the child should be eating from the family pot 4–5 times in a day. He should take only 2–3 breastfeeds (while going to sleep) and mostly eat everyday household food and seasonal fruits. The child should be given one cooked egg everyday. At one year of age, although the baby weighs on an average about 10 kg, but his caloric and nutritional needs are about one-half of his mother. By 18 months, the child can eat family food and is able to use his fingers and spoon to feed himself. Avoid introduction of junk food, cola drinks and tinned juices to establish healthy eating habits. Toddlers should not be offered nuts, candies, popcorn, roasted Bengal gram because of potential risk of choking.

The child should not be forced fed, instead he should be encouraged to self feed. The child is likely to create some mess by spilling the food but he will soon learn to self-feed without any fuss. Mother should be relaxed and show due patience while feeding the toddler. The child may eat a bit, play in-between and then eat again. The food should be offered when child is hungry and not tired or sleepy. Avoid use of distractions (like TV, laptop, videogames, picture book, etc.) and use of various silly pranks while feeding the child. The meal times should be a pleasant experience for the child and not a tug of war between him and the rest of the family. The practice of washing hands before and after feeding should be strictly followed at an early age so that it becomes a useful habit later in life.

WEIGHT GAIN

Most newborns loose up to 5–7% of body weight during the first 2 to 3 days of life. The weight remains stationary during next one to two days and birth weight is regained by the end of first week. Preterm babies lose more weight compared to term babies while babies with intrauterine growth retardation (IUGR) may not lose any weight especially when fed early and adequately. There is rapid weight gain during first year of life **(see Box)**.

Most babies double their birth weight by 4–5 months, triple it by one year and quadruple it by 2 years of age. The weight should be recorded on a Road-to-Health card during first 5 years of life. The trend or slope of the weight curve is more important than its location on the chart. The growth curve of healthy child should be directed upwards or it should run parallel to the 50th percentile line. In general boys weigh more than girls at all ages except during 10–12 years of age when girls are usually heavier than boys because of early onset of adolescence or sexual maturation.

Weight gain velocity	
Age	**Weight gain**
0–4 months	1.0 kg/month (30 g/day)
5–8 months	0.75 kg/month (25 g/day)
9–12 months	0.5 kg/month (20 g/day)
1–3 years	2.25 kg/year
4–9 years	2.75 kg/year
10–18 years	
Girls	4.0 – 5.0 kg/year
Boys	6.0 – 7.0 kg/year

Average weight can be calculated by the formula weight in kg = (Age in years + 4) × 2.

Weight Record (*see* Road-to-Health card)

WHITE SPOTS ON THE FACE

Preschool children are prone to develop ill-defined hypopigmented or white patches with fine scales (pityriasis alba) on the face. These are more common in summer but their exact cause is unknown. There is a wrong belief that they occur due to worm infestation or nutritional deficiency. They are benign and disappear spontaneously. Mother should scrub the face with soap and water at least twice a day. Local application of an antibiotic cream and mild emollient is usually followed by recovery. It may take several weeks for the lesions to resolve. When skin patches are milky or chalky white in color and involve the eyelids or lips, consultation should be sought with a dermatologist to rule out vitiligo or leucoderma.

WHITE SPOTS ON THE NAILS

White spots on the nails are common in children. They occur due to minor day-to-day trauma to the nails. Following a minor injury to nail/s, white spots appear after about 6 weeks when both child as well as mother cannot the recall the nature or mode of injury. There is no scientific evidence for the myth that they occur due to deficiency of calcium or zinc. They do not need any treatment and disappear spontaneously.

WHOOPING COUGH (Pertussis)

It is a highly contagious infection caused by Gram-positive bacilli *Bordetella pertussis* which is transmitted by droplets which are disseminated through coughing, talking and crying. The disease can occur at any age including neonates. The symptoms appear after an incubation period (time taken from exposure to onset of symptoms) of 7–14 days. There are 3 distinct stages of the disease. The first stage is characterized by fever, watering from nose, cough and irritation of throat which lasts for 7–10 days. This is followed by paroxysmal stage which lasts for 2–4 weeks. There are severe and prolonged bouts of cough wherein face becomes suffused and flushed or blue (*kali khansi*) and bout of cough terminates with a long drawn inspiratory sound or "whoop". The cough is usually followed by vomiting with expulsion of thick tenacious mucus. The bouts of cough may be triggered by intake of fluids, milk and food. During the *convalescent stage*, the bouts of cough become less frequent, appetite and general condition gradually improves.

Common complications include middle ear infection (acute otitis media), pneumonia, pneumothorax, bronchiectasis and flaring of latent tuberculosis. Paroxysms of cough may lead to development of hernia, rectal prolapse and subconjunctival bleeding in the eye/s. Because of prolonged course and frequent occurrence of vomiting, the child may become malnourished.

Treatment The disease is life-threatening in infants and they should preferably admitted in the hospital. Erythromycin is given for 2 weeks to reduce the period of infectivity. Steam inhalation or cold humidification is useful to reduce viscosity of mucus and facilitate expulsion of phlegm. Nebulization with salbutamol or oral bronchodilators may reduce bouts of coughing. Cough suppressants and antihistaminics should be avoided as they can worsen the cough. The child should be given balanced nutritious diet. It is best to feed the child after the bout of cough.

Prevention DTP (diphtheria, tetanus and pertussis) vaccine is useful to prevent pertussis. Three doses of DTP at 4–8 weeks intervals are given during first 6 months of life followed by boosters at the age of 18 months and 4½ years. Due to increasing incidence of whooping cough in older children, a DTP vaccine with low content of diphtheria toxoid and low dose of acellular pertussis antigen (Tdap or Boostrix) is available for administration of booster doses in children above 6 years of age.

Wheezy Child (*see* Bronchial Asthma)

WILMS' TUMOR

It is one of the most common tumor of the kidney in preschool children. There is gradual enlargement of abdomen due to growth of the tumor. The associated symptoms include fever, vomiting, loss of appetite, pallor, abdominal pain, high blood pressure and passage of blood in urine (hematuria). The diagnosis is confirmed by skiagrams of abdomen and imaging studies like computed tomography (CT) and magnetic resonance imaging (MRI). In advanced cases, the tumor may infiltrate into adjoining tissues or spread to a distant site (metastasize) especially liver and lungs. The standard modalities of treatment include surgical excision, chemotherapy (actinomycin D and vincristine) and radiotherapy depending upon the stage of the disease. When early and aggressive management protocol is followed, more than 90% patients of Wilms' tumor are curable.

WILSON DISEASE

It is a genetic or metabolic disorder which is associated with excessive deposition of copper in the liver, basal ganglia of brain, kidneys and cornea of eyes. The symptoms usually start after the age of 5 years with enlargement of liver, tremors, dystonia, behaviour changes, speech difficulties and fall in school grades. A rusty-brown arc or ring (Kayser-Fleischer ring) may be seen along the upper or lower border of cornea. The disease is progressive if diagnosis is delayed. Early treatment wih oral d-penicillamine is curative as it effectively binds copper and excretes it. The dietary intake of copper should be restricted by avoiding intake of copper-rich foods like liver, shellfish, nuts and chocolates. The child must be given supplements of vitamin B_6 and zinc.

WINDY BABY

Excessive wind or gas and flatulence are extremely common in newborn babies and infants. Babies swallow wind while feeding and during bouts of crying. Bottle fed babies are likely to swallow more air if hole in the teat is too small or too big. If a feeding bottle is not tilted properly, the baby may swallow air rather than milk. In breastfed babies, intake of lentils with covering (kidney beans, *urad dal*, black *chana,* white *chana*) and cruciferous vegetables (cauliflower, cabbage, turnips, raddish, kale, mustard leaves etc.) by the nursing mother is associated with flatulence in the mother and excessive wind in her suckling infant. Milk digestion in general is associated with greater production of gas because of excessive content of lactose. If a baby is not burped properly after a feed, the wind travels down in the intestines with excessive passage of gas from bottom. When wind gets "blocked" the baby may develop bouts of intestinal colic. Crying leads to further swallowing of air with worsening of flatulence.

Excessive wind or gas should be considered as normal during early infancy and there is no need for any concern and anxiety. Proper technique of feeding and effective burping (eructation of swallowed air) reduces the risk of flatulence. The child should be placed in the right lateral position after the feed. Placing the child in a tummy position with hips raised facilitates the expulsion of gas from the bottom. When wind is "blocked" and child cries due to colic, application of *hing* (asafoetida) around the navel and administration of antispasmodic drops or concoction of fennel seeds (*saunf*), carom seeds (*ajwain*) and cardamom (*elaichi*) provides prompt relief.

WORM INFESTATIONS

Worm infestations are common in children living in poor environmental sanitation conditions and having poor sense of personal hygiene. The eggs of worms are passed in feces contaminating the soil and growing vegetables. Infection occurs through fecal-oral route by eating mud (pica) or taking raw vegetables without peeling and proper washing. Larvae of some worms like hookworms enter the body by piercing through skin of children walking bare feet. Eating infected pork and beef without proper cooking may lead to infection by tapeworms. Drinking contaminated water and taking infected food may lead to development acute amebic dysentery and giardiasis. Due to high risk of infestation in children, it is a good idea to deworm them periodically every 6 months or so. The preventive strategies should be practiced as a safeguard against development of worm infestations **(see Box)**.

Prevention of worm infestations

- Daily bath and strict personal cleanliness should be maintained. The under garments should be changed daily.
- Ensure that the child washes hands with soap and water after defecation and before taking food.
- Nails should be trimmed in children twice a week and kept clean.
- Children need supervision to prevent eating of mud. Toys and hands should be kept clean.
- Salads and raw vegetables should be thoroughly washed with running water and taken after peeling.
- The water used for drinking should be clean and protected against contamination with excreta.
- Avoid taking raw pork which should be properly cooked before eating.
- Children should wear shoes while playing outdoors.
- Wear a tight underwear at night so that child has no direct access to anus for itching to prevent autoinfection.

Threadworms (Pinworms)

These worms are most common but do not cause any serious health hazards. They are white in color, small in size and thin like a thread (about 1.0 cm long). Female worms which are loaded with eggs wriggle out of anus at night and cause anal itching and sleeplessness. In girls, the worms may enter the vaginal orifice causing the child to suddenly wake up at night with unexplained episodes of shrieking. You may be able to see the wriggling threadworms by examining the stretched anal orifice under bright light at night.

Itching can be relieved by local application of a soothing cream or bland oil (avoid mustard oil which is highly irritant). A number of medications (mebendazole, albendazole) are available and course must be repeated after 2 weeks to break the cycle of re-infection. Auto-infection can be prevented by wearing a tight underwear at night (so that anus is not directly accessible for itching) and by keeping the nails trimmed and clean. It is desirable to treat all the members of the family simultaneously to prevent cross infection.

Roundworms (*Ascaris lumbricoides*)

These worms are round in shape and large in size (male worm is about 15–20 cm long while female worm measures 25–35 cm). The common symptoms include episodes of abdominal pain, excessive appetite (as if the worms are eating the food), failure to thrive and pallor despite good appetite. Teeth grinding during sleep is not due to worm infestation although it is commonly believed so by the parents. The larvae of worms may travel into the lungs and produce wheezing and asthma-like symptoms. Heavy infestation may lead to intestinal obstruction because of formation of a ball of worms. At times the worms may be passed in the feces or vomited out when infestation is heavy.

The infestation can be treated by a single dose of albenda-zole 400 mg or mebendazole 100 mg twice a day for 3 days. In susceptible children (poor sanitation and lack of personal hygiene), regular deworming can be advised every 6 months. Preventive measures should be followed to prevent reinfection.

Hookworms (*Ancylostoma duodenale*)

These are tiny dark-pink worms which are not visible in the stools on naked eye examination (male worm is about 8 mm and female 12 mm in size). The infection occurs by penetration of larvae through the soles of feet. These worms are attached to the gut (duodenum) and suck blood. The child develops vague upper abdominal discomfort and loss of appetite. The child looks pale, sickly and puffy. Specific antiworm medications (levamisole, albendazole) are available. Anemia should be treated by administration of iron and intake of iron-rich foods.

Tapeworms (*Taenia solium, Taenia saginata*)

These are extremely long (2–3 meters) and flat worms. Most infestations do not produce any symptoms. Infection occurs by taking improperly cooked or processed pork or beef. Intake of vegetables contaminated with eggs of tapeworms may lead to development of cysticercosis (nodules in the muscles or brain causing convulsions). Cysticercosis may occur in vegetarians who do not consume any pork or beef. Cysticercosis is diagnosed by CT scan or MRI of brain and biopsy of muscle nodule. Adult tapeworm is treated by administration of niclosamide and quinacrine. Cysticercosis of brain is treated with anticonvulsants and specific medications like albendazole and praziquantel.

X-LINKED DISORDERS

X-linked or sex-linked disorders are transmitted through defective genes which are located in the X-chromosome. In X-linked recessive disorders, girls (XX) are the carriers of the defective gene (they do not suffer from the disease because they have 2 X) while boys (XY) suffer from the disease. The common X-linked disorders (where mother is a carrier while males suffer from the disease) include hemophilia, Duchenne muscular dystrophy, G6PD deficiency and Bruton disease (hereditary agammaglobulinemia). When mother is having an X-linked disorder (carrier) 25% sons will be affected and 25% will be normal, while 25% daughters would be carriers and 25% will be normal. But when father is suffering from an X-linked disorder, all daughters will be carriers while all sons will be normal.

X-SYNDROME

Metabolic syndrome X is characterized by abdominal obesity, insulin resistance, elevated blood levels of insulin, lipid abnormalities, atherosclerosis, essential hypertension, impaired fasting glucose or impaired glucose tolerance, type 2 diabetes mellitus and coronary heart disease. Polycystic ovaries or poly-cystic ovarian disease (PCOD) may be associated with metabolic syndrome X in adolescent girls. People who carry excess fat in their tummy (apple-shaped) instead of hips, buttocks and thighs (pear-shaped) are more likely to develop type 2 diabetes mellitus, high blood pressure and heart disease. Waist circumference of >90 cm in men or >80 cm in women or waist to hip ratio of more than 1.0 in men or more than 0.85 in women is highly suggestive of metabolic syndrome X and adverse health consequences.

XEROPHTHALMIA

Xerophthalmia or dryness of eyes occurs due to vitamin A deficiency. The initial symptom is poor dark adaptation and inability to see after sunset (night blindness). The outer covering of eyes (conjunctiva and cornea) become dry, lustreless and wrinkled in both the eyes. Bitot spots may appear as chalky–gray nodules on the outer angle of eyes. It may lead to softening of cornea with ulceration and blindness. The condition occurs in malnourished children especially after a bout of measles or prolonged diarrhea. The condition is managed as a medical emergency, under the guidance of an ophthalmologist by administration of vitamin A and local therapy. Vitamin A is administered through intramuscular route (25,000 iu <6 months, 50,000 iu in 6–12 months, and 100,000 iu >12 months) in two doses 24 hours apart followed by another dose after 15 days. The condition can be prevented by intake of calorie-dense nutritious diet and consuming vitamin A rich foods like green leafy vegetables, carrots, papaya, mango, eggs, milk and dairy products.

YAWNING

A yawn is a reflex consisting of a long deep breath of air with open mouth, bulging of eardrums and stretching of limbs. It is physiological and spontaneous and usually occurs before going to sleep or on waking up. Yawning may be a symptom of over-work, tiredness and sleepiness or boredom. In humans yawning is "contagious" and is often triggered by watching others yawn. It is important to remember that during newborn period yawning, sneezing and hiccups are physiological responses and their presence should be considered as an indicator that the baby is healthy.

YOGA

Yoga refers to union of body and mind, a state of complete awareness and peace with the help of certain physical and mental exercises and postures. It is useful for achieving mental peace, poise, enthusiasm and self confidence to face the challenges of modern society which is riddled with unrest and mental stress. Every school should introduce yoga and yogic practices as a part of core curriculum to promote our heritage.

YO-YO DIETING

Yo-yo dieting and bingeing are commonly practiced by adolescent girls and it may have several adverse effects on health. A consistent lifestyle of increased physical activity and healthy eating of plenty of green vegetables and seasonal fruits with avoidance of junk foods and fried food items is more conducive to sound health. Frequent spells of fasting or missing the breakfast leads to slowing down of metabolism with excessive laying down of fat during the periods of bingeing. The initial aggressive calorie reduction of foods leads to loss of both muscle and body fat. During bingeing the weight is regained by laying down of extra fat rather than muscles. There may be episodes of repeated loss and regain of body weight (weight cycling or yo-yo effect) which adversely affects the health and well being.

ZEN HEALING

Zen refers to Buddhist philosophy of contemplation of one's essential nature to awaken the power within or create self-awareness. Medicine and meditation come from the same root, one heals the body physically and the other spiritually. Health is not merely absence of disease but boundless energy, enthusiasm, happiness, peace of mind, success and loving relationship, which cannot be achieved only by having a sound body unless the mind is tranquil and peaceful. The secret of good health is governed by moderation, regularity, rest and mental peace, chakra balancing, healthy life style and physical activity all in a balance.

ZINC

Zinc is emerging as an important trace mineral required for production of a large number of metalloenzymes. It has an important biological role for promotion of physical growth, sexual maturation and integrity of immune system. Zinc is useful for prevention and treatment of acute and persistent diarrhea and respiratory infections. Zinc supplements during pregnancy are credited to enhance fetal growth in women belonging to poor socioeconomic group. Zinc supplements are useful to promote the growth of infants with intrauterine growth retardation.

ZOONOSIS

Zoonosis is a Greek word (zoon: animal, nosos: disease) which refers to diseases transmitted through animals or vertebrates. Human beings and animals have lived in harmony and with interdependence for ages, and in return animals have shown faith and concern toward human beings but have also transmitted several diseases. Children come in direct contact with household pets as well as the excreta of stray, wild or domestic animals. The infection may be transmitted directly from the animal to the human being or with the help of another vector such as mosquitoes, fleas and ticks. The common zoonosis include *Dogs*: Rabies, hydatid disease, visceral larva migrans, *Cats*: Toxoplasmosis, visceral larva migrans, cat scratch disease, rabies, *Rats*: Plague, rat bite fever, leptospirosis, tularemia, *Cattle*: Anthrax, brucellosis, leptospirosis, *T. saginata* and *Pigs*: *T. solium*, cysticercosis, Japanese encephalitis and swine flu.

Glossary of English and Hindi Names of Foodstuffs

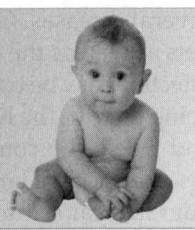

Cereals, Grains, and Split Lentils (Pulses and Dals)

English name	Hindi name
Arrow root	*Arraroot, paniphal, tikora*
Barley	*Jaon*
Bengal gram, brown chickpeas	*Chana*
Black lentil, horse bean	*Kali dal, urad dal*
Broken wheat grains	*Dalia*
Buckwheat flour	*Kuttu ka atta*
Corn	*Makai*
Finger millet	*Ragi, mandua*
Flax seed or linseed	*Alsi ke beej*
Foxtail millet	*Kangani*
Great millet	*Jowar*
Green gram	*Moong dal*
Kidney beans	*Rajma*
Maize	*Bhutta*
Oats	*Jai, javie*
Olive	*Jaitune*
Pearl millet	*Bajra*
Pigeon peas	*Arhar or toor dal*
Puffed rice	*Kumura, murmura*
Quinoa (prounced as keen-wah)	*Maraiyo, bathua*
Rape seeds or canola	*Gingli*
Red lentil	*Masoor dal, malka masoor*
Refined wheat flour	*Maida*
Rice	*Chawal*
Safflower seeds	*Kusum ke beej*
Semolina	*Suji, rava*
Sesame seeds	*Til ka beej*

Sorghum	*Jawar, juar*
Soya beans	*Bhatma*
Split Bengal gram	*Chana dal*
Split Bengal gram flour	*Besan*
Split yellow lentils	*Moong dhuli dal*
Sunflower seeds	*Surajmukhi ke beej*
Tapioca	*Simla aloo*
Water chestnut	*Singhara*
White chickpeas	*White chana, kabuli chana*
Whole wheat flour	*Gehun ka atta*
Whole wheat grains	*Gehun*

Vegetables

English name	Hindi name
Amaranth	*Chaulai, chaurai saag*
Artichokes	*Hari phul gobi*
Ash gourd	*Safed kaddu, petha*
Asparagus	*Shalwar, musli*
Aurbergines, brinjal, egg plant	*Baingan*
Beet root	*Chakundar*
Bitter gourd	*Karela*
Bitter gourd	*Karela*
Black-eyed peas, cow peas	*Lobia*
Bottle gourd	*Lauki, ghiya*
Broccoli	*Hari phoolgobi*
Brussels sprout	*Chhoti gobi*
Cabbage	*Bandgobi, pattagobi*
Capsicum, bell pepper	*Simla mirch*
Carrot	*Gajar*
Cauliflower	*Phulgobi*
Celery	*Ajamoda*
Cluster beans	*Gowaar phali*
Colocasia	*Kachalu*
Colocasia roots	*Arbi*
Coriander	*Dhania*
Cucumber	*Kheera, kakri*
Curry leaves, sweet neem	*Kadi patta*
Drumsticks	*Saijan*

(contd.)

(*contd.*)

Elephant foot yam	*Jimikand*
Fenugreek	*Methi*
French beans	*France beans*
Garlic	*Lehsun*
Gherkins, ivy gourd	*Kundru, thendli*
Ginger	*Adrak*
Green mustard	*Sarson ka saag*
Green peas	*Mattar*
Horseradish	*Horseradish*
Indian gooseberry	*Amla*
Indian round gourd, apple gourd, baby pumpkin	*Tinda*
Kale	*Karam ka saag*
Knol khol	*Gand gobi, kathgobi*
Lettuce	*Kasmisaag, salad patta*
Lime	*Nimbu*
Linseed	*Alsi*
Lotus root or stem	*Bhein, kamal kakri*
Mint leaves	*Pudina*
Mushrooms	*Goochi, khumban*
Okra, lady's finger	*Bhindi*
Onions	*Piyaaj*
Pointed gourd	*Parwal*
Potatoes	*Aloo*
Pumpkin	*Kaddu*
Radish	*Mooli*
Ridged gourd	*Turai, tori*
Snake gourd	*Chichinga, padwal*
Spinach	*Palak*
Squash	*Kumhadda*
Sweet potatoes	*Shakarkandi*
Tomatoes	*Tamatar*
Turnips	*Shalgum*
Watercress	*Jal kumbhi, peni saag*
White goose foot	*Bathua saag*
Yam, taro	*Sooran*

Fresh Fruits

English name	Hindi name
Apple	*Seb, sabe*
Avocado	*Makhanphal*
Bael, stone apple, Bengal quince	*Bael, sriphal*
Banana	*Kela*
Berries	*Gilaus, cherries*
Cantaloupe	*Sarda*
Cranberries	*Kheet*
Custard apple	*Seetaphal, shareefa*
Figs	*Anjeer*
Fresh coconut	*Nariyal*
Grape fruit	*Chakothra*
Grapes	*Angoor*
Guava	*Amrud*
Honey dew melon, musk-melon, cantaloupe	*Sarda*
Indian gooseberry	*Amla*
Jackfruit	*Kathal*
Jambul	*Jamun*
Jujube	*Ber*
Lemon	*Nimboo*
Loquat	*Lokat*
Lychee, litchi	*Leechee*
Mango	*Aam*
Melon	*Kharbooza*
Mulberry or black berry	*Shehtooth*
Natal plum	*Karonda*
Olives	*Zaitoon*
Orange	*Sangtra*
Papaya	*Papita*
Peach	*Aadoo*
Pear	*Nashpati*
Persimmon or caci	*Japani phal, ramphal*
Phalsa (Grewia asiatica)	*Falsa*
Pineapple	*Ananas*

(contd.)

(*contd.*)

Plum	*Alubukhara*
Pomegranate	*Anar*
Raspberry	*Raspari*
Sapota, sapodilla	*Chickoo*
Strawberries	*Jharberi, stroberri*
Sweet lemon	*Mausambi*
Tangerine, mandarin	*Kinnow, keenu*
Water melon	*Tarbooz*

Dry Fruits and Nuts

English name	Hindi name
Almonds	*Badaam*
Apricot	*Khurmani, khubani*
Cashew nut	*Kaaju*
Chia seeds (sweet basil seeds)	*Sabja seeds or flooda seeds*
Cudpahnut	*Chironji, charoli, piyala*
Dates	*Khajur*
Dry dates	*Chhuara*
Dry plum	*Jardaloo*
Flax seeds	*Alsi*
Fox nuts	*Makhana*
Ground nuts, pea nuts	*Mungphali*
Hazelnuts	*Pahadi badaam, akhrot ka phal*
Melon seeds	*Magaz*
Pine nuts	*Chilgozey, nioze*
Pistachio	*Pista*
Prunes	*Dried alubukhara*
Pumpkin seeds	*Kaddu ke beej, magaz*
Raisins, currants	*Kishmish*
Sesame seeds	*Til*
Sultanas	*Munakka*
Sunflower seeds	*Suryamukhi ke beej, chironji or charoli*
Walnut	*Akhroat*

Indian Spices

English name	Hindi name
Aloe vera	*Kanwaar paatha, bol*
Alum	*Fitkari*
Anise (Aniseeds)	*Saunf choti*
Asafoetida	*Hing*
Black cardamom	*Badi elaichi*
Black cummin seeds	*Kala jeera*
Black rock salt	*Kala namak*
Caraway seeds	*Shah jeera*
Carom seeds, thymol seeds, omum, oregano	*Ajwain*
Celery	*Amjud*
Cinnamon	*Dalchini*
Cloves	*Laung*
Coconut dry	*Sukha nariyal or copra*
Coriander powder	*Dhania*
Cummin seeds	*Jeera*
Dill	*Sowa*
Dry fenugreek	*Kasoori methi*
Dry ginger	*Saunth*
Fennel or aniseeds	*Saunf*
Fenugreek seeds	*Methi*
Garcinia indica	*Kokum*
Ginger aromatic	*Saunth*
Green cardamom	*Chhoti elaichi*
Holy basil	*Tulsi*
Indian bay leaf	*Tejpata*
Jaggery	*Gurh*
Kokum	*Bhirinda*
Long pepper	*Pippali, mug*
Mace	*Javitri*
Mango powder	*Amchoor*
Mint leaves	*Pudina*
Nigella seeds	*Kalonji*
Nutmeg	*Jaiphal*
Onion seeds, black	*Kalonji*

(contd.)

(*contd.*)

Pandanus water	*Kewda water*
Pepper corn	*Kali mirch*
Pomegranate seeds	*Anardaana*
Poppy seeds	*Khas khas*
Psyllium husk	*Isabgol*
Rock candy	*Mishri*
Rock salt	*Sendha namak*
Rose water	*Gulab jal*
Sage	*Kamarkas*
Table salt	*Namak*
Tamarind	*Imli*
Turmeric	*Haldi*
Vanilla	*Vanilla*
Vetiver, screwpine essence	*Kewda*
Vinegar	*Sirka*
White pepper	*Safed mirch, dakni mirch*